Cardiovascular Disease

Editors

NIKHIL K. CHANANI
SHANNON E.G. HAMRICK

CLINICS IN PERINATOLOGY

www.perinatology.theclinics.com

Consulting Editor
LUCKY JAIN

March 2016 • Volume 43 • Number 1

ELSEVIER

1600 John F. Kennedy Boulevard • Suite 1800 • Philadelphia, Pennsylvania, 19103-2899

http://www.theclinics.com

CLINICS IN PERINATOLOGY Volume 43, Number 1
March 2016 ISSN 0095-5108, ISBN-13: 978-0-323-41657-3

Editor: Kerry Holland
Developmental Editor: Casey Jackson

Clinics in Perinatology (ISSN 0095-5108) is published quarterly by Elsevier Inc., 360 Park Avenue South, New York, NY 10010-1710. Months of issue are March, June, September, and December. Business and Editorial Offices: 1600 John F. Kennedy Blvd., Ste. 1800, Philadelphia, PA 19103-2899. Customer Service Office: 3251 Riverport Lane, Maryland Heights, MO 63043. Periodicals postage paid at New York, NY and additional mailing offices. Subscription prices are $290.00 per year (US individuals), $502.00 per year (US institutions), $340.00 per year (Canadian individuals), $614.00 per year (Canadian institutions), $420.00 per year (international individuals), $614.00 per year (international institutions), $100.00 per year (US students), and $195.00 per year (Canadian and international students). International air speed delivery is included in all Clinics subscription prices. All prices are subject to change without notice. **POSTMASTER:** Send address changes to *Clinics in Perinatology*, Elsevier Health Sciences Division, Subscription Customer Service, 3251 Riverport Lane, Maryland Heights, MO 63043. **Customer Service: Telephone: 1-800-654-2452** (U.S. and Canada); **1-314-447-8871** (outside U.S. and Canada). **Fax: 1-314-447-8029. E-mail: journalscustomerservice-usa@elsevier.com** (for print support); **journalsonlinesupport-usa@elsevier.com** (for online support).

Reprints. For copies of 100 or more, of articles in this publication, please contact the Commercial Reprints Department, Elsevier Inc., 360 Park Avenue South, New York, NY 10010-1710. Tel. 212-633-3874; Fax: 212-633-3820; E-mail: reprints@elsevier.com.

Clinics in Perinatology is also publilshed in Spanish by McGraw-Hill Interamericana Editores S.A., P.O. Box 5-237, 06500 Mexico D.F., Mexico.

Clinics in Perinatology is covered in *MEDLINE/PubMed (Index Medicus) Current Contents, Excepta Medica, BIOSIS and ISI/BIOMED.*

Contributors

CONSULTING EDITOR

LUCKY JAIN, MD, MBA
Richard W Blumberg Professor and Interim Chair, Emory University School of Medicine, Department of Pediatrics, Executive Medical Director and Interim Chief Academic Officer, Children's Healthcare of Atlanta, Atlanta, Georgia

EDITORS

NIKHIL K. CHANANI, MD
Assistant Professor of Pediatrics, Division of Cardiology, Sibley Heart Center Cardiology, Emory University and Children's Healthcare of Atlanta, Atlanta, Georgia

SHANNON E.G. HAMRICK, MD
Associate Professor of Pediatrics, Divisions of Neonatology and Cardiology, Emory University and Children's Healthcare of Atlanta, Atlanta, Georgia

AUTHORS

DAVID M. AXELROD, MD
Clinical Assistant Professor, Division of Pediatric Cardiology, Department of Pediatrics, Stanford University Medical Center, Palo Alto, California

MOHAMAD AZHAR, PhD
Department of Cell Biology and Anatomy, University of South Carolina School of Medicine, Columbia, South Carolina

WENDY M. BOOK, MD
Professor of Medicine, Division of Cardiology, Department of Medicine; Director, Emory Adult Congenital Heart Center, Emory University School of Medicine, Atlanta, Georgia

WILLIAM L. BORDER, MBChB, MPH
Children's Healthcare of Atlanta; Department of Pediatrics, Emory University School of Medicine, Atlanta, Georgia

VALERIE Y. CHOCK, MD
Clinical Associate Professor, Division of Neonatology, Department of Pediatrics, Stanford University Medical Center, Palo Alto, California

ERIN McMANUS CONNOCK, MA
Children's Hospital of Philadelphia, Philadelphia, Pennsylvania

JEANNE CRIBBEN, MSOT
Children's Hospital of Philadelphia, Philadelphia, Pennsylvania

MARY T. DONOFRIO, MD
Professor of Pediatrics; Director, Fetal Heart Program, Division of Cardiology; Division of Fetal and Transitional Medicine, Children's National Health System, Washington, DC

GEORG HANSMANN, MD, PhD, FESC, FAHA
Department of Pediatric Cardiology and Critical Care, Hannover Medical School, Hannover, Germany

CAMDEN HEBSON, MD
Assistant Professor of Pediatrics, Departments of Medicine and Pediatrics, The Sibley Heart Center, Emory University School of Medicine, Atlanta, Georgia

EDGAR JAEGGI, MD, FRCPC
Labatt Family Heart Centre, Hospital for Sick Children, University of Toronto, Toronto, Ontario, Canada

HEIDI E. KARPEN, MD
Assistant Professor of Pediatrics, Emory University School of Medicine, Atlanta, Georgia

ROBERTA L. KELLER, MD
Associate Professor of Pediatrics, Neonatology, Department of Pediatrics, UCSF Benioff Children's Hospital, University of California San Francisco, San Francisco, California

LAZAROS KOCHILAS, MD, MSCR
Children's Healthcare of Atlanta; Associate Professor of Pediatrics, Emory University School of Medicine, Atlanta, Georgia

PETRA KOEHNE, MD, PhD
Department of Neonatology, Charité University Medical Center, Berlin, Germany

BEATRICE LATAL, MD MPH
Child Development Center, University Children's Hospital Zurich, Zurich, Switzerland

RACHELLE LESSEN, MS, RD
Children's Hospital of Philadelphia, Philadelphia, Pennsylvania

AMY JO LISANTI, PhD, RN, CCNS
Children's Hospital of Philadelphia, Philadelphia, Pennsylvania

ERICKA S. McLAUGHLIN, DO
Children's Healthcare of Atlanta; Department of Pediatrics, Emory University School of Medicine, Atlanta, Georgia

BARBARA MEDOFF-COOPER, PhD, RN, FAAN
Professor, University of Pennsylvania, School of Nursing; The Children's Hospital of Philadelphia, Philadelphia, Pennsylvania

ANITA J. MOON-GRADY, MD
Professor of Clinical Pediatrics; Director, Fetal Cardiovascular Program, UCSF Benioff Children's Hospitals, University of California San Francisco, San Francisco, California

ANNIKA ÖHMAN, MD
Labatt Family Heart Centre, Hospital for Sick Children, University of Toronto, Toronto, Ontario, Canada

MATTHEW E. OSTER, MD, MPH
Children's Healthcare of Atlanta; Assistant Professor of Pediatrics, Emory University School of Medicine, Atlanta, Georgia

V. MOHAN REDDY, MD
Professor of Surgery; Chief, Division of Pediatric Cardiothoracic Surgery, University of California San Francisco Medical Center, Stanford, California

HANNES SALLMON, MD
Department of Neonatology, Charité University Medical Center, Berlin, Germany

LAURA SANAPO, MD
Fetal Medicine Fellow, Division of Fetal and Transitional Medicine, Children's National Health System, Washington, DC

ANITA SARAF, MD, PhD
Cardiovascular Fellow, Division of Cardiology, Department of Medicine, Emory University School of Medicine, Atlanta, Georgia

BRIAN A. SCHLOSSER, BS, RDCS, RDMS, FASE
Children's Healthcare of Atlanta, Atlanta, Georgia

DAVID TEITEL, MD
Medical Director, Pediatric Heart Center, UCSF Benioff Children's Hospital San Francisco; Chief of Pediatric Cardiology; Professor of Pediatrics, UCSF, San Francisco, California

STEPHANIE M. WARE, MD, PhD
Department of Pediatrics, Herman B Wells Center for Pediatric Research, Indiana University School of Medicine; Department of Medical and Molecular Genetics, Indiana University School of Medicine, Indianapolis, Indiana

Contents

Chronic medical conditions account for most nonobstetrical pregnancy-related maternal complications. Preconception counseling of women with cardiovascular disease can be aided by an understanding of cardiovascular physiology in pregnancy and risk scores to guide management.

Advances in ultrasound technology and specialized training have allowed clinicians to diagnose congenital heart disease in utero and counsel families on perinatal outcomes and management strategies, including fetal cardiac interventions and fetal surgery. This article gives a detailed approach to fetal cardiac assessment and provides the reader with accompanying figures and video clips to illustrate unique views and sweeps invaluable to diagnosing congenital heart disease. We demonstrate that using a sequential segmental approach to evaluate cardiac anatomy enables one to decipher the most complex forms of congenital heart disease. Also provided is a review of fetal cardiac intervention and surgery from the fetal cardiologist's perspective.

Cardiovascular malformations (CVMs) are the most common birth defect, occurring in 1% to 5% of all live births. Genetic, epigenetic, and environmental factors all influence the development of CVMs, and an improved understanding of the causation of CVMs is a prerequisite for prevention. Cardiac development is a complex, multistep process of morphogenesis that is under genetic regulation. Although the genetic contribution to CVMs is well recognized, the genetic causes of human CVMs are still identified infrequently. This article discusses the key genetic concepts characterizing human CVMs, their developmental basis, and the critical developmental and genetic concepts underlying their pathogenesis.

Advances in fetal echocardiography have improved prenatal diagnosis of congenital heart disease (CHD) and allowed better delivery and perinatal management. Some newborns with CHD require urgent intervention after delivery. In these cases, delivery close to a pediatric cardiac center may be considered, and the presence of a specialized cardiac team in the delivery room or urgent transport of the infant should be planned in advance. Delivery planning, monitoring in labor, rapid intervention at birth if needed, and avoidance of iatrogenic preterm delivery have the potential to improve outcomes for infants with prenatally diagnosed CHD.

Screening for critical congenital heart disease (CCHD) was added to the United States Recommended Uniform Screening Panel in 2011. Since that time, CCHD screening with pulse oximetry has become nearly universal for newborns born in the United States. There are various algorithms in use. Although the goal of the screening program is to identify children who may have CCHD, most newborns who have a low oxygen saturation will not have CCHD. Further study is needed to determine optimal guidelines for CCHD screening in special settings such as the neonatal intensive care unit, areas in high altitude, and home births.

Heart defects are the most common congenital malformation. Approximately 8,000 infants per year in the United States require diagnosis in the newborn period to avoid severe injury or death. It is incumbent on the neonatologist and pediatrician to expeditiously detect the presence of symptomatic heart disease so that infants can be stabilized before cardiovascular decompensation. Evaluating infants and further categorizing them into the particular pathophysiology are necessary to stabilize them in anticipation of more definitive care by the pediatric cardiac team.

Cardiac arrhythmias are an important aspect of fetal and neonatal medicine. Premature complexes of atrial or ventricular origin are the main cause of an irregular heart rhythm. The finding is typically unrelated to an identifiable cause and no treatment is required. Tachyarrhythmia most commonly relates to supraventricular reentrant tachycardia, atrial flutter, and sinus tachycardia. Several antiarrhythmic agents are available for the perinatal treatment of tachyarrhythmias. Enduring bradycardia may result from sinus node dysfunction, complete heart block and nonconducted atrial bigeminy as the main arrhythmia mechanisms. The management and outcome of bradycardia depend on the underlying mechanism.

A patent ductus arteriosus (PDA) is associated with several adverse clinical conditions. Several strategies for PDA treatment exist, although data regarding the benefits of PDA treatment on outcomes are sparse. Moreover, the optimal treatment strategy for preterm neonates with PDA remains subject to debate. It is still unknown whether and when PDA treatment should be initiated and which approach (conservative, pharmacologic, or surgical) is best for individual patients (tailored therapies). This article reviews the current strategies for PDA treatment with a special focus on recent developments such as oral ibuprofen, high-dose regimens, and the use of paracetamol (oral, intravenous).

Both protein and energy malnutrition are common in neonates and infants with congenital heart disease (CHD). Neonates with CHD are at increased risk of developing necrotizing enterocolitis (NEC), particularly the preterm population. Mortality in patients with CHD and NEC is higher than for either disease process alone. Standardized feeding protocols may affect both incidence of NEC and growth failure in infants with CHD. The roles of human milk and probiotics have not yet been explored in this patient population.

Newborn infants with complex congenital heart disease are at risk for developmental delay. Developmental care practices benefit prematurely born infants in neonatal intensive care units. Cardiac intensive care units until recently had not integrated developmental care practices into their care framework. Interdisciplinary developmental care rounds in our center have helped in the promotion of developmentally supportive care for infants before and after cardiac surgery. This article discusses basic principles of developmental care, the role of each member of the interdisciplinary team on rounds, common developmental care practices integrated into care from rounds, and impacts to patients, families, and staff.

The premature neonate with congenital heart disease (CHD) represents a challenging population for clinicians and researchers. The interaction between prematurity and CHD is poorly understood; epidemiologic study suggests that premature newborns are more likely to have CHD and that fetuses with CHD are more likely to be born premature. Understanding the key physiologic features of this special patient population is paramount. Clinicians have debated optimal timing for referral for cardiac surgery, and management in the postoperative period has rapidly advanced. This article summarizes the key concepts and literature in the care of the premature neonate with CHD.

Beatrice Latal

Survival after bypass surgery in moderate and severe congenital heart disease (CHD) has increased dramatically. Although cardiac outcome is often very good, these children are at increased risk of developmental impairments in all developmental domains. Risk factors for developmental impairment include a genetic disorder, preterm birth, longer intensive care stay, poorer socioeconomic environment, and more complex forms of CHD. Health care providers, patients, and parents must be aware and informed about noncardiac sequelae and tertiary centers performing open-heart surgery in neonates and infants must establish a neurodevelopmental follow-up program to provide regular neurodevelopmental assessments. These allow for individual counseling and early detection and treatment of developmental problems.

Roberta L. Keller

Pulmonary hypertension in the perinatal period can present acutely (persistent pulmonary hypertension of the newborn) or chronically. Clinical and echocardiographic diagnosis of acute pulmonary hypertension is well accepted but there are no broadly validated criteria for echocardiographic diagnosis of pulmonary hypertension later in the clinical course, although there are significant populations of infants with lung disease at risk for this diagnosis. Contributing cardiovascular comorbidities are common in infants with pulmonary hypertension and lung disease. It is not clear who should be treated without confirmation of pulmonary vascular disease by cardiac catheterization, with concurrent evaluation of any contributing cardiovascular comorbidities.

PROGRAM OBJECTIVE

The goal of *Clinics in Perinatology* is to keep practicing perinatologists, neonatologists, obstetricians, practicing physicians and residents up to date with current clinical practice in perinatology by providing timely articles reviewing the state of the art in patient care.

TARGET AUDIENCE

Perinatologists, neonatologists, obstetricians, practicing physicians, residents and healthcare professionals who provide patient care utilizing findings from *Clinics in Perinatology.*

LEARNING OBJECTIVES

Upon completion of this activity, participants will be able to:
1. Review management and delivery techniques for the mother with cardiovascular disease.
2. Discuss treatment methods for arrhythmias and patent ductus arteriosus in the neonate.
3. Recognize and identify outcomes for preterm infants with congenital heart disease.

ACCREDITATION

The Elsevier Office of Continuing Medical Education (EOCME) is accredited by the Accreditation Council for Continuing Medical Education (ACCME) to provide continuing medical education for physicians.

The EOCME designates this enduring material for a maximum of 15 *AMA PRA Category 1 Credit*(s)™. Physicians should claim only the credit commensurate with the extent of their participation in the activity.

All other health care professionals requesting continuing education credit for this enduring material will be issued a certificate of participation.

DISCLOSURE OF CONFLICTS OF INTEREST

The EOCME assesses conflict of interest with its instructors, faculty, planners, and other individuals who are in a position to control the content of CME activities. All relevant conflicts of interest that are identified are thoroughly vetted by EOCME for fair balance, scientific objectivity, and patient care recommendations. EOCME is committed to providing its learners with CME activities that promote improvements or quality in healthcare and not a specific proprietary business or a commercial interest.

The planning committee, staff, authors and editors listed below have identified no financial relationships or relationships to products or devices they or their spouse/life partner have with commercial interest related to the content of this CME activity:
David M. Axelrod, MD; Mohamad Azhar, PhD; Wendy M. Book, MD; William L. Border, MBChB, MPH; Nikhil K. Chanani, MD; Valerie Y. Chock, MD; Erin McManus Connock, MA; Jeanne Cribben, MSOT; Mary T. Donofrio, MD; Anjali Fortna; Shannon E.G. Hamrick, MD; Georg Hansmann, MD, PhD, FESC, FAHA; Camden Hebson, MD; Kerry Holland; Edgar Jaeggi, MD, FRCPC; Lucky Jain, MD, MBA; Heidi E. Karpen, MD; Roberta L. Keller, MD; Petra Koehne, MD, PhD; Beatrice Latal, MD, MPH; Rachelle Lessen, MS, RD; Amy Jo Lisanti, PhD, RN, CCNS; Ericka S. McLaughlin, DO; Barbara Medoff-Cooper, PhD, RN, FAAN; Anita J. Moon-Grady, MD; Palani Murugesan; Annika Öhman, MD; Matthew E. Oster, MD, MPH; V. Mohan Reddy, MD; Hannes Sallmon, MD; Laura Sanapo, MD; Anita Saraf, MD, PhD; Brian A. Schlosser, BS, RDCS, RDMS, FASE; Megan Suermann; David Teitel, MD; Stephanie M. Ware, MD, PhD.

The planning committee, staff, authors and editors listed below have identified financial relationships or relationships to products or devices they or their spouse/life partner have with commercial interest related to the content of this CME activity:
Lazaros Kochilas, MD, MSCR is a consultant/advisor for Novartis AG. His spouse/partner has stock ownership in, and an employment affiliation with, United HealthCare Services, Inc.

UNAPPROVED/OFF-LABEL USE DISCLOSURE

The EOCME requires CME faculty to disclose to the participants:
1. When products or procedures being discussed are off-label, unlabelled, experimental, and/or investigational (not US Food and Drug Administration [FDA] approved); and
2. Any limitations on the information presented, such as data that are preliminary or that represent ongoing research, interim analyses, and/or unsupported opinions. Faculty may discuss information about pharmaceutical agents that is outside of FDA-approved labelling. This information is intended solely for CME and is not intended to promote off-label use of these medications. If you have any questions, contact the medical affairs department of the manufacturer for the most recent prescribing information.

TO ENROLL

To enroll in the *Clinics in Perinatology* Continuing Medical Education program, call customer service at 1-800-654-2452 or sign up online at http://www.theclinics.com/home/cme. The CME program is available to subscribers for an additional annual fee of $235 USD.

METHOD OF PARTICIPATION

In order to claim credit, participants must complete the following:
1. Complete enrolment as indicated above.
2. Read the activity.
3. Complete the CME Test and Evaluation. Participants must achieve a score of 70% on the test. All CME Tests and Evaluations must be completed online.

CME INQUIRIES/SPECIAL NEEDS

For all CME inquiries or special needs, please contact elsevierCME@elsevier.com.

CLINICS IN PERINATOLOGY

Erratum

Information has appeared incorrectly in the article "Donor Human Milk for Preterm Infants: What It Is, What It Can Do, and What Still Needs to Be Learned" (2014, volume 41, pages 437 – 450). The author stated that "The HTST procedure used by Prolacta Bioscience uses a temperature of 72°C for 16 seconds." That is not the process used nor was it at the time this article published. The process used is proprietary and is in keeping with the requirements of the Milk Pasteurization Ordinance which sets forth the requirements for dairy pasteurization.

Clin Perinatol 43 (2016) xv
http://dx.doi.org/10.1016/j.clp.2016.01.015
0095-5108/16/$ – see front matter © 2016 Elsevier Inc. All rights reserved.

perinatology.theclinics.com

Foreword

The Journey to Adult Congenital Heart Disease

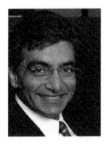

Lucky Jain, MD, MBA
Consulting Editor

The growing number of births to mothers who themselves had significant congenital heart disease marks a remarkable milestone in our journey of caring for these complex patients (**Fig. 1**).[1] One such patient at our institution was a survivor of single-ventricle physiology, complete with the usual share of complications such as pulmonary hypertension. The large-scale planning required to manage this pregnancy, and to take it beyond the threshold of viability, was pretty remarkable. Equally fascinating was the depth of understanding of the complex physiologic interactions of the mother and fetus.[2] In the end, the delivery was early but relatively free of complications, and the newborn blossomed under the care of our neonatology team, unencumbered by the limits of intrauterine oxygen and nutrient delivery. I remember the sight of this young mom holding her precious baby for a few fleeting moments before being whisked away to the NICU. This story makes me giddy with joy, to see the remarkable collaborative work between a large team of talented providers, including pediatric and adult cardiologists, neonatologists, perinatologists, and elaborate support services linked to these specialties. It also makes me proud to have been a part of this journey and to have participated in care of these patients early on in their lives: the journey of near certain death for a baby with complex congenital heart, to a similar patient 20 years later giving birth to a healthy child is pretty amazing!

This remarkable journey of pediatric cardiology has been fueled by an intense grounding of the subspecialty in fundamentals of physiology, and a partnership between surgical and medical teams like none other. Biomedical engineering has also played a key role in refining care, as has the ability to image hearts noninvasively from early on in fetal life.

Yet, pregnant or not, many adult congenital heart patients don't do that well, particularly patients with Eisenmenger physiology, severe pulmonary hypertension, significant ventricular outflow obstruction, and ventricular dysfunction.[3] Pregnancy, labor, and the rigors of delivery increase the hemodynamic stress on the cardiovascular

Clin Perinatol 43 (2016) xvii–xix
http://dx.doi.org/10.1016/j.clp.2015.12.002
0095-5108/16/$ – see front matter © 2016 Published by Elsevier Inc.

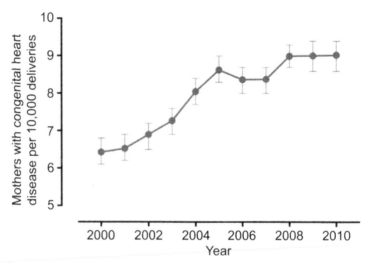

Fig. 1. The rise in pregnancies to women who themselves had congenital heart disease. (*From* Thompson JL, Kuklina EV, Bateman BT, et al. Medical and obstetric outcomes among pregnant women with congenital heart disease. Obstet Gynecol 2015;126(2):350; with permission.)

system and place women with heart disease at increased risk of complications, including heart failure and death. Systematic assessment of pregnancy risk in these women, ideally before conception, is essential in optimizing maternal and fetal outcomes.[4] The American College of Cardiology and American Heart Association have put forth comprehensive guidelines for management of adult congenital heart patients, including recommendations for appropriate transition of care from pediatric to adult providers.[5] These guidelines call for a smooth handoff of the care of these patients to adult providers, and many centers now have adult congenital heart clinics staffed by pediatric and adult specialists.

There is much to celebrate, but the job is not done yet. In this issue of *Clinics in Perinatology*, Drs Hamrick and Chanani have put together a state-of-the-art compilation of articles related to congenital heart disease covering the entire spectrum of malformations and their management. They point to areas ripe for further refinement and development. I want to thank the editors, authors, and our publishing team at Elsevier, led by Kerry Holland and Casey Jackson, for bringing together another superb issue of the *Clinics in Perinatology* for you. I also want to thank you, the loyal readers, for another successful year of learning together. We look forward to 2016 being another banner year for us!

Lucky Jain, MD, MBA
Emory University School of Medicine
Department of Pediatrics
Children's Healthcare of Atlanta
2015 Uppergate Drive
Atlanta, GA 30322, USA

E-mail address:
ljain@emory.edu

REFERENCES

1. Thompson JL, Kuklina EV, Bateman BT, et al. Medical and obstetric outcomes among pregnant women with congenital heart disease. Obstet Gynecol 2015; 126(2):346–54.
2. Roos-Hesselink JW, Ruys PT, Johnson MR. Pregnancy in adult congenital heart disease. Curr Cardiol Rep 2013;15(9):401.
3. Bhatt AB, DeFaria Yeh D. Pregnancy and adult congenital heart disease. Cardiol Clin 2015;33(4):611–23.
4. Moghbeli N, Pare E, Webb G. Practical assessment of maternal cardiovascular risk in pregnancy. Congenit Heart Dis 2008;3(5):308–16.
5. Gerardin JF, Menk JS, Pyles LA, et al. Compliance with adult congenital heart disease guidelines: are we following the recommendations? Congenit Heart Dis 2015. http://dx.doi.org/10.1111/chd.12309.

Preface

Perinatal Cardiovascular Disease

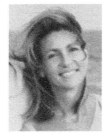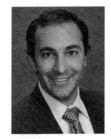

Shannon E.G. Hamrick, MD   Nikhil K. Chanani, MD

Editors

The impact of cardiovascular disease on an infant extends from the preconception period to well beyond childhood. For our issue focused on cardiovascular health we sought to encompass the breadth of knowledge that would be the most relevant for the bedside clinician. The initial interaction for a family of a child with heart disease may begin as a fetus or as a parent. In addition, for neonatal clinicians, medical decisions and family counseling often occur with very little warning. We hoped to assemble material that would allow a clinician to quickly peruse this issue, find the relevant reference, and then be prepared to help a family during a critical junction.

    The interaction between cardiology and perinatology/neonatology has also become increasingly complex and encompasses genetics, diagnostics, interventions, counseling, routine stabilization, and day-to-day care of both mother and baby. Thus, we have included articles spanning maternal cardiac disease (pregnancy in the adult congenital population), genetics, fetal diagnosis and intervention, to the specifics of newborn care (delivery room management, congenital heart disease screening, recognition of the undiagnosed congenital heart lesion after birth, arrhythmia treatment, nutrition and intestinal complications, developmentally appropriate care, care specific to the preterm newborn), to more long-term issues such as pulmonary hypertension and neurodevelopmental outcomes. Furthermore, as the field continues to evolve with deeper genetic analysis and innovative treatment modalities, our authors also reflect on many of these cutting-edge tools. Even though many of us won't have access to some of these interventions, this issue will help to keep the practitioner current and relevant as well. Ultimately, the goal is to establish a foundation for a healthy adult. It is hoped, whether in the middle of the night as an emergency reference or during the

Clin Perinatol 43 (2016) xxi–xxii
http://dx.doi.org/10.1016/j.clp.2015.12.001
0095-5108/16/$ – see front matter © 2016 Published by Elsevier Inc.

perinatology.theclinics.com

day as a reliable guide, this issue of *Clinics in Perinatology* will be an important bedside tool for anyone that participates in the care of a patient with perinatal heart disease.

Shannon E.G. Hamrick, MD
Divisions of Neonatology and Cardiology
Emory University and
Children's Healthcare of Atlanta
Emory Children's Center
316 F 3rd Floor
Atlanta, GA 30322, USA

Nikhil K. Chanani, MD
Division of Cardiology
Sibley Heart Center Cardiology
Emory University and
Children's Healthcare of Atlanta
2835 Brandywine Road, Suite 300
Atlanta, GA 30341, USA

E-mail addresses:
sehamri@emory.edu (S.E.G. Hamrick)
chananin@kidsheart.com (N.K. Chanani)

Risk Assessment and Management of the Mother with Cardiovascular Disease

 CrossMark

Camden Hebson, MD[a,b], Anita Saraf, MD, PhD[c],
Wendy M. Book, MD[d],*

KEYWORDS

- Congenital heart disease • Maternal health • Pregnancy • Preconception counseling

KEY POINTS

- Cardiovascular disease is the most common nonobstetrical contributor to maternal mortality in developed countries.
- Preexisting cardiovascular conditions are increasingly common in women of childbearing age and contribute to both maternal and fetal complications.
- Women with congenital heart defects are making up an increasing proportion of pregnancies.
- Prepregnancy counseling is recommended at every opportunity for women with underlying cardiovascular conditions, as many pregnancies are unplanned.
- Antenatal and perinatal management by a team experienced in cardiovascular disease is recommended for women with underlying congenital heart defects and other cardiovascular conditions.

Funding: Dr W.M. Book receives funding from the Centers for Disease Control and Prevention CDC-RFA-DD12-1207 cooperative agreement. Dr A. Saraf has received funding from the American Heart Association Post-Doctoral Fellowship grant and the NRSA Individual Post Doctoral Fellowship Grant by the National Institutes of Health.

[a] Department of Medicine, The Sibley Heart Center, Emory University School of Medicine, 1365 Clifton Road Northeast, Clinic A, 2nd Floor, Cardiology, Atlanta, GA 30322, USA; [b] Department of Pediatrics, The Sibley Heart Center, Emory University School of Medicine, 1365 Clifton Road Northeast, Clinic A, 2nd Floor, Cardiology, Atlanta, GA 30322, USA; [c] Division of Cardiology, Department of Medicine, Emory University School of Medicine, 1365 Clifton Road Northeast, Atlanta, GA 30322, USA; [d] Division of Cardiology, Department of Medicine, Emory Adult Congenital Heart Center, Emory University School of Medicine, 1365 Clifton Road Northeast, Clinic A, 2nd Floor, Cardiology, Atlanta, GA 30322, USA
* Corresponding author.
E-mail address: wbook@emory.edu

Advances in medical care, particularly cardiac surgery, over the past half century have led to significant improvements in outcomes for children with chronic medical conditions. Children with structural heart defects, both genetic and acquired, have seen a profound improvement in survival.[1,2] With anticipated adult survival for most children with cardiovascular conditions, an increasing number of women of childbearing age are seeking pregnancy-related advice from physicians in multiple specialties.

MATERNAL MORTALITY: IMPACT OF CARDIOVASCULAR DISEASE

Maternal cardiovascular disease is an increasingly common cause of pregnancy-related maternal and fetal morbidity and mortality.[3] In general, maternal mortality has been declining over the past 50 years as improvements in recognizing and treating obstetric complications have improved. However, in recent years, nonobstetrical complications related to medical and mental health problems have increased[3,4] accounting for approximately two-thirds of maternal deaths.[3] In the United States, cardiovascular causes are the most common cause of pregnancy-related mortality, accounting for 15% of all deaths,[4] with similar trends noted in the United Kingdom. Recent increases in US maternal mortality over the past decade to 17.8 per 100,000 live births[4] emphasize the need to address chronic maternal conditions and risk factors before pregnancy.

CONGENITAL HEART DEFECTS: REPAIRED, NOT CURED

Advances in congenital heart disease (CHD) have resulted in a growing population of adults with CHD,[1,2] including an increasing number of women of childbearing potential. Congenital heart defects are a heterogeneous group of cardiac conditions ranging from mild CHD with minimal hemodynamic consequences to complex defects with abnormal circulations, even after palliative surgeries. Therefore, women with CHD face a higher risk of pregnancy-related cardiovascular events and death, varying by CHD type and repair.[5] Deliveries for women with CHD have increased[6] in comparison with the general population by 34.9% from 1998 to 2007, compared with 21.3% in the general population.[5] In the Western hemisphere, CHD is the most common form of heart disease complicating pregnancy.[7–9]

PRECONCEPTION COUNSELING FOR THE WOMAN WITH CARDIOVASCULAR DISEASE

- Counseling should occur at every opportunity in women of childbearing potential.
- Counseling should include maternal, fetal, and neonatal risk assessment.
- Counseling should include contraception.
- Counseling should include genetic risks.

Prepregnancy counseling has been identified as a top recommendation by the Center for Maternal and Child Enquiries[10] to decrease adverse pregnancy-related outcomes in women with preexisting medical illness. Because more than half of pregnancies are unplanned, women of childbearing age with cardiovascular conditions should be offered prepregnancy counseling at each office visit, by knowledgeable providers. Prepregnancy counseling should include an informed discussion regarding risk assessment of the mother, genetic considerations (discussed further in McLaughlin ES, Schlosser BA, Border WL: Fetal diagnostics and fetal intervention, in this issue), management recommendations, and discussion regarding contraception and/or alternatives to pregnancy when appropriate. Before planned pregnancy, good communication among a multidisciplinary team with experience in managing cardiovascular disease and pregnancy is critical to develop a management plan individualized to the woman's particular cardiac condition. Maternal cardiovascular health should be optimized before pregnancy to ensure the best outcome for mother and baby. Close communication between the perinatologist and a cardiologist experienced in managing cardiovascular disease and pregnancy is essential.

DETERMINING MATERNAL CARDIOVASCULAR RISK
Hemodynamic Changes in Normal Pregnancy

There are 2 major cardiovascular physiologic changes that must occur during pregnancy:

- Decrease in vascular resistance (systemic and pulmonary)
- Increase in cardiac output (CO)

These changes are vital to support the needs of the mother and fetus. With the decrease in vascular resistance, systemic blood pressure decreases, with nadir around the end of the second trimester. This decrease in vascular resistance occurs despite increasing CO; it is only during labor and delivery that blood pressure actually elevates. During pregnancy, there is a 50% increase in intravascular volume, with a steady increase until delivery. This additional preload, combined with an average 20% increase in heart rate by the third trimester, leads to the overall increase in CO. Hemodynamic changes in pregnancy are summarized in **Table 1**. Women with certain congenital heart lesions that limit CO or predispose to elevated pulmonary vascular resistance are at the highest risk of poor outcomes and complications. Severe valvular stenosis, myocardial injury, cardiomyopathy, Eisenmenger syndrome, and palliated single ventricle disease (reliant on passive pulmonary blood flow) are all examples. Women who are marginally compensated at baseline have particular difficulty tolerating the volume shifts that occur during normal pregnancy.

Maternal Risk Stratification

Three predictive tools can help determine cardiac complication risk in pregnant women with CHD: World Health Organization (WHO) classification, Cardiac Disease

Table 1
Summary of hemodynamic changes during normal pregnancy, labor and delivery, and postpartum

Hemodynamic Parameter	Change During Normal Pregnancy	Change During Labor and Delivery[a]	Change During Post Partum
Blood volume	↑ 50%	↑	↓
Heart rate	↑ 10–15 beats/min	↑	↓
CO	↑ 50% (by third trimester)	↑	↓
Systolic blood pressure	↓ 10–20 mm Hg	↑	↓
Stroke volume	↑ First and second trimesters	↑	↓
Systemic vascular resistance	↓	↑	↓
Basal oxygen consumption	↑	↑	↓

[a] More drastic changes noted with general anesthesia compared with caudal anesthesia and when patients are lying supine versus on the side.

Adapted from Naderi S, Raymond R. Pregnancy and heart disease. Cleveland Clinic Center for Continuing Education. Available at: http://www.clevelandclinicmeded.com/medicalpubs/diseasemanagement/cardiology/pregnancy-and-heart-disease/; and Metcalfe J, Ueland K. Maternal cardiovascular adjustments to pregnancy. Prog Cardiovasc Dis 1974;16(4):364.

in Pregnancy (CARPREG) score, and ZAHARA score. The 2011 European Society of Cardiology task force recommended the WHO classification based on its superior performance in predicting risk.[11] The scores are summarized in **Tables 2** and **3**.

The WHO classification[12] was formed from expert opinion and covers both anatomic and physiologic conditions. Risk stratification ranges from similar to the general population (class I) to contraindicated (class IV) (see **Table 2**). The ZAHARA[13] risk score is based on a large retrospective study of more than 700 women with CHD. The scoring system is weighted based on each individual risk factor (see **Table 3**). The CARPREG[14] risk score was derived from a prospective study of women with both acquired and CHD. Four main risk factors were highlighted, with each one being worth 1 point:

1. Left ventricular (LV) systolic dysfunction (ejection fraction [EF] <40%)
2. Left heart obstruction (mitral valve area <2 cm^2, aortic valve area <1.5 cm^2, peak LV outflow gradient >30 mm Hg)
3. Previous cardiac event (clinical heart failure, transient ischemic attack, arrhythmia, or stroke)
4. New York Heart Association (NYHA) function class greater than 2, or cyanosis

Based on point total, the risk of a cardiac event during pregnancy is predicted to be 4% (0 points), 27% (1 point), and 62% (≥2 points).

Table 2
WHO classification of risk of pregnancy in cardiac disease

WHO Class 1[a]	WHO Class 2[b]	WHO Class 3[c]	WHO Class 4[d]
Mild PS	ASD unoperated, if otherwise well	Mechanical valve	Pulmonary hypertension, all causes
Restrictive or closed VSD or PDA	Repaired TOF	Systemic right ventricle	Severe systemic ventricular dysfunction (severe symptoms or EF <30%)
Repaired ASD	Most arrhythmias	Fontan	Previous peripartum cardiomyopathy with any residual LV dysfunction
Repaired TAPVR	Coarctation repair	Cyanotic heart disease (current)	Severe left heart obstruction
PACs, PVCs	Native or tissue valvular disease not WHO 4[e]	Other complex CHD	Marfan syndrome with root >4 cm
	Marfan syndrome, no root dilation[e]	—	—

Abbreviations: ASD, atrial septal defect; EF, ejection fraction; LV, left ventricle; PAC, premature atrial contractions; PDA, patent ductus arteriosus; PS, pulmonary stenosis; PVC, premature ventricular contractions; TAPVR, total anomalous pulmonary venous return; TOF, tetralogy of Fallot; VSD, ventricular septal defect.
  [a] WHO 1: Risk of pregnancy *not detectably higher* than general population.
  [b] WHO 2: *Small increased risk* of maternal morbidity or mortality.
  [c] WHO 3: *Significantly increased risk* of morbidity and mortality; expert joint cardiology and obstetrics preconception counseling needed.
  [d] WHO 4: *Pregnancy contraindicated.*
  [e] Can be WHO 2 or 3, depending on physician judgment and individual patient modifiers.[12]

Table 3
ZAHARA classification is based on a large retrospective study of more than 700 women with CHD; the scoring system is weighted based on importance of each individual risk factor

ZAHARA Risk Score for Cardiac Events[a] During Pregnancy			
Risk Factor	Points	Total Points	Risk (%)
At least moderate systemic AV valve regurgitation	0.75	0	2.9
At least moderate subpulmonary AV valve regurgitation	0.75	0.51–1.5	7.5
NYHA class >1[b]	0.75	1.51–2.5	17.5
Cyanotic heart disease (regardless if now corrected)	1.0	2.51–3.5	43.1
Prior arrhythmia[c]	1.5	>3.5	70.0
Cardiac medications before pregnancy	1.5	—	—
Left heart obstruction (PG >50 mm Hg)	2.5	—	—
Mechanical valve	4.25	—	—

Abbreviations: AV, atrioventricular; NYHA, New York Heart Association; PG, peak gradient.
[a] Cardiac events: arrhythmia requiring treatment, cerebrovascular accident, congestive heart failure requiring treatment, myocardial infarction, SBE (subacute bacterial endocarditis), death.
[b] CHD + any significant and resultant dyspnea/shortness of breath with exertion.
[c] Prior arrhythmia requiring medical treatment (ablation, medications, cardioversion, and so forth).
Data from Drenthen W, Boersma E, Balci A, et al, ZAHARA Investigators. Predictors of pregnancy complications in women with congenital heart disease. Eur Heart J 2010;31:2124–32.

When comparing the different risk scores, patterns emerge. The authors' group has compared the different risk scores in a higher-acuity patient population (n = 113 patients, 53% NYHA functional class >1, 59% ZAHARA score >1.5; Hebson C, Book W and Lindley K, unpublished data, 2015). The cardiac event rate was 33%. The best correlating area under the curve (AUC) for maternal cardiac risk came from the ZAHARA score (AUC 0.82) compared with the WHO classification (AUC 0.69) and CARPREG score (AUC 0.71).

In general, preexisting maternal cardiovascular disease should be addressed before conception, including problems such as hypertension, obesity, atherosclerotic disease, heart failure, arrhythmias, thromboembolic events, and CHD (including residual lesions). Maternal functional class is predictive of a poor outcome during pregnancy.[9] Women with functional class III to IV symptoms, regardless of cause, should be strongly discouraged from becoming pregnant.[11] In addition, patients with mechanical valves, pulmonary arterial hypertension, and aortic aneurysms are at highest risk. Prevention requires that the provider recognize the risk and clearly communicate this with patients, including discussion of appropriate contraception. A comprehensive discussion regarding contraception options for women with CHD is beyond the scope of this article; interested readers are referred to a review by Silversides and colleagues.[15]

Assessment of Fetal Risk

Although studies are limited, attempts at predicting fetal risk in women with cardiac disease have been made. Overall fetal mortality, among those born to women with cardiac disease, is 1.7%. There is an additional perinatal mortality rate of 2.3% (higher than in the general population [0.5%]). Both prematurity and low birth weight have been linked to advanced maternal WHO class.[16] On the other hand, in a recent prospective study by Balci and colleagues,[17] none of the published risk scores (ZAHARA, CARPREG, WHO) accurately predicted poor neonatal outcome. However, NYHA classification has been linked to outcomes: if asymptomatic, the risk is close to baseline, whereas the risk of poor fetal outcome reaches 30% if a woman has severe symptoms during pregnancy.[18] In the presence of maternal cardiac disease, the rate of prematurity is around 16%.[19] Based on the CARPREG study,[14] there was a 20% rate of neonatal complications (prematurity in 17%, small for gestational age in 4%, and fetal and neonatal death rates of 1% each). Risk factors for poor outcomes included NYHA functional class greater than 2, cyanosis, aortic or mitral stenosis, active smoking, multiple gestations, and use of an anticoagulant besides aspirin. In a study by Khairy and colleagues,[20] the percentage of neonates with an adverse outcome was 28%, including prematurity (21%), small for gestational age (8%), intrauterine fetal demise (3%), and intraventricular hemorrhage and neonatal death (1.4% each). The investigators found that LV outflow tract gradient greater than 30 mm Hg independently predicted poor neonatal outcome with an odds ratio of 7.5.

Inheritance of congenital heart disease
In a study of more than 6000 pregnancies (parent or sibling with CHD), the incidence of any cardiac defect in the newborn was 2.7%.[21] One-third of the patients had the same defect as the parent or sibling. An older study of 837 children found an incidence closer to 10%.[22] A third study from the United Kingdom involving almost 400 children found a recurrence risk of 4.1% in offspring and 2.1% in siblings. Recurrence risk was greater if the mother had CHD versus the father (5.7% vs 2.2%).[23] In the CARPREG study, cardiac defects were present in 7% of live births among the cohort.[7,14] Given these studies, the often-quoted incidence of CHD in women who themselves have a congenital cardiac defect is around 5%.

Cardiac medications in pregnancy
Approximately one-third of women with chronic cardiovascular conditions take medications during pregnancy, with beta-blockers (BBs) being the most common followed by angiotensin-converting enzyme inhibitors (ACE-Is), diuretics, and antiplatelet agents.[24] BBs are associated with the highest risk of low birth weight and ACE-Is with the highest risk of fetal malformations.[24] **Table 4** provides an overview of current Food and Drug Administration classification of medications during pregnancy, with notations regarding specifics of a certain trimester, and use during lactation. Use of all medications during pregnancy should include a comprehensive assessment balancing potential risk versus benefit to both mother and baby. In some circumstances, alternative and safer medications may be substituted during pregnancy.

Management of the woman with cardiovascular disease during pregnancy
Initial assessment of the mother should occur as soon as pregnancy is established and include discussion of goals of care, identification of subspecialty needs for mother and baby, and development of a management plan. Any potentially teratogenic medications should be discontinued if feasible and safe, with an alternative medication initiated, either before conception or as soon as the woman learns she is pregnant. The timing and frequency as well as the type of cardiovascular assessment will vary by the cardiac condition.

Understanding the onset of abnormal cardiovascular signs and symptoms during pregnancy requires an understanding of the normal physiology and normal signs and symptoms in pregnancy. Pregnancy is a high-output, low-resistance uteroplacental circulation, which permits an increase in circulating volume and CO.[25] In the setting of a normal cardiovascular system, this high-output, low-resistance circulation can be sustained throughout pregnancy without compromise to maternal health. In the presence of underlying cardiovascular abnormalities, augmentation of CO may be limited

Table 4
Medication type, usage, potential toxicity, and pregnancy/lactation classification

Medication	Use	Major Effects	Pregnancy[a]	Lactation[a]
Antiarrhythmic				
Adenosine	Arrhythmia (SVT)	None reported	C	L1
Digoxin	Arrhythmia, CHF	Low birth weight, prematurity	C	L2
Lidocaine	Arrhythmia, anesthesia	Neonatal CNS depression	B	L2
Procainamide	Arrhythmia	None reported	C	L3
Sotolol	Arrhythmia	Placental and fetal growth retardation	B	L4
Antihypertensive				
BBs	Hypertension Heart failure Cardiomyopathy	Bradycardia IUGR (atenolol) Transient hypoglycemia	C	Atenolol: L3 Labetolol: L3 Metprolol: L3 Propranolol: L2
ACE-Is	Hypertension Heart failure Cardiomyopathy	Teratogenicity	D	L2-L4
Calcium channel blockers	Hypertension Arrhythmia	None reported Nifedipine is preferred	C	Nifedapine: L2 Amlodipine: L3 Diltiazem: L3 Verapamil: L2

(continued on next page)

Table 4
(continued)

Medication	Use	Major Effects	Pregnancy[a]	Lactation[a]
Aldomet (Methyldopa)	Hypertension	None reported	B	L2
Hydralazine	Hypertension, heart failure	Fetal distress with maternal hypotension	B	L2
Clonidine	Hypertension	Maternal rebound tachycardia. None to fetus	B	—
Nitrates	Hypertension	Fetal distress with maternal hypotension	C	Isosorbide dinitrate: L3
Diuretics				
Loop diuretics	Diuretic	Intravascular volume depletion; impairs placental perfusion	Lasix: C Torsemide: B	L3
Thiazide diuretics	Diuretic	Intravascular volume depletion; impairs placental perfusion	B	L3
Anticoagulants				
Warfarin	Mechanical valve, hypercoagulable state, DVT, AF, Eisenmenger syndrome	Teratogenicity restricted to first trimester and at doses >5 mg/d. Crosses placenta, should not be used near time of delivery	X	L2
Low-molecular-weight heparin	Mechanical valve, hypercoagulable state, DVT, AF, Eisenmenger syndrome	Hemorrhage, unclear effects on maternal bone mineral density	B	L3
Unfractionated heparin	Mechanical valve, hypercoagulable state, DVT, AF, Eisenmenger syndrome	Maternal osteoporosis, hemorrhage, thrombocytopenia, thrombosis	C	L1
Fondaparinux	HIT in pregnancy	None reported	B	No data

Antiplatelets				
Aspirin	Antiplatelet	<100 mg during pregnancy	<100 mg: C >100 mg: D	L3 risk of Reye syndrome with higher doses
Clopidogrel	Antiplatelet for MI, TIA	None reported	B	L3
Glycoprotein IIB/IIIA inhibitors	Antiplatelet	Limited data, none reported	B	No data

Pregnancy classification: A, Adequate and well-controlled studies have failed to demonstrate a risk to the fetus in the first trimester of pregnancy (and there is no evidence of risk in later trimesters); B, Animal reproduction studies have failed to demonstrate a risk to the fetus and there are no adequate and well-controlled studies in pregnant women; C, Animal reproduction studies have shown an adverse effect on the fetus and there are no adequate well-controlled studies in humans, but potential benefits may warrant use of the drug in pregnant women despite potential risks; D, There is positive evidence of human fetal risk based on adverse reaction data from investigational or marketing experience or studies in humans, but potential benefits may warrant use of the drug in pregnant women despite potential risks; X, Studies in animals or humans have demonstrated fetal abnormalities and/or there is a positive evidence of human fetal risk based on adverse reaction data from investigational or marketing experience, and the risks involved in use of the drug in pregnant women clearly outweigh potential benefits; N, The Food and Drug Administration has not classified the drug.

Lactation classification: L1, COMPATIBLE: drug that has been taken by a large number of breastfeeding mothers without any observed increase in adverse effects in the infant. Controlled studies in breastfeeding women fail to demonstrate a risk to the infant and the possibility of harm to the breastfeeding infant is remote; or the product is not orally bioavailable in an infant. L2, PROBABLY COMPATIBLE: drug that has been studied in a limited number of breastfeeding women without an increase in adverse effects in the infant and/or the evidence of a demonstrated risk that is likely to follow use of this medication in a breastfeeding woman is remote. L3, PROBABLY COMPATIBLE. There are no controlled studies in breastfeeding women; however, the risk of untoward effects to a breastfed infant is possible or controlled studies show only minimal nonthreatening adverse effects. Drugs should be given only if the potential benefit justifies the potential risk to the infant. (New medications that have absolutely no published data are automatically categorized in this category, regardless of how safe they may be.) L4, POSSIBLY HAZARDOUS: There is positive evidence of risk to a breastfed infant or to breast milk production, but the benefits of use in breastfeeding mothers may be acceptable despite the risk to the infant (eg, if the drug is needed in a life-threatening situation or for a serious disease for which safer drugs cannot be used or are ineffective). L5, HAZARDOUS: Studies in breastfeeding mothers have demonstrated that there is significant and documented risk to the infant based on human experience or it is a medication that has a high risk of causing significant damage to an infant. The risk of using the drug in breastfeeding women clearly outweighs any possible benefit from breastfeeding. The drug is contraindicated in women who are breastfeeding an infant.

Abbreviations: AF, atrial fibrillation; CNS, central nervous system; DVT, deep vein thrombosis; HIT, heparin-induced thrombocytopenia; IUGR, intrauterine growth retardation; MI, myocardial infarction; SVT, supraventricular tachycardia; TIA, transient ischemic attack.

a Food and Drug Administration's classification of risk.

Data from Hale TW, Rowe HE. Medications and mothers' milk, 16th edition. Amarillo, TX: Hale Publishing; 2014; and Powrie RO, Greene RF, Camnn W, editors. Appendix: Medications and their relative risk to breastfeeding infants. de Swiet's Medical Disorders in Obstetric Practice, 5th edition. Oxford, UK: Wiley-Blackwell; 2010.

either because of obstruction in the circulation or inability to accommodate an increasing plasma volume or both. At each visit, the provider should document functional class, symptoms of heart failure, arrhythmias, and/or thromboembolic complications. Physical examination findings (neck veins, murmurs, gallops, hepatomegaly, edema) should be outlined at baseline and then at each subsequent visit. Signs and symptoms of normal pregnancy may overlap with those of cardiac disease, making assessment more challenging.[26] For patients at higher risk, an electrocardiogram should be obtained at each visit. Echocardiography should be used when indicated for higher-risk patients in whom dynamic changes during pregnancy will be poorly tolerated.

MATERNAL CARDIOVASCULAR COMPLICATIONS OF PREGNANCY
Arrhythmias

Although there is an increase in premature ventricular and atrial contractions during normal pregnancy,[27] arrhythmias are even more common in the presence of underlying maternal cardiovascular disease, particularly CHD. In a review of 87 pregnancies in 73 women, Silversides and colleagues[28] found that 44% of women in normal sinus rhythm at baseline but with a history of tachyarrhythmia before pregnancy had a recurrence of their tachyarrhythmia. Atrial fibrillation and flutter were most likely to occur (50%–52%), with ventricular tachycardia less likely but frequent (27%). Tachyarrhythmia was associated with a higher risk of adverse fetal events in comparison with women who did not have recurrence.[28] For unstable patients with tachycardia, cardioversion may be performed as in the nonpregnant state. Bradycardia in general is poorly tolerated in women with underlying cardiac disease, limiting the ability to meet CO demands of pregnancy, because CO depends on the product of stroke volume (SV) and heart rate. For symptomatic bradycardias, pacemaker implantation during pregnancy may be needed.[11]

Coronary Artery Disease

Coronary disease in women of childbearing age is uncommon but may occur in women with risk factors, including diabetes, hypertension, late repair of coarctation of the aorta, and prior repair of congenital coronary anomalies. Women with CAD are at an increased risk of ischemic complications during pregnancy, including angina, ventricular arrhythmia, and cardiac arrest. In one study, women with ischemic complications had a high rate of obstetric (16%) and fetal/neonatal (30%) events.[29]

Heart Failure

Dilated cardiomyopathy
Women with preexisting dilated cardiomyopathy have a high rate of cardiovascular events during pregnancy. In one study, 39% of pregnancies were complicated by one or more cardiac events (atrial fibrillation/flutter [14%], ventricular tachycardia [3%], heart failure [25%] and transient ischemic attack [3%]).[30] Women with cardiomyopathy should be counseled on the high risk of adverse events with pregnancy.

Development of heart failure during pregnancy
Heart failure is the most common major cardiovascular complication during pregnancy. Women with cardiomyopathy, pulmonary hypertension, and/or poor functional class (≥3) are at greatest risk. Development of heart failure typically occurs during the late second trimester or after birth, during times of greatest volume shifts. Development of heart failure is associated with maternal mortality, preeclampsia, and adverse maternal and perinatal outcome, including fetal death.[31] Postpartum heart failure is

most commonly associated with peripartum cardiomyopathy but may also be seen in mitral regurgitation (14%), cardiomyopathies (11%), tetralogy of Fallot (6%), and other underlying cardiac conditions.[31] The diagnosis of heart failure relies on clinical evaluation and echocardiography. In select situations, B-type natriuretic peptide (BNP) measurements in pregnancy may supplement clinical assessment. In a study by Kampman and colleagues,[32] N-terminal pro-B–type BNP levels less than 128 pg/mL at 20 weeks' gestation had a negative predictive value of 96.9%, whereas levels more than this had a positive predictive value for adverse cardiovascular events.

In general, the onset of heart failure signs and symptoms heralds the need for delivery. By definition, heart failure identifies a cardiovascular system that is no longer able to meet circulatory hemodynamic demands. Medication should be initiated, including diuresis for fluid retention; delivery should be planned as soon as feasible and safe for the mother and baby. In rare situations, prolonged hospitalization with aggressive management of heart failure may be an option to allow maturing the fetus to a viable age.

Peripartum cardiomyopathy (PPCM) by definition occurs in women with no prior history of cardiac disease. A recent European Society of Cardiology working group has updated the definition to "idiopathic cardiomyopathy presenting with LV systolic dysfunction toward the end of pregnancy or in the months following delivery where no other etiology is found."[33] Typically LVEF is less than 45%. Although the cause of PPCM is unclear, deficient antioxidant response, increased blood levels of immunoglobulins (autoimmune), and inflammatory markers have been demonstrated previously. Likely multiple pathways can lead to the same phenotype. Women with a history of PPCM are at high risk for adverse outcomes with future pregnancies and should be counseled at each opportunity.[33,34]

SPECIFIC CARDIAC CONDITIONS
Congenital Heart Disease

An in-depth discussion of the impact of specific maternal congenital heart defects and diagnoses on pregnancy management is beyond the scope of this article.[35–37] **Tables 5** and **6** provide an overview of maternal risk and management recommendation. Cardiac conditions associated with high maternal and fetal complications in which pregnancy is considered contraindicated are listed in the **Box 1** later.

A discussion of a few common and critical specific diagnoses follows.

Coarctation of the aorta is associated with a risk as high as 30% for hypertensive complications during pregnancy[38,39] and even higher risk with small aortic diameter (<15 mm) by cardiac MRI.[40]

Table 5	
Management recommendations generally considered beneficial by consensus expert opinion	
Condition	**Management Recommendations**
Severe pulmonary stenosis	Repair before pregnancy
Severe aortic or mitral stenosis	Repair/valve replacement before surgery
Ebstein anomaly with cyanosis	Repair before pregnancy
Symptomatic pulmonary regurgitation with RV dilatation	Pulmonary valve replacement before pregnancy
Marfan syndrome with aorta >45 mm	Surgery before pregnancy
SVT during pregnancy	Vagal manuevers, adenosine

Abbreviations: RV, right ventricle; SVT, supraventricular tachycardia.

Table 6	
Recommendations that may be beneficial, based on expert opinion	
Condition	Management Considerations: May Be Beneficial
Asymptomatic pulmonary regurgitation with RV dilatation	Pulmonary valve replacement before pregnancy
Mild-moderate aortic stenosis	Image aorta before pregnancy
Bicuspid valve aortopathy with aorta >50 mm	Consider surgery before pregnancy
Univentricular heart, Fontan palliation	Anticoagulation during pregnancy and post partum
Symptomatic mitral stenosis (mitral valve area >1.5 cm^2)	Consider balloon valvuloplasty in select candidates after team discussion of risks and benefits

Abbreviation: RV, right ventricle.

Valvular heart disease is associated with the significant maternal morbidity and mortality and, thus, deserves special discussion.

Prosthetic heart valves

A recent study from the prospective worldwide Registry of Pregnancy and Cardiac disease (ROPAC) described the pregnancy outcomes of 212 women with a mechanical heart valve (MHV), 134 patients with a tissue heart valve (THV), and 2620 other patients without a prosthetic valve. Women with a prosthetic heart valve had an increased maternal mortality (MHV 1.4%, THV 1.5%) compared with 0.2% in women with no heart valve. Mechanical valve thrombosis is a potentially fatal complication during pregnancy, with the highest risk during the first trimester and when off of warfarin. Hemorrhagic events were also more common in women in ROPAC, occurring in 23% of women with MHV versus roughly 5% of those with THV or no heart valve.[41] Although heparin use in the first trimester is associated with a higher rate of

Box 1
High maternal risk, WHO class IV, pregnancy contraindicated
Eisenmenger syndrome
Transposition of the great arteries, systemic RV with moderate dysfunction and/or severe tricuspid regurgitation
Univentricular heart with or without Fontan palliation and any of the following: • Decreased ventricular function • Moderate to severe atrioventricular valve regurgitation • Cyanosis • Protein-losing enteropathy
Ehlers-Danlos type IV (high risk aortic dissection)
Coarctation of the aorta, repaired or unrepaired, with significant obstruction
Turner syndrome with dilated aorta (>27 mm/m^2)
Current or prior type B aortic dissection
Heart failure of any cause with functional class III or IV
Abbreviation: RV, right ventricle.

valve thrombosis, vitamin K antagonist use in the first trimester compared with heparin was associated with a higher rate of miscarriage (28.6% vs 9.2%, P<.001) and late fetal death (7.1% vs 0.7%, P = .016).[41] Options for anticoagulation management in pregnancy are discussed in further detail in the 2011 European Society of Cardiology guidelines,[11] including discussion of specific situations in which warfarin continuation is reasonable. Women with MHVs should undergo extensive counseling regarding the risks of pregnancy and need for centralization of care at an experienced multidisciplinary center.[41]

Aortic stenosis
Severe aortic stenosis (AS) is associated with high maternal risk for development of heart failure, chest pain, and sudden death; therefore, intervention is recommended before pregnancy. Women with moderate or severe AS who become symptomatic during pregnancy are more likely to require cardiac interventions late after pregnancy than those who have never been pregnant.[42–45] Given the significant potential for both maternal and obstetric complications with mechanical valves during pregnancy, counseling at the time of valve replacement surgery is imperative, with consideration of the tissue valve.

LABOR AND DELIVERY

Maternal cardiac patients benefit from a multidisciplinary team including a high-risk obstetrician, cardiologist, and an obstetric anesthesiologist. Overall, maternal mortality during labor and delivery is low, even among patients with high-risk lesions, such as Fontan circulation.[46] However, cardiac and obstetric complications during and after delivery are high and include pulmonary edema, arrhythmias, and hemorrhage. Timing and mode of delivery should be discussed in advance with patients and their families, in addition to possible complications that might arise, in order to prepare patients for the emotional rigors of a high-risk delivery. Antenatal planning with the multidisciplinary team also allows for creation of a delivery plan during both elective and emergency scenarios of labor and delivery, thereby creating a realistic appreciation for possible complications should patients decompensate. This planning is specifically important in complex congenital lesions, lesions requiring anticoagulation with heparin, mechanical valves, and Eisenmenger syndrome. Furthermore, per current guidelines, primary cesarean delivery should be considered for patients on oral anticoagulants in preterm labor, women with severe heart failure, aortic root-diameter of greater than 45 mm, patients with Marfan syndrome with an aortic root diameter of greater than 40 mm, and patients with acute or chronic aortic dissection.[11,47]

Hemodynamic Changes of Labor and Delivery

The potential for decompensation in patients with high-risk cardiovascular lesions is significant during labor and delivery, mainly because of the rapid fluctuations in maternal hemodynamic parameters.[48] Although contractions add approximately 300 to 500 mL of blood to the maternal circulation, the pain and anxiety associated with labor further adds approximately 50% to 60% to the cardiac output, heart rate, and blood pressure. These hemodynamic changes in conjunction with changes in vascular collagen, increase the risk of aortic dissection, particularly among women with aortopathy, such as Marfan syndrome, and vascular type 4 Ehlers-Danlos syndrome. Similarly, the risk of pulmonary edema increases early after delivery among patients with mitral and AS due to rapid fluid shifts. In these cases, the duration of labor is shortened with the use of forceps or vacuum assistance.[49] The risk of pulmonary edema in stenotic valvular lesions further increases postpartum, when pressure on the inferior vena cava from a term uterus is relieved. After delivery, CO and SV increase dramatically, further straining the heart and creating hemodynamic problems in those women limited by a fixed CO due to anatomic obstruction. Within the next 1 to 6 weeks after delivery, other hemodynamic parameters, including heart rate, cardiac output, and stroke volume, will return to prepregnancy values. In general, the use of central venous lines or pulmonary arterial catheters is not pervasive in the United States, Canada, or Europe to monitor hemodynamic changes and is only carried out in a small subset of unstable high-risk patients. Vasoactive drugs are used if needed through peripheral access via the antecubital fossa.[50]

Mode of Delivery

Although often discussed, cardiac conditions rarely influence the mode of delivery, with the exception of significant aortic pathology or dissection. Vaginal delivery is preferred over cesarean delivery in most patients with stable cardiac disease[51] and can be achieved for higher-risk patients with a judicious use of maternal positioning and analgesia. However, the overall use of cesarean delivery for delivery in cardiac patients ranges from 21% to 55% in different countries, which is significantly higher than the normal population.[52] This preference is guided mostly by concerns for need of emergent cesarean delivery due to sudden hemodynamic compromise in labor and delivery. However, vaginal delivery with an effective epidural causes less drastic hemodynamic changes and is associated with a lower incidence of complications, including hemorrhage, infection, and thrombosis, as compared with cesarean deliveries.[50] Institutions that have a lower cesarean delivery rate in women with heart disease make a concerted effort to prevent surgical intervention unless absolutely necessary.

A 2013 meta-analysis investigated the safety of vaginal delivery versus caesarean delivery in 29,262 patients with CHD in 113 studies.[53] This study found no increase in maternal or fetal complications based on cesarean versus vaginal delivery alone, irrespective of the severity of the cardiac pathology. Patients with NYHA class III and IV had the highest rate of complications, including death, and benefited from a shorter trial of labor with delivery under good analgesic control. Similarly, a study on planned cesarean delivery outcomes from the ROPAC investigators reviewed 1262 deliveries in the Netherlands.[52] In this study, there was no difference in maternal mortality (1.8% vs 1.5%), heart failure (8.8% vs 8.2%), or hemorrhage (6.2% vs 5.1%) in those with elective versus emergency cesarean delivery, indicating that emergency cesarean delivery may be a viable option if vaginal delivery fails. However, other UK studies indicate that the relative risk (RR) for mortality for all elective cesarean deliveries is 2.3 when compared with vaginal delivery, and the RR climbs to 12 for emergency cesarean delivery, when compared with vaginal delivery in cardiac patients.[46,54] When feasible, vaginal delivery has neonatal benefits with respect to greater gestational time and greater birth weight. Institutions that carry out higher rates of vaginal deliveries in high-risk cardiac patients implement a careful management plan composed of close monitoring with an escalating scale of invasive monitoring, which provides accurate, dynamic information to guide vasoactive therapy.[46,50] Patients with intracardiac shunts are continually evaluated with pulse oximetry if patients are pushing during the second stage of labor. Increases in intrathoracic pressures related to the Valsalva maneuver can accentuate right to left shunts, leading to hypoxia and stress in the fetus. For this reason, in some institutions, limited pushing is allowed during the second stage of labor to avoid effects of Valsalva. To manage analgesia, low-dose epidural is implemented in all women in labor and forceps and vacuum are used as needed to assist with delivery. Additional recommendations for cardiac monitoring during labor and delivery include

- Continuous telemetry monitoring for patients predisposed to arrhythmias and to ischemia
- Defibrillator pads for patients at risk for poorly tolerated tachyarrhythmias
- Pulse-oximetry for intracardiac shunts or cyanotic heart disease
- Intra-arterial catheter to monitor blood pressure in high-risk women during hemodynamic changes associated with uterine contractions
- Central venous catheter in unstable patients for monitoring and for vasoactive drug infusions
- Intrapulmonary catheter, rarely used during high-risk deliveries, considered for titration of pulmonary vasodilatory agents in patients with pulmonary hypertension
- Echocardiography if needed to evaluate real-time cardiac performance during circulatory instability

Advantages to a planned cesarean delivery in high-risk patients include experienced daytime staff with sufficient monitoring and fewer changes in maternal hemodynamics by eliminating labor contractions. Maternal heart disease has been associated with postpartum hemorrhage, but this was not isolated to assisted delivery or prolonged second stage of labor.[55]

Anesthetics

1. Neuroaxial (spinal and epidural) causes blockade of the sympathetic chain below the level at which anesthesia is applied, causing vasodilation in the lower body.[56] Although there are few absolute contraindications to using regional anesthesia in structural cardiac lesions, there is a relative contraindication for patients with high-grade AS, certain spinal surgeries, increased intracranial pressures, and severe hypovolemia and some skeletal abnormalities.[57] Other absolute contraindications include moderate or severe bleeding diathesis, including anticoagulation and infection at the site of insertion.
2. General anesthesia allows controlled manipulation of the respiratory and cardiovascular parameters and facilitates transesophageal echocardiography during delivery.[57] Intubation during general anesthesia allows for maintaining higher end-expiratory pressures, thereby decreasing pulmonary edema. However, complications from general anesthesia can be severe, including failed intubations, tachycardia, and respiratory complications. Opioids are often used to induce general anesthesia and blunt sympathetic response.[58]

Guidelines for management of a parturient with cardiac disease are limited. Most of the evidence comes from smaller studies and case reports and is influenced by anecdotal evidence. Therefore, most obstetricians guide treatment based on personal experience and a multidisciplinary approach.

IMPACT OF MATERNAL HEART DISEASE ON THE DEVELOPING FETUS

Congenital anomalies are the leading cause of death in infancy, and CHD makes up 30% to 50% of these cases. Reasons to screen for CHD include determining prognosis, appropriate birth institution and level of care needed for postpartum care, determining route of delivery, and enlisting subspecialists to aid with care. As an example, patients with ductal-dependent circulations can receive intravenous prostaglandins soon after birth while still hemodynamically stable rather than waiting for symptoms related to ductal closure (shock, severe cyanosis). Despite the theoretic benefits, proof of improved outcome due to prenatal diagnosis has only been shown in certain patient populations, such as patients who are candidates for biventricular repair and patients with hypoplastic left heart syndrome. Please refer to the article (Sanapo L, Moon-Grady AJ, Donofrio MT: Perinatal and delivery management of the infant with congenital heart disease, in this issue) for further discussion regarding perinatal and delivery room management.

The best modality for screening for CHD during the prenatal period is dedicated fetal echocardiography. This modality provides a superior evaluation of the cardiac anatomy compared with the anatomic fetal ultrasound done during the second trimester by obstetrics. The optimal time for fetal echocardiography is between 18 and 22 weeks. Acoustic windows are optimal; based on findings, there is time for further evaluation (including genetic testing) to aid decision making and family planning. Although the anatomy is visualized as well as possible by echocardiography, some lesions can be missed, including small ventricular septal defects, atrial septal defects, partial anomalous pulmonary venous return, and coronary anomalies. A transthoracic echocardiogram after birth should be used if concern remains or to confirm known findings from the fetal echocardiogram. Indications for fetal echocardiogram are listed in the Best Practices (**Box 2**) later. See the article (Sanapo L, Moon-Grady AJ, Donofrio MT: Perinatal and delivery management of the infant with congenital heart disease, in

---

Box 2
Indications for obtaining a fetal echocardiogram

Cardiac or noncardiac anomaly on obstetric ultrasound

Fetal hydrops

Known concerning genetic mutation (aneuploidy, and so forth)

Fetal arrhythmia or frequent ectopy

Increased nuchal translucency ($\geq$3 mm)

Monochorionic twins

Maternal diabetes diagnosed by the first trimester

Uncontrolled maternal phenylketonuria

Maternal SSA/SSB autoantibodies

Maternal teratogen exposure (thalidomide, retinoic acid, NSAID during the third trimester)

Suspicion of fetal myocarditis

Assisted reproduction technology used

Congenital heart disease in a first-degree relative

First- or second-degree relative with a genetic disorder associated with congenital heart disease (Down, Noonan, Holt-Oram syndromes, and so forth)

Maternal rubella syndrome

Abbreviation: NSAID, nonsteroidal antiinflammatory drug.
  Adapted from Donofrio MT, Moon-Grady AJ, Hornberger LK, et al, American Heart Association Adults With Congenital Heart Disease Joint Committee of the Council on Cardiovascular Disease in the Young and Council on Clinical Cardiology, Council on Cardiovascular Surgery and Anesthesia, and Council on Cardiovascular and Stroke Nursing. Diagnosis and treatment of fetal cardiac disease: a scientific statement from the American Heart Association. Circulation 2014;129:2189.

this issue) for further discussion regarding both diagnostic and therapeutic options for evaluating fetuses with suspected CHD.

There is a low risk of CHD (1%–2%) in the following conditions, and fetal echocardiography is only sometimes indicated: exposure to certain maternal medications (lithium, nonsteroidal antiinflammatory drugs before the third trimester, and so forth), CHD in a second-degree relative, fetal intra-abdominal venous anomaly, and anomaly of the umbilical cord. In total, about 4% of patients with CHD have an identifiable syndrome. Chromosomal abnormalities and genetic syndromes associated with CHD are listed later (**Tables 7** and **8**), along with recurrence risk.[21]

Genetic Counseling and Testing for Women with Congenital Heart Disease

As women with CHD survive to childbearing age, the predicting likelihood of successful pregnancy becomes an essential part of a physician's duties. To predict the risk of disease recurrence, formal genetic counseling can be invaluable.

During a genetic counseling session, topics such as disease transmission, penetrance and expressivity of disease, severity of disease (risk for morbidity and mortality, hospitalization, health care cost, and so forth), and the role of artificial insemination, surrogacy, and early diagnosis via embryo biopsy may all be discussed. The specifics of testing, including timing and risks, may also be reviewed.

Counseling before and after genetic testing is essential, including the risk of the procedure (fetal loss), psychological risks (anxiety for the parents), limits of genetic testing, possibility of finding variants of unknown significance, the possibility of identifying consanguinity or nonpaternity, and that negative testing does not rule out all genetic disease. The increasing importance of post-test counseling has become

Table 7
Chromosomal abnormalities and association with CHD

Chromosome Abnormality	Percentage of Individuals with Heart Defects (%)	Types of Congenital Heart Defects Observed
Down syndrome	40–50	Complete AV canal, VSD, ASD
Trisomy 18	>90	ASD, VSD, PDA, TOF, DORV, D-TGA, CoA, BAV
Trisomy 13	80	ASD, VSD, PDA, HLHS, atrial isomerism
Wolf-Hirschorn syndrome (4p deletion)	50–60	ASD, VSD, PDA, aortic atresia, dextrocardia, TOF
Cri-du-chat (5p deletion)	30–60	VSD, ASD, PDA
Jacobsen syndrome	55	HLHS, valvar AS, VSD, CoA, truncus arteriosus
DiGeorge syndrome	75	IAA-B, truncus arteriosus, isolated aortic arch anomalies, TOF, VSD
Turner syndrome	25–35	CoA, BAV, valvar AS, HLHS

Abbreviations: ASD, atrial septal defect; AV, atrioventricular; BAV, bicuspid aortic valve; CoA, coarctation; D-TGA, D-transposition of the great arteries; DORV, double outlet right ventricle; HLHS, hypoplastic left heart syndrome; IAA-B, Interrupted aortic arch, type B; PDA, patent ductus arteriosus; TOF, tetralogy of Fallot; VSD, ventricular septal defect.

Data from Roos-Hesselink JW, Kerstjens-Frederikse WS, Meijboom FJ, et al. Inheritance of congenital heart disease. Neth Heart J 2005;13:88–91; and Gill HK, Splitt M, Sharland GK, et al. Patterns of recurrence of congenital heart disease: an analysis of 6640 consecutive pregnancies evaluated by detailed fetal echocardiography. J Am Coll Cardiol 2003;42:923–9.

Table 8
Recurrence risks for offspring of patients with CHD

CHD	Offspring Recurrence Rate (Nonsyndromic)	Associated Syndromes
Any CHD in either parent	5%	—
Atrial septal defect	3%–5%	Holt-Oram
Ventricular septal defect	2%–5%	—
Atrioventricular septal defect	10%–14%	Down syndrome
Pulmonary stenosis, supravalvar pulmonary stenosis	3%–5%	Noonan, Alagille, Williams
Tetralogy of Fallot	3%–5%	22q11
Aortic valve stenosis, bicuspid aortic valve	12%–20% in affected mother, 5% in affected father	Scheie syndrome
Coarctation	4%–10%, higher likelihood if associated with BAV	Turner syndrome
Ebstein anomaly	6%	—
D-TGA	2%	None
L-TGA	3%–5%	None

Abbreviations: BAV, bicuspid aortic valve; D-TGA, D-transposition of the great arteries; L-TGA, L-transposition of the great arteries.

Data from Roos-Hesselink JW, Kerstjens-Frederikse WS, Meijboom FJ, et al. Inheritance of congenital heart disease. Neth Heart J 2005;13:88–91; and Oyen N, Poulsen G, Wohlfahrt J, et al. Recurrence of discordant congenital heart defects in families. Circ Cardiovasc Genet 2010;3:122–8.

apparent as genetic testing becomes more sensitive; it is often impossible to discuss all the potential findings ahead of time.

SUMMARY

- Women with preexisting medical conditions should have prepregnancy counseling by doctors with experience in managing their disorder.
- Women with medical disorders in pregnancy should be managed in a coordinated multidisciplinary clinic, avoiding poor communication between subspecialists responsible for their care.
- There should be adequate critical care support for the management of a pregnant woman who develops complications. Plans should be in place for provision of critical care on delivery units or maternity care on critical care units, depending on the most appropriate setting for the situation.

REFERENCES

1. Moons P, Bovijn L, Budts W, et al. Temporal trends in survival to adulthood among patients born with congenital heart disease from 1970 to 1992 in Belgium. Circulation 2010;122:2264–72.
2. Marelli AJ, Mackie AS, Ionescu-Ittu R, et al. Congenital heart disease in the general population: changing prevalence and age distribution. Circulation 2007;115:163–72.
3. Knight M, Kenyon S, Brocklehurst P, et al. Saving lives, improving mothers care lessons learned to inform future maternity care from the UK and Ireland

confidential enquiries into maternal deaths and morbidity 2009-2012. Oxford national perinatal epidemiology unit, University of Oxford; 2014.

4. CDC - Pregnancy mortality surveillance system - maternal and infant health - reproductive health. Available at: www.cdc.gov; http://www.cdc.gov/reproductivehealth/maternalinfanthealth/pmss.html. Accessed November 9, 2015.

5. Opotowsky AR, Siddiqi OK, D'Souza B, et al. Maternal cardiovascular events during childbirth among women with congenital heart disease. Heart 2012;98: 145–51.

6. Thompson JL, Kuklina EV, Bateman BT, et al. Medical and obstetric outcomes among pregnant women with congenital heart disease. Obstet Gynecol 2015; 126:346–54.

7. Siu SC, Sermer M, Colman JM, et al, Cardiac Disease in Pregnancy (CARPREG) Investigators. Prospective multicenter study of pregnancy outcomes in women with heart disease. Circulation 2001;104:515–21.

8. Roos-Hesselink JW, Ruys TPE, Stein JI, et al, ROPAC Investigators. Outcome of pregnancy in patients with structural or ischaemic heart disease: results of a registry of the European Society of Cardiology. Eur Heart J 2013;34:657–65.

9. Warnes CA. Pregnancy and delivery in women with congenital heart disease. Circ J 2015;79(7):1416–21.

10. O'Herlihy C. Reviewing maternal deaths to make motherhood safer: 2006–2008. BJOG 2011;118:1403–4.

11. Regitz-Zagrosek V, Blomstrom Lundqvist C, Borghi C, et al, ESC Committee for Practice Guidelines. ESC guidelines on the management of cardiovascular diseases during pregnancy: the task force on the management of cardiovascular diseases during pregnancy of the European Society of Cardiology (ESC). Eur Heart J 2011;32:3147–97.

12. Thorne S, MacGregor A, Nelson-Piercy C. Risks of contraception and pregnancy in heart disease. Heart 2006;92:1520–5.

13. Drenthen W, Boersma E, Balci A, et al, ZAHARA Investigators. Predictors of pregnancy complications in women with congenital heart disease. Eur Heart J 2010; 31:2124–32.

14. Siu SC, Sermer M, Harrison DA, et al. Risk and predictors for pregnancy-related complications in women with heart disease. Circulation 1997;96:2789–94.

15. Silversides CK, Sermer M, Siu SC. Choosing the best contraceptive method for the adult with congenital heart disease. Curr Cardiol Rep 2009;11:298–305.

16. Mahle WT, Clancy RR, McGaurn SP, et al. Impact of prenatal diagnosis on survival and early neurologic morbidity in neonates with the hypoplastic left heart syndrome. Pediatrics 2001;107:1277–82.

17. Balci A, Sollie-Szarynska KM, van der Bijl AGL, et al, ZAHARA-II Investigators. Prospective validation and assessment of cardiovascular and offspring risk models for pregnant women with congenital heart disease. Heart 2014;100: 1373–81.

18. Gilboa SM, Salemi JL, Nembhard WN, et al. Mortality resulting from congenital heart disease among children and adults in the United States, 1999 to 2006. Circulation 2010;122:2254–63.

19. Drenthen W, Pieper PG, Roos-Hesselink JW, et al. Outcome of pregnancy in women with congenital heart disease: a literature review. J Am Coll Cardiol 2007;49:2303–11.

20. Khairy P, Ouyang DW, Fernandes SM, et al. Pregnancy outcomes in women with congenital heart disease. Circulation 2006;113:517–24.

21. Gill HK, Splitt M, Sharland GK, et al. Patterns of recurrence of congenital heart disease: an analysis of 6,640 consecutive pregnancies evaluated by detailed fetal echocardiography. J Am Coll Cardiol 2003;42:923–9.
22. Whittemore R, Wells JA, Castellsague X. A second-generation study of 427 probands with congenital heart defects and their 837 children. J Am Coll Cardiol 1994;23:1459–67.
23. Burn J, Brennan P, Little J, et al. Recurrence risks in offspring of adults with major heart defects: results from first cohort of British collaborative study. Lancet 1998; 351:311–6.
24. Ruys TPE, Maggioni A, Johnson MR, et al. Cardiac medication during pregnancy, data from the ROPAC. Int J Cardiol 2014;177:124–8.
25. Hunter S, Robson SC. Adaptation of the maternal heart in pregnancy. Br Heart J 1992;68:540–3.
26. Villablanca AC. Heart disease during pregnancy. Which cardiovascular changes are normal or transient? Postgrad Med 1998;104:183–4, 187–92.
27. Shotan A, Ostrzega E, Mehra A, et al. Incidence of arrhythmias in normal pregnancy and relation to palpitations, dizziness, and syncope. Am J Cardiol 1997; 79:1061–4.
28. Silversides CK, Harris L, Haberer K, et al. Recurrence rates of arrhythmias during pregnancy in women with previous tachyarrhythmia and impact on fetal and neonatal outcomes. Am J Cardiol 2006;97:1206–12.
29. Burchill LJ, Lameijer H, Roos-Hesselink JW, et al. Pregnancy risks in women with pre-existing coronary artery disease, or following acute coronary syndrome. Heart 2015;101:525–9.
30. Grewal J, Siu SC, Ross HJ, et al. Pregnancy outcomes in women with dilated cardiomyopathy. J Am Coll Cardiol 2009;55:45–52.
31. Ruys TPE, Roos-Hesselink JW, Hall R, et al. Heart failure in pregnant women with cardiac disease: data from the ROPAC. Heart 2014;100:231–8.
32. Kampman MAM, Balci A, van Veldhuisen DJ, et al, ZAHARA II Investigators. N-terminal pro-B-type natriuretic peptide predicts cardiovascular complications in pregnant women with congenital heart disease. Eur Heart J 2014; 35:708–15.
33. Kampman MAM, Balci A, Groen H, et al, ZAHARA II Investigators. Cardiac function and cardiac events 1-year postpartum in women with congenital heart disease. Am Heart J 2015;169:298–304.
34. Hoes MF, van Hagen I, Russo F, et al. Peripartum cardiomyopathy: Euro Observational Research Program. Neth Heart J 2014;22:396–400.
35. Colman JM, Sermer M, Seaward PG, et al. Congenital heart disease in pregnancy. Cardiol Rev 2000;8:166–73.
36. Foster E, Graham TP, Driscoll DJ, et al. Task force 2: special health care needs of adults with congenital heart disease. J Am Coll Cardiol 2001;37:1176–83.
37. Sermer M, Colman J, Siu S. Pregnancy complicated by heart disease: a review of Canadian experience. J Obstet Gynaecol 2003;23:540–4.
38. Drenthen W, Pieper PG, van der Tuuk K, et al, Zahara Investigators. Cardiac complications relating to pregnancy and recurrence of disease in the offspring of women with atrioventricular septal defects. Eur Heart J 2005;26:2581–7.
39. Beauchesne LM, Connolly HM, Ammash NM, et al. Coarctation of the aorta: outcome of pregnancy. J Am Coll Cardiol 2001;38:1728–33.
40. Jimenez-Juan L, Krieger EV, Valente AM, et al. Cardiovascular magnetic resonance imaging predictors of pregnancy outcomes in women with coarctation of the aorta. Eur Heart J Cardiovasc Imaging 2014;15:299–306.

41. van Hagen IM, Roos-Hesselink JW, Ruys TPE, et al, ROPAC Investigators and the EORP Team. Pregnancy in women with a mechanical heart valve: data of the European Society of Cardiology Registry of Pregnancy and Cardiac Disease (ROPAC). Circulation 2015;132(2):132–42.

42. Tzemos N, Silversides CK, Colman JM, et al. Late cardiac outcomes after pregnancy in women with congenital aortic stenosis. Am Heart J 2009;157:474–80.

43. Heuvelman HJ, Arabkhani B, Cornette JMJ, et al. Pregnancy outcomes in women with aortic valve substitutes. Am J Cardiol 2013;111:382–7.

44. Henriquez DD, Roos-Hesselink JW, Schalij MJ, et al. Treatment of valvular heart disease during pregnancy for improving maternal and neonatal outcome. Cochrane Database Syst Rev 2011;(5):CD008128.

45. Arabkhani B, Heuvelman HJ, Bogers AJJC, et al. Does pregnancy influence the durability of human aortic valve substitutes? J Am Coll Cardiol 2012;60:1991–2.

46. Canobbio MM, Mair DD, van der Velde M, et al. Pregnancy outcomes after the Fontan repair. J Am Coll Cardiol 1996;28:763–7.

47. Hiratzka LF, Bakris GL, Beckman JA, et al, Society for Vascular Medicine. 2010 ACCF/AHA/AATS/ACR/ASA/SCA/SCAI/SIR/STS/SVM guidelines for the diagnosis and management of patients with thoracic aortic disease: executive summary. A report of the American College of Cardiology Foundation/American Heart Association Task Force on Practice Guidelines, American Association for Thoracic Surgery, American College of Radiology, American Stroke Association, Society of Cardiovascular Anesthesiologists, Society for Cardiovascular Angiography and Interventions, Society of Interventional Radiology, Society of Thoracic Surgeons, and Society for Vascular Medicine. Catheter Cardiovasc Interv 2010;76:E43–86.

48. Bridges EJ, Womble S, Wallace M, et al. Hemodynamic monitoring in high-risk obstetrics patients, I. Expected hemodynamic changes in pregnancy. Crit Care Nurse 2003;23:53–62.

49. Gelson E, Gatzoulis M, Johnson M. Valvular heart disease. BMJ 2007;335:1042–5.

50. Dob DP, Yentis SM. Practical management of the parturient with congenital heart disease. Int J Obstet Anesth 2006;15:137–44.

51. Silversides CK, Colman JM, Sermer M, et al. Early and intermediate-term outcomes of pregnancy with congenital aortic stenosis. Am J Cardiol 2003;91:1386–9.

52. Ruys TPE, Roos-Hesselink JW, Pijuan-Domènech A, et al, ROPAC Investigators. Is a planned caesarean section in women with cardiac disease beneficial? Heart 2015;101:530–6.

53. Asfour V, Murphy MO, Attia R. Is vaginal delivery or caesarean section the safer mode of delivery in patients with adult congenital heart disease? Interact Cardiovasc Thorac Surg 2013;17:144–50.

54. Wildsmith JA. Confidential enquiries into maternal deaths, 1997–1999. Br J Anaesth 2003;90:257–8.

55. Robertson JE, Silversides CK, Mah ML, et al. A contemporary approach to the obstetric management of women with heart disease. J Obstet Gynaecol Can 2012;34:812–9.

56. Tihtonen K, Kööbi T, Yli-Hankala A, et al. Maternal hemodynamics during cesarean delivery assessed by whole-body impedance cardiography. Acta Obstet Gynecol Scand 2005;84:355–61.

57. Turnbull J, Bell R. Obstetric anaesthesia and peripartum management. Best Pract Res Clin Obstet Gynaecol 2014;28:593–605.
58. Orme RMLE, Grange CS, Ainsworth QP, et al. General anaesthesia using remifentanil for caesarean section in parturients with critical aortic stenosis: a series of four cases. Int J Obstet Anesth 2004;13:183–7.

Fetal Diagnostics and Fetal Intervention

Ericka S. McLaughlin, DO[a,b,*], Brian A. Schlosser, BS, RDCS, RDMS[a],
William L. Border, MBChB, MPH[a,b]

KEYWORDS

- Fetal echocardiography • Congenital heart disease • Fetal diagnostics
- Fetal intervention • Sequential segmental analysis

KEY POINTS

- Expectations for the accurate diagnosis of congenital heart disease in fetuses have increased significantly.
- Improved ultrasound technology allows for detailed anatomic and physiologic assessment of the fetal heart.
- Consistent application of a sequential segmental approach to the fetal echocardiogram ensures an accurate and comprehensive diagnosis to allow for appropriate perinatal management.

 Video content accompanies this article at http://www.perinatology.theclinics. com/

INTRODUCTION

Congenital heart disease (CHD) is the most common type of birth defect; however, it is one of the most frequently missed abnormalities by prenatal ultrasound.[1] With advances in the fetal diagnosis of CHD and the availability of fetal therapies, it has become crucial to improve the screening of obstetric patients and correctly diagnose fetuses with CHD in utero. The fetal diagnosis of CHD impacts the prenatal and postnatal care of mothers and fetuses. Although the benefits of fetal diagnosis have been controversial, recent studies suggest that an accurate fetal diagnosis and actions taken as a result of a fetal diagnosis may improve morbidity and mortality, specifically for fetuses with critical CHD.[2–5]

Disclosures: None.
[a] Children's Healthcare of Atlanta, The McGill Building, 2835 Brandywine Road, Suite 300, Atlanta, GA 30341, USA; [b] Department of Pediatrics, Emory University School of Medicine, Atlanta, GA, USA
* Corresponding author. The McGill Building, 2835 Brandywine Road, Suite 300, Atlanta, GA 30341.
E-mail address: mclaughline@kidsheart.com

Clin Perinatol 43 (2016) 23–38
http://dx.doi.org/10.1016/j.clp.2015.11.003
0095-5108/16/$ – see front matter © 2016 Elsevier Inc. All rights reserved.

perinatology.theclinics.com

RATES OF FETAL DIAGNOSIS

The reported rates of fetal diagnosis of CHD vary greatly among regions and institutions. A recent study found that in the United States, the prenatal diagnosis rate of CHD was 26% in 2006 and increased to 42% in 2012.[6] These data are similar to previously reported data from other centers.[7,8] The rate of fetal diagnosis of CHD is affected by the type of cardiac lesion, ultrasound practice, and training of the examiner.[7,8] Other factors, however, have been postulated to affect the fetal diagnosis of CHD, including maternal body habitus, maternal socioeconomic status, ethnicity, and geographic region of care.

OBSTETRIC SCREENING

Prenatal diagnosis of CHD requires a multidisciplinary approach. It requires access to timely prenatal care, efficient screening by trained sonographers, reliable interpretation, and the ability to refer to a pediatric cardiologist. A mother receiving prenatal care in the United States will almost universally receive a routine obstetric ultrasound.[7] Despite having universal obstetric screening, rates of prenatal diagnosis of CHD vary greatly and remain low in certain areas.

The current guidelines from the American Institute of Ultrasound in Medicine, the American College of Radiology, and the American College of Obstetrics and Gynecology recommend that women should have a detailed anatomy screening ultrasound between 18 and 20 weeks of estimated gestational age, unless there is an indication for one earlier.[9] The cardiac examination was initially limited to a four-chamber view of the heart. More recently, it has also included evaluation of the outflow tracts. Studies have shown that the four-chamber view can detect greater than 50% of serious cardiac malformations, but additional evaluation of the outflow tracts, including the "three-vessel" view, increases detection rates to 90%.[10] This suggests that by following current guidelines, along with a more detailed assessment of the heart in a systematic fashion, an institution can significantly improve their rates of prenatal diagnosis of CHD.

FETAL ECHOCARDIOGRAPHY

Fetal echocardiography provides a detailed assessment of the structure and function of the fetal cardiovascular system to ensure an accurate diagnosis and guide prenatal counseling and perinatal management. Although obstetric screening has expanded its evaluation of the fetal heart, the fetal echocardiogram provides a dedicated fetal cardiac examination to include all cardiac structures and can further focus on the counseling regarding the pathophysiology of the cardiac lesion and future treatment options.

Indications for Fetal Echocardiography

Indications for fetal echocardiography are divided into maternal and fetal factors (**Box 1**). Recently, the American Heart Association published a complete list of indications for fetal echocardiography.[11] The leading indication for referral for a fetal echocardiogram is an abnormal obstetric screening ultrasound.[12] Conversely, of those fetuses with CHD who had a fetal echocardiogram, only 10% of those patients were referred for an identifiable risk factor.[13] Therefore, all fetuses should at least undergo a comprehensive screening ultrasound by a trained professional.

Timing of Fetal Echocardiogram

The timing of the fetal echocardiogram should be determined by the reason for referral. Although fetal echocardiography can be performed in the first trimester, the optimal

---

Box 1
Indications for fetal echocardiography

Maternal Indications

Maternal disease
    Diabetes mellitus, particularly pregestational
    Autoimmune disorders
    Phenylketonuria

First-degree relative with congenital heart disease

Maternal infection
    Rubella

Maternal medication use[a]

Exposure to teratogens

Use of assisted-reproductive technology

Fetal Indications

Abnormal screening ultrasound

Abnormal nuchal translucency

Suspected arrhythmia

Presence of extracardiac fetal anomalies

Abnormal karyotype

Monochorionic twins

Hydrops fetalis

   [a] An extensive list of maternal medications is found in the American Heart Association Scientific Statement on Diagnosis and Treatment of Fetal Cardiac Disease.

---

time to visualize the fetal anatomy from a transabdominal approach is between 18 and 22 weeks gestation. An echocardiogram before this time frame is difficult, secondary to patient size and movement, and leads to an incomplete assessment. Because the primary indication for a fetal echocardiogram is an abnormal obstetric screening ultrasound, most patients are referred after their 18- to 20-week obstetric ultrasound. After 30 weeks gestation, images are difficult to obtain secondary to bone shadowing and increased fetal mass compared with amniotic fluid volume.

Equipment

The recommended equipment used for fetal echocardiography should have the capability to perform two-dimensional imaging, M-mode, and Doppler. Because the patient is often moving and has a fast heart rate, equipment with good spatial and temporal resolution is preferred. Axial resolution of 1 mm or less is important to detect subtle findings within the fetal heart. Image magnification is also important for better identification of the size and structure of the fetal heart. Generally, transabdominal studies should be performed with a curvilinear transducer, or a suitable phased-array transducer, in the 3- to 8-MHz range.

COMPLETE FETAL ECHOCARDIOGRAM

Several organizations have published practice guidelines to standardize the fetal cardiac examination.[9,14,15] A complete fetal cardiac checklist has been compiled in **Box 2**. It is recommended that for the first fetal echocardiogram a patient encounters, they receive a

Box 2	
Fetal cardiac checklist	
Feature	Checklist
Anatomic and biometric examination	Fetal number and position
	Cardiothoracic ratio
	Biparietal diameter
	Femur length
	Abdominal arrangement
	Umbilical cord assessment
Imaging/sweeps	Transverse abdominal view
	Four-chamber view
	Outflow sweep (five-vessel)
	Long-axis view/sweep
	Short-axis sweep (three-vessel)
	Caval long-axis view
	Aortic arch view
	Ductal arch view
Doppler assessment	Inferior vena cava
	Hepatic veins
	Ductus venosus
	Superior vena cava
	Pulmonary veins
	Foramen ovale
	Atrioventricular valves
	Semilunar valves
	Ductus arteriosus
	Aortic arch
	Umbilical artery
	Umbilical vein
	Middle cerebral artery
Measurements	Atrioventricular valve annulus
	Semilunar valve annulus
	Main pulmonary artery
	Branch pulmonary arteries
	Aortic arch and isthmus
	Right/left ventricular length
	Ventricular short axis diameter
Rhythm and rate	M-mode of atrial and ventricular wall motion
	Doppler examination of atrial and ventricular flow patterns

complete cardiac anatomic scan. Imaging the fetus is difficult secondary to fetal movement and positioning, making it difficult to perform an assessment of every structure that is recommended. However, the list in **Box 2** should be used as a recommended goal for every study. Each fetal echocardiogram should include careful imaging of the fetal cardiac anatomy, using a series of standardized sweeps in transverse and longitudinal imaging planes. Sweeps through the fetal heart should always be attempted, and often require a gentle slide of the transducer, rather than simply tilting. Transverse views should be obtained as close to perpendicular to the long axis of the fetus as possible. A complete fetal echocardiogram includes appropriate cardiac measurements, and normal ranges for fetal cardiac structures and z scores have been reported based on gestational age.

The complete fetal cardiovascular assessment also requires the use of color and pulsed Doppler. Color flow imaging and Doppler evaluation are essential parts of the necessary fetal echocardiography components. They are used to confirm the patency of the ventricular inflows and outflows, to assess the competency of valves, to confirm the systemic and pulmonary venous connections, to assess flow through both arches, and to confirm or rule out atrial or ventricular septal defects.

SEQUENTIAL SEGMENTAL APPROACH

CHD is complex and includes a wide variety of lesions. The authors suggest that using a sequential segmental approach, rather than blindly obtaining a set of standard echocardiographic views, guides the operator to think more in terms of anatomic relationships and results in more accurate and complete diagnoses. The sequential segmental approach provides a logical framework to evaluate and describe the heart, which is essential with complex CHD. Multiple imaging planes are used to evaluate the fetal heart. Depending on the institution preference or fetal position, these imaging planes and sweeps may be performed in a varying order. By using the sequential segmental approach, the operator can think about the heart in a systematic fashion and then the order of the imaging planes becomes less important.

The sequential segmental approach describes the heart using the three main cardiac segments (atrial, ventricular, and great arteries), and the connections between each segment, including the atrioventricular and ventriculoarterial connections.[16] In this approach, the main segments are defined by their most consistent anatomic features, and not their relationship to one another or their relationship in space. The systemic and pulmonary venous returns are also defined, and additional intracardiac abnormalities, such as ventricular septal defects. By using this approach, the authors suggest that "complex" CHD then becomes "simple" to diagnose and decreases the likelihood of error.

Historically, there have been many approaches to describe the congenitally malformed heart. Currently, there are two major classification systems that describe the heart based on morphologic features using a systematic approach. These classification systems have been proposed by Drs Anderson and Van Praagh; however, the details of each system are not described here.[17,18] Instead, the authors give the fetal scanner a practical approach to the fetal cardiac examination.

Fetal Position and Abdominal Arrangement

After determining the lie of the fetus, and subsequently ascertaining the left and right sides of the fetus, a careful transverse sweep of the fetal chest and abdomen is performed to determine abdominal arrangement and cardiac axis (Video 1). This overall view also allows the scanner to assess for the presence of pleural, pericardial, and peritoneal fluid collections, and to evaluate for evidence of skin edema.

The abdominal sweeps give an assessment of abdominal arrangement or situs, with careful attention paid to the location of the abdominal aorta and inferior vena cava, and the liver and stomach (**Fig. 1**). Because the abdominal (visceral) situs almost always corresponds to the atrial situs, this can help to determine the atrial arrangement and the presence of heterotaxy syndrome, also known as isomerism.

During each fetal echocardiogram, the umbilical cord should be evaluated. There are known associations between CHD and umbilical cord abnormalities. Also, umbilical artery and vein Doppler abnormalities are associated with fetal circulatory compromise, cardiac dysfunction, and certain types of CHD. Therefore, a complete fetal echocardiogram should include the structure of the umbilical cord and Doppler assessment of the umbilical vein and artery.

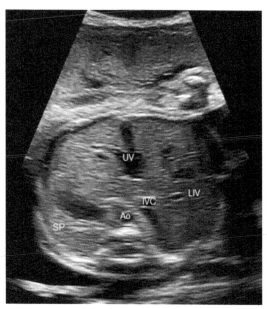

Fig. 1. Transverse abdominal view demonstrating the normal cross-sectional anatomy below the diaphragm. The liver is located on the right and stomach bubble and spleen are on the left. Here one can see the umbilical vein on the anterior aspect of the abdomen. The aorta is anterior to the spine with the inferior vena cava located anterior and slightly rightward to the aorta. Ao, aorta; IVC, inferior vena cava; LIV, liver; SP, spleen; UV, umbilical vein.

Atrial Arrangement

Instead of proceeding to a standard fetal view, the next step in the sequential segmental approach is to determine the atrial arrangement or situs. Each atrial segment is characterized as a morphologic right or left atrium, so there are four possibilities of atrial arrangement: (1) usual (situs solitus), (2) mirror-image (situs inversus), (3) right isomerism, and (4) left isomerism. The abdominal arrangement can often predict the corresponding atrial arrangement; however, to definitively define the morphology of an atrium, one should investigate the atrial appendages. Although not always optimally imaged, the shape of the atrial appendage is important and is the most reliable morphologic feature of the atrium. The morphologic right atrial appendage is a triangular-shaped structure with a broad base, where the pectinate muscles extend out of the appendage. A morphologic left atrial appendage is more "finger-shaped" with a narrow base, and with the pectinate muscles confined to the appendage. The left atrium can also usually be recognized by its presence anterior to the coronary sinus. In fetal echocardiography, the atrial appendages are best seen in four-chamber and short-axis views (**Fig. 2**).

An additional important feature at the atrial level is the presence and size of the foramen ovale. It is particularly important to use color and pulsed-wave Doppler to interrogate the direction of flow at the atrial septum. Normally, the flow is from right-to-left. However, in certain forms of CHD, this flow can be left-to-right; become restrictive; or there can even be premature closure of the foramen, which may be detrimental for the patient or be an indication for fetal cardiac intervention. The atrial septum can also be evaluated for the presence of additional defects, such as a primum atrial septal defect.

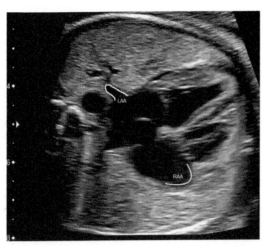

Fig. 2. Four-chamber view demonstrating the atrial appendages. This heart has usual atrial arrangement. The appendages are outlined to delineate how the right atrial appendage is a triangular-shaped structure with a broad base and the left atrial appendage is "finger-shaped" with a narrow base. This figure also demonstrates the normal shape of the atrial septum in utero, as it bows from right to left. LAA, left atrial appendage; RAA, right atrial appendage.

Note that atrial arrangements are not determined by their connections to the systemic or pulmonary veins, which can vary in their connections to the atria. In addition to the three main cardiac segments, the pulmonary and systemic venous connections need to be carefully documented. The pulmonary veins are visualized from multiple views, in particular the short-axis, long-axis, and four-chamber views (Video 2). Often, it is difficult to identify all four pulmonary veins, but effort should be made to visualize as many as possible with both color and pulsed-wave Doppler. The systemic venous connection and ductus venosus can ideally be visualized in the caval long-axis view (**Fig. 3**, Videos

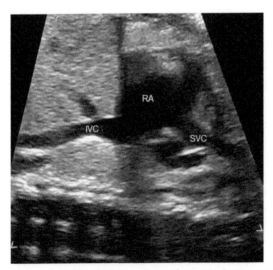

Fig. 3. Bicaval view. This is the view used to evaluate the systemic venous connections. Here one sees the superior vena cava and inferior vena cava entering the right atrium. IVC, inferior vena cava; RA, right atrium; SVC, superior vena cava.

3 and 4). The relationship of the inferior vena cava to the aorta is best visualized in the transverse abdominal view and if abnormalities are identified in this view, then isomerism (heterotaxy) should be suspected.

Atrioventricular Connections

The atrioventricular connection refers to the connection between the atria and ventricles, which can be concordant (meaning the right atrium corresponds with the right ventricle) or discordant (meaning the right atrium corresponds with the left ventricle). Note that atrioventricular valves correspond with their respective ventricles (eg, the tricuspid valve goes along with a morphologic right ventricle and the mitral valve with a morphologic left ventricle). The atrioventricular valves can also be absent or form a single common valve.

In fetal echocardiography, it is important to determine if there are one or two valves, the size and structure of the valve, and the function of the valve. The four-chamber view is an ideal view to determine much of this information; however, additional views, such as the long-axis and short-axis views, can also be helpful (**Figs. 4** and **5**). Color Doppler of the atrioventricular valves is used to assess flow across the valve and degree of regurgitation (Video 5).

Ventricular Arrangement

In conjunction with the atrioventricular morphology, it is important to determine the number of ventricles, size, function, and the anatomic morphology of the ventricles. It is important to determine the morphology of the ventricle because the right and left ventricles are formed and function differently. There are certain morphologic features that help to distinguish whether a ventricle is a morphologic right ventricle versus a morphologic left ventricle. The morphologic right ventricle shows a moderator band in its cavity and has coarse trabeculations, particularly along the interventricular septum. The atrioventricular valve associated with the right ventricle is the tricuspid valve, which is generally more apically displaced and is known to have chordal

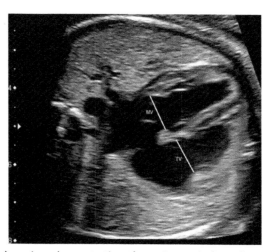

Fig. 4. Four-chamber view demonstrating the atrioventricular valves. In this view, one can evaluate the crux of the heart and insertion of the atrioventricular valves. One can also assess the overall size and morphology of the mitral valve and tricuspid valve. MV, mitral valve; TV, tricuspid valve.

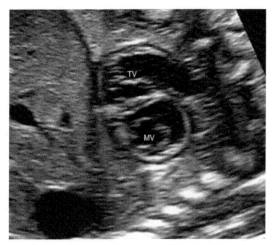

Fig. 5. Short-axis view of the atrioventricular valves. This view is used as an additional image of the atrioventricular valves en face to help determine the morphology and function of the valve. MV, mitral valve; TV, tricuspid valve.

attachments to the ventricular septum. The morphologic left ventricle shows a smoother, less trabeculated ventricular cavity and is associated with the mitral valve, which has no chordal attachments to the ventricular septum. These features can typically be identified in the four-chamber view and confirmed on the long- and short-axis views (**Fig. 6**, Videos 6 and 7).

The position of the right ventricle can often help determine the ventricular looping, a developmental designation. In general, if the primitive right ventricle loops to the right during development, the ventricles are designated as D-looped or have right-handed topology. If the primitive right ventricle loops to the left, the ventricles are L-looped or

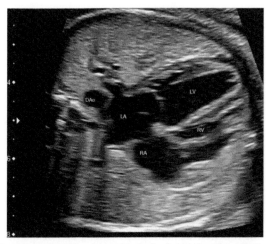

Fig. 6. Four-chamber view. This view is used to help determine the relationship between the atria and ventricles and the morphology and function of the right and left ventricles. DAo, descending aorta; LA, left atrium; LV, left ventricle; RA, right atrium; RV, right ventricle.

have left-handed topology. There are rare instances when the looping of the ventricle is difficult to determine, as in the case of complex single ventricle or ventricles with an "upstairs-downstairs" configuration.

Ventriculoarterial Connections

The ventriculoarterial connection refers to the connection between the ventricular body and the great arteries. It is important to denote the number of valves, their location in comparison with the ventricle, the presence of an infundibulum, and the shape and function of the semilunar valve. By convention, the semilunar valve that opens to the aorta is called the aortic valve and the valve that opens to the pulmonary artery is called the pulmonary valve. In the instance where there is one vessel, this valve is called a common arterial valve. The relationship of the great arteries to the ventricles is described in four ways: (1) concordant, (2) discordant, (3) double-outlet, or (4) single-outlet. Double outlet refers to a heart where both arteries seem to arise from one ventricle, often with the presence of bilateral infundibulums, and is characterized by the degree of ventricular septal override. A single outlet refers to any heart where there is one outlet from the heart, as seen in a common arterial trunk, pulmonary atresia, and aortic atresia.

The ventriculoarterial connections are assessed using the outflow tract sweep, which sweeps anteriorly and superiorly from the four-chamber view (Video 8). The ventriculoarterial connections can also be assessed in the long-axis view and sweep (**Fig. 7**). Complete interrogation of the ventriculoarterial connections includes measurements of the valves, color, and Doppler. The semilunar valves normally have three cusps; however, they can range from having one cusp to having multiple, particularly in the case of a common arterial trunk. It is also important to characterize the shape of these valves and whether they are stenotic, atretic/functionally atretic, or dilated. One should determine the direction of flow from the ventricle to the great artery and quantify the amount of stenosis or regurgitation at the valvar level.

Coronary arteries can be identified on fetal echocardiography. In certain types of cardiac pathology it is important to identify the location, size, and flow of the coronary arteries. These are seen best in the short-axis view.

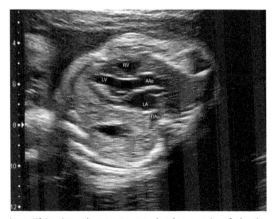

Fig. 7. Long-axis view. This view demonstrates the long axis of the heart. Here one sees the left atrium entering the left ventricle and its connection to the ascending aorta. In this image one also sees the size and relationship of the right ventricle. AAo, ascending aorta; DAo, descending aorta; LA, left atrium; LV, left ventricle; RV, right ventricle.

Relationship of the Great Arteries

The great artery connections, spatial positions, and size are important to determine. Care must be taken to ensure that the main pulmonary artery bifurcates into the right and left branches. The aorta is distinguished by demonstrating the take-off of the carotid and subclavian arteries. In a normal heart, the ventricular outflow tracts cross, with the aorta being posterior and rightward to the pulmonary artery at the base of the heart. If the great arteries course in a parallel fashion, one should consider certain types of CHD, such as transposition of the great arteries or double-outlet right ventricle. In the fetal echocardiogram, this view is obtained by sweeping from the four-chamber view anteriorly and superiorly (see Video 8). Even more superior to this view is the three-vessel view, which is a transverse view of the upper mediastinum, where a discrepancy in size and relationship of the great arteries can suggest CHD (**Fig. 8**). Normally, in the three-vessel view the pulmonary artery is largest, followed by the aorta, and lastly the superior vena cava, which is the smallest.

It is also important to evaluate the aortic arch and ductal arch in the long axis. The ductus arteriosus is an important structure to visualize in the fetal cardiac examination, and it is key to differentiate between the true aortic arch and the ductal arch (**Figs. 9 and 10**). The size of the arches, directionality of blood flow, and their relationship to one another and the trachea can all be obtained from these images. Measurements should be taken of the aortic arch with special attention paid to the aortic isthmus to evaluate for possible coarctation.

Additional Malformations

The sequential segmental approach focuses on the basic morphology of the heart; however, it is important to determine if there are additional cardiac abnormalities, including atrial and ventricular septal defects. It is also important to recognize extracardiac malformations or associated anomalies.

ASSESSMENT OF FETAL CARDIAC RHYTHM

Each fetal echocardiogram should include an assessment of the fetal heart rate and rhythm. This is performed by measuring the cardiac cycle length from M-mode

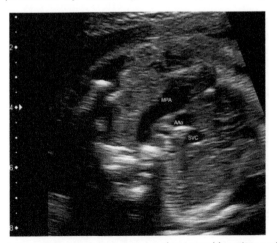

Fig. 8. Three-vessel view. This image demonstrates the normal location and size discrepancy at the three-vessel view of the main pulmonary artery, ascending aorta, and the superior vena cava. AAo, ascending aorta; MPA, main pulmonary artery; SVC, superior vena cava.

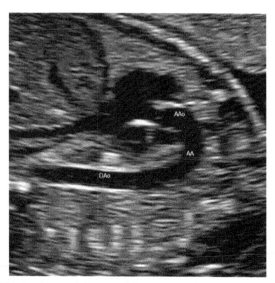

Fig. 9. True arch. This is a long axis image of the aortic arch. This image shows the ascending aorta, the true aortic arch, and the descending aorta. AA, true aortic arch; AAo, ascending aorta; DAo, descending aorta.

interrogation of the atrium and ventricle or by using simultaneous Doppler assessment of the mitral inflow and aortic outflow or the superior vena cava and the ascending aorta. The normal fetal heart rate ranges from 120 to 180 beats per minute at mid-gestation. A more detailed approach is provided in the article (see Jaeggi E, Öhman A: Fetal and Neonatal Arrhythmias, in this issue).

LIMITATIONS OF FETAL ECHOCARDIOGRAPHY

There are some limitations to fetal echocardiography. Minor valve abnormalities, atrial septal defects, partial anomalous pulmonary venous return, and coronary anomalies

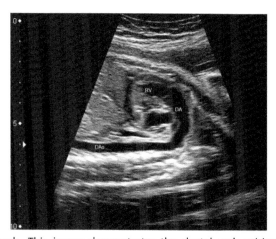

Fig. 10. Ductal arch. This image demonstrates the ductal arch arising from the right ventricle and connecting to the descending aorta. DA, ductal arch; DAo, descending aorta; RV, right ventricle.

are difficult to diagnose. Also, given the equal ventricular pressures, a tiny ventricular septal defect can be missed because there may be minimal shunting between the chambers. CHD that results from failure of a normal fetal structure to disappear, such as a patent ductus arteriosus, obviously cannot be detected until the fetus is delivered and the fetal circulation has transitioned to newborn circulation. Therefore, coarctation of the aorta is also difficult to diagnose.

FETAL INTERVENTIONS

The term fetal intervention covers a broad array of procedures and maneuvers intended to alter the natural course of a condition in utero to improve postnatal outcome. The boundaries between the disciplines involved in these procedures are, by necessity, blurred. It is essential to have a multidisciplinary team involved in every step of the process: from the prenatal assessment and counseling, to surgery/intervention, and finally to the postnatal care. Team members typically include perinatologists; fetal surgeons; fetal cardiologists; anesthesiologists; obstetricians; neonatologists; and support staff, such as social workers, bioethicists, and spiritual support services. This requires a tremendous allocation of resources and expertise and has led to the development of specialized fetal centers of excellence that can provide this care. Discussed next are some of the common interventions that typically involve the fetal cardiologist.

Fetal Cardiac Catheterization

One of the fetal cardiac lesions that have garnered the most attention in this arena is that of critical aortic stenosis. This arose from the observation that in a certain subset of these fetuses, critical aortic stenosis led to left ventricular dysfunction and later left ventricular hypoplasia, with resultant postnatal expression as hypoplastic left heart syndrome. For most cardiologists, the key is being able to identify who might benefit from a fetal procedure, be able to counsel the family regarding risks and benefits, and communicate effectively with a center of excellence that provides the service. The group at Boston Children's Hospital has reported outcomes after in utero aortic balloon valvuloplasty, where procedural success was obtained in 74% of fetuses and more than 30% went on to biventricular circulation at birth, and an additional 8% were later converted to a biventricular circulation.[19] These investigators came up with a "threshold score" that accurately predicted biventricular outcome. This score is derived by assigning points for specific preintervention cardiac measurements determined from a fetal echocardiogram, such as left ventricular dimensions and annulus measurements. Scores ranged from 0 to 5. In their cohort of fetal patients, a threshold score greater than or equal to four had 100% sensitivity, 53% specificity, 38% positive predictive value, and 100% negative predictive value for identifying fetuses that had a biventricular outcome from the time of birth without an intermediate stage 1 procedure. Suffice it to say, in a fetal patient with critical aortic stenosis, who has left ventricular dysfunction and evidence of flow abnormalities, such as retrograde flow in the transverse arch and left-to-right shunting at the atrial level, it has been our practice to discuss fetal intervention with parents and offer the option of consultation with a fetal intervention center.

Another abnormality that has provided impetus for fetal intervention is that of an intact or highly restrictive atrium septum in the setting of hypoplastic left heart syndrome. This leads to a high left atrial pressure in utero, with subsequent damage to the pulmonary vasculature, resulting in significant mortality and morbidity after birth.[20] The procedure entails the creation of an adequate atrial septal defect either by balloon atrial septostomy or by placement of an interatrial stent, which can be technically difficult because the atrial septum is often thick in this setting. However, promising technical successes have been reported.[21]

Finally, pulmonary atresia with intact ventricular septum has also been the target of fetal intervention, with pulmonary valve perforation and valvuloplasty. This is more controversial because it encompasses a wide spectrum of disease and varied grades of right heart hypoplasia, which may be amenable to staged approaches after birth. However, in the setting of severe tricuspid insufficiency and impending hydrops, it has been shown to be effective.[22]

Fetal Surgery

Fetal surgeries can be closed, where the procedure is undertaken using catheters, needles, or trochars that are inserted through the wall of the uterus, or they can be open requiring a hysterotomy and exposure of the fetus. Discussed next are a few selected surgeries that impact the heart and typically require fetal cardiology consultation.

Twin-twin transfusion syndrome is one of the closed interventions requiring fetal cardiology input. It is a condition that occurs in 9% to 15% of monochorionic twin pregnancies and if left untreated, carries a high mortality.[23,24] However, the broad variability in progression of the disorder makes patient selection somewhat problematic. The Quintero staging system is the most widely used scale to assess severity of twin-twin transfusion syndrome. It entails assessment of the maximal vertical amniotic fluid pocket in donor and recipient sacs, the presence of the bladder in the donor twin, the presence of critical Doppler findings, and the presence of hydrops.[25] The fetal cardiologist plays an important role in the fetal cardiac evaluation, especially in the setting of cardiac dysfunction or the development of right ventricular outflow tract obstruction. More recently, other staging systems that incorporate more sophisticated cardiac measurements have been used to provide more fidelity to the assessment, such as the Cincinnati staging system and the Children's Hospital of Philadelphia scoring system.[26,27] The Cincinnati staging system focuses on the severity of cardiac involvement of the recipient twin and takes into account severity of atrioventricular valve regurgitation, ventricular wall hypertrophy, and ventricular function as measured by the myocardial performance index. These more sophisticated "cardiac" scoring systems are additive to the Quintero staging system; however, their practical application in determining if and when to perform a fetal procedure varies between centers.

An example of an open fetal surgery where cardiology input is required is that of large congenital cystic adenomatoid malformations of the lung. These lesions can result in cardiovascular compromise by compressing the heart and resulting in hydrops. In selected cases (usually in the setting of hydrops), microcystic or solid lung lesions can be removed with open fetal surgery.[28] Fetal cardiologists can help during these procedures by providing live assessment of cardiac function and fetal stability during surgery and help in resuscitation of the fetus if required.

Another fetal surgical procedure that often requires cardiology input is that of ex utero intrapartum treatment or the EXIT procedure. This is when the mother undergoes general anesthesia with neuromuscular blockade, a hysterotomy is performed, and the fetus is partially delivered. The fetus thus remains on maternal "bypass" while surgeons can perform fetal intubation, tracheostomy, or tumor resection without the concern for significant fetal hypoxia. The fetal cardiologist provides live assessment of fetal cardiac function during the early parts of the procedure, and then continues with transthoracic echocardiography on the fetal chest while the airway is established. Because the fetus is given neuromuscular blockade, it is very difficult to assess clinically, and the echocardiographer provides valuable information regarding fluid status and cardiac function of the fetus.

SUMMARY

This article provides a user-friendly cardiocentric approach toward the practice of fetal echocardiography, which should lead to thoughtful and purpose-driven diagnostic studies. In the modern era, expectations are high for screening, timely referral, and accurate diagnosis of CHD. By using a sequential segmental approach, a sonographer and interpreter ensure accurate and complete fetal cardiac evaluation. Also summarized are some of the areas where fetal diagnosticians and fetal interventionalists/surgeons interface, and help to improve the natural history of a fetal condition. This is indeed a team sport and one cannot emphasize enough the importance of good relationships and communication with all physicians and practitioners involved in the care of the mother and fetus, to ensure that sound decisions are made in the best interests of both patients.

SUPPLEMENTARY DATA

Supplementary data related to this article are found at http://dx.doi.org/10.1016/j.clp. 2015.11.003.

REFERENCES

1. Yagel S, Weissman A, Rotstein Z, et al. Congenital heart defects: natural course and in utero development. Circulation 1997;96(2):550–5.
2. Kumar RK, Newburger JW, Gauvreau K, et al. Comparison of outcome when hypoplastic left heart syndrome and transposition of the great arteries are diagnosed prenatally versus when diagnosis of these two conditions is made only postnatally. Am J Cardiol 1999;83(12):1649–53.
3. Mahle WT, Clancy RR, McGaurn SP, et al. Impact of prenatal diagnosis on survival and early neurologic morbidity in neonates with the hypoplastic left heart syndrome. Pediatrics 2001;107(6):1277–82.
4. Tworetzky W, McElhinney DB, Reddy VM, et al. Improved surgical outcome after fetal diagnosis of hypoplastic left heart syndrome. Circulation 2001;103(9): 1269–73.
5. Morris SA, Ethen MK, Penny DJ, et al. Prenatal diagnosis, birth location, surgical center, and neonatal mortality in infants with hypoplastic left heart syndrome. Circulation 2014;129(3):285–92.
6. Quartermain MD, Pasquali SK, Hill KD, et al. Variation in prenatal diagnosis of congenital heart disease in infants. Pediatrics 2015;136(2):e378–85.
7. Friedberg MK, Silverman NH, Moon-Grady AJ, et al. Prenatal detection of congenital heart disease. J Pediatr 2009;155(1):26–31.e1.
8. Pinto NM, Keenan HT, Minich LL, et al. Barriers to prenatal detection of congenital heart disease: a population-based study. Ultrasound Obstet Gynecol 2012;40(4): 418–25.
9. American Institute of Ultrasound in Medicine. AIUM practice guideline for the performance of an antepartum obstetric ultrasound examination. J Ultrasound Med 2003;22(10):1116–25.
10. Kirk JS, Riggs TW, Comstock CH, et al. Prenatal screening for cardiac anomalies: the value of routine addition of the aortic root to the four-chamber view. Obstet Gynecol 1994;84(3):427–31.

11. Donofrio MT, Moon-Grady AJ, Hornberger LK, et al. Diagnosis and treatment of fetal cardiac disease: a scientific statement from the American Heart Association. Circulation 2014;129(21):2183–242.

12. Wright L, Stauffer N, Samai C, et al. Who should be referred? an evaluation of referral indications for fetal echocardiography in the detection of structural congenital heart disease. Pediatr Cardiol 2014;35(6):928–33.

13. Stumpflen I, Stumpflen A, Wimmer M, et al. Effect of detailed fetal echocardiography as part of routine prenatal ultrasonographic screening on detection of congenital heart disease. Lancet 1996;348(9031):854–7.

14. Rychik J, Ayres N, Cuneo B, et al. American society of echocardiography guidelines and standards for performance of the fetal echocardiogram. J Am Soc Echocardiogr 2004;17(7):803–10.

15. Lee W, Allan L, Carvalho JS, et al. ISUOG consensus statement: what constitutes a fetal echocardiogram? Ultrasound Obstet Gynecol 2008;32(2):239–42.

16. Anderson RH, Shirali G. Sequential segmental analysis. Ann Pediatr Cardiol 2009;2(1):24–35.

17. Shinebourne EA, Macartney FJ, Anderson RH. Sequential chamber localization: logical approach to diagnosis in congenital heart disease. Br Heart J 1976; 38(4):327–40.

18. Van Praagh R. Terminology of congenital heart disease. Glossary and commentary. Circulation 1977;56(2):139–43.

19. McElhinney DB, Marshall AC, Wilkins-Haug LE, et al. Predictors of technical success and postnatal biventricular outcome after in utero aortic valvuloplasty for aortic stenosis with evolving hypoplastic left heart syndrome. Circulation 2009; 120(15):1482–90.

20. Rychik J, Rome JJ, Collins MH, et al. The hypoplastic left heart syndrome with intact atrial septum: atrial morphology, pulmonary vascular histopathology and outcome. J Am Coll Cardiol 1999;34(2):554–60.

21. Marshall AC, Levine J, Morash D, et al. Results of in utero atrial septoplasty in fetuses with hypoplastic left heart syndrome. Prenat Diagn 2008;28(11):1023–8.

22. Tulzer G, Arzt W, Franklin RC, et al. Fetal pulmonary valvuloplasty for critical pulmonary stenosis or atresia with intact septum. Lancet 2002;360(9345):1567–8.

23. Sebire NJ, Snijders RJ, Hughes K, et al. The hidden mortality of monochorionic twin pregnancies. Br J Obstet Gynaecol 1997;104(10):1203–7.

24. Robyr R, Lewi L, Salomon LJ, et al. Prevalence and management of late fetal complications following successful selective laser coagulation of chorionic plate anastomoses in twin-to-twin transfusion syndrome. Am J Obstet Gynecol 2006; 194(3):796–803.

25. Quintero RA, Morales WJ, Allen MH, et al. Staging of twin-twin transfusion syndrome. J Perinatol 1999;19(8 Pt 1):550–5.

26. Rychik J, Tian Z, Bebbington M, et al. The twin-twin transfusion syndrome: spectrum of cardiovascular abnormality and development of a cardiovascular score to assess severity of disease. Am J Obstet Gynecol 2007;197(4):392.e1–8.

27. Crombleholme TM, Lim FY, Habli M, et al. Improved recipient survival with maternal nifedipine in twin-twin transfusion syndrome complicated by TTTS cardiomyopathy undergoing selective fetoscopic laser photocoagulation. Am J Obstet Gynecol 2010;203(4):397.e1–9.

28. Adzick NS. Open fetal surgery for life-threatening fetal anomalies. Semin Fetal Neonatal Med 2010;15(1):1–8.

Genetic and Developmental Basis of Cardiovascular Malformations

Mohamad Azhar, PhD[a],*, Stephanie M. Ware, MD, PhD[a,b],*

KEYWORDS

- Congenital heart defects • Congenital heart disease • Development • Gene dosage

KEY POINTS

- Phenotypic heterogeneity (different phenotypes/same genetic cause) and locus heterogeneity (different genetic cause/same phenotype) are common in CVM.
- Genes important for syndromic CVM may also cause nonsyndromic CVM.
- An understanding of the genes and pathways required for critical stages of heart formation informs the approach to genetic testing and diagnosis.
- The same gene or genetic locus may cause different types of CVMs (phenotypic heterogeneity).
- Mouse models are important tools to investigate the complex genetics of CVMs.

INTRODUCTION

The underlying causes of cardiovascular malformations (CVMs) can include cytogenetic abnormalities, single-gene disorders, environmental causes, or (most commonly) the causes can be multifactorial (**Table 1**). Chromosomal abnormalities account for 12% to 14% of all live-born cases and 20% to 33% of fetal cases of congenital CVMs, indicating that the proper genetic control of cardiac development is

Disclosure: The authors have nothing to disclose.
Funding: Supported in part by Riley Children's Foundation, Showalter Trust, Center of Excellence in Cardiovascular Research Fund, and the National Institutes of Health Grant (R01HL126705-01) (M. Azhar); and by an American Heart Association Established Investigator Award, Burroughs Wellcome Foundation, March of Dimes, and Indiana University Health - Indiana University School of Medicine Strategic Research Initiative (S.M. Ware).
[a] Department of Cell Biology & Anatomy, University of South Carolina School of Medicine, 6439 Garners Ferry Road, Columbia, SC 29208, USA; [b] Department of Medical and Molecular Genetics, Indiana University School of Medicine, 1044 West Walnut Street, Indianapolis, IN 46202, USA
* Corresponding authors.
E-mail addresses: mazhar@iu.edu; stware@iu.edu

Table 1
Causes of CVMs

Cause	Example	Characteristic CVMs
Environmental/teratogenic	Lithium chloride	Ebstein anomaly
Genetic		
Chromosomal	Trisomy 21	Atrioventricular canal defect
Contiguous gene/CNV	22q11.2 deletion syndrome	Conotruncal malformations
Single gene	Noonan syndrome	Pulmonary valve stenosis
Epigenetic		
DNA methylation	De novo SMAD2 mutations	Conotruncal malformations LV obstructions Heterotaxy

Abbreviation: CNV, copy number variant.

essential.[1–4] CVMs can occur as isolated findings, as part of a well-defined syndrome, or in conjunction with additional extracardiac anomalies not formally recognized as a syndrome.[5] The designation of CVMs as isolated can be problematic because many important distinguishing features of syndromic conditions, such as developmental delay or dysmorphic features, may not be apparent at initial evaluation. As a result, syndromic cases of CVM may be underestimated. In addition, the traditionally cited incidence for CVMs of ~1% of live births likely also underestimates the scope and impact of disease. Taking into account high rates of CVMs in spontaneous abortuses, common malformations such as bicuspid aortic valve (BAV) (present in 1.2% of the population), and latent cardiac diseases such as aortic dilatation, which are not included in the birth incidence of CVMs, genetically mediated CVMs are likely much more common than was previously thought. When considering the cause of CVMs, as opposed to the proportion of CVM cases that manifest as disease at birth, the incidence increases to approximately 5%.

Recently, we summarized the overall progress in the molecular genetic analyses of CVMs and current recommendations for clinical application of genetic testing. In particular, we reviewed the utility and limitations of chromosomal microarray analyses (CMAs) and the emerging clinical roles for whole-exome sequencing and other next-generation sequencing (NGS) technologies.[6] Readers with an interest in the current clinical testing approaches for CVMs are referred there. This article focuses on common genetic and developmental themes across the wide variety of CVMs and the ability of animal models and knowledge of cardiac developmental biology to affect the understanding of, and approach to, CVMs.

THE GENETIC BASIS OF CARDIOVASCULAR MALFORMATIONS

Epidemiologic studies suggest that a syndromic form of CVM is identifiable in approximately 20% to 30% of cases.[4] Known genetic causes are extremely heterogeneous, encompassing not only mutations in cardiac relevant genes but also more complex chromosomal abnormalities, submicroscopic duplications/deletions, and whole-chromosome aneuploidies (see **Table 1**). As noted earlier, CVMs can be isolated or can occur as part of a well-recognized genetic syndrome, and this distinction may be subtle.

Inheritance patterns for many CVM-associated genetic conditions are well characterized (reviewed in Ref.[6]) (**Table 2**). Genetic syndromic conditions associated with

Table 2
Examples of common syndromes with CVMs caused by single-gene mutations

Gene	Syndromes	Common Cardiac Anomalies
CHD7, SEMA3E	CHARGE syndrome	ASD, VSD, TOF
FBN1	Marfan syndrome	Aortic dilation
JAG1, NOTCH2	Alagille syndrome	PS, peripheral PS, TOF
KMT2D	Kabuki syndrome	ASD, VSD, TOF, CoA
PTPN11, KRAS, NRAS, HRAS, RAF1, SOS1, NF1, CBL, BRAF, SHOC2, MAP2K1, MAP2K2	Rasopathies: Noonan, Cardiofaciocutaneous, Costello syndromes	PS, HCM
SKI	Shprintzen-Goldberg syndrome	Aortic dilatation
TBX5	Holt-Oram syndrome	ASD, VSD, AVSD, conduction system disease
TFAP2b	Char syndrome	PDA
TGFB2, TGFBR1, TGFBR2, SMAD3	Loeys-Dietz syndrome types 1–4	Aortic dilatation
TGFB3	Rienhoff syndrome	Aortic dilatation
ZIC3	X-linked heterotaxy syndrome	Heterotaxy

Abbreviations: ASD, atrial septal defect; AVSD, atrioventricular septal defect; CHARGE, Coloboma of the eye, Heart defects, Atresia of the choanae, Retardation of growth and/or development, Genital and/or urinary abnormalities, and Ear abnormalities and deafness; CoA, coarctation of the aorta; HCM, hypertrophic cardiomyopathy; PDA, patent ductus arteriosus; PS, pulmonic stenosis; TOF, tetralogy of Fallot; VSD, ventricular septal defect.

CVMs are most commonly *de novo* or autosomal dominant. For dominantly inherited conditions, such as Noonan or Holt-Oram syndromes, the individual recurrence risk for offspring with the syndrome is 50%. Importantly, not all patients with a particular syndrome have associated heart defects and the proportion can vary by syndrome. Furthermore, the presence or severity of a CVM in the parent does not predict the severity in the child.

Isolated CVMs may be inherited as autosomal dominant, autosomal recessive, or X-linked conditions, but are most commonly sporadic with multifactorial causes (**Table 3**). Like other conditions inherited as a complex trait, isolated CVMs may show familial clustering with reduced penetrance.[7] For these reasons, recurrence risks for isolated CVMs can be difficult to assign. Consistent evidence of high heritability of isolated CVMs indicates that a strong genetic component exists, even for defects occurring without an obvious mode of inheritance.[8]

GENE DOSAGE AS A MECHANISM FOR CARDIOVASCULAR MALFORMATION

Gene dosage is an important concept underlying genetic disease, including birth defects. For many genes, a missing (deletion) or extra (duplication) copy of that gene results in no phenotypic consequences. In contrast, dosage-sensitive genes produce abnormal phenotypes in the absence of 2 functional genes. Aneuploidies such as trisomy 21 and Turner syndrome show that proper chromosome number is required for normal development. CVMs, including atrioventricular septal defect (AVSD), are seen in approximately 50% of individuals with Down syndrome. Likewise, up to 50% of patients with Turner syndrome have a CVM, most commonly a defect in the left

Table 3
Genes causing isolated heart defects

Gene	Protein
ETS1	V-Ets avian erythroblastosis virus E26 oncogene homolog 1
TGFB2, TGFB3	Transforming growth factor ligand 2, 3
TGFBR1, TGFBR2	Transforming growth factor receptor 1, 2
SMAD2, SMAD3	Mothers against decapentaplegic, drosophila, homologs 2, 3
HAND1, HAND2	Heart and neural crest derivatives expressed 1, 2
GATA4, GATA5, GATA6	GATA binding protein 4–6
TBX1	T-box 1
TBX20	T-box 20
CITED2	Cbp/P300-interacting transactivator, with Glu/Asp-rich carboxy-terminal domain, 2
MESP1	Mesoderm posterior 1 homolog
IRX4	Iroquois homeobox 4
MYOCD	Myocardin
Nkx2-5, Nkx2-6	NK2 homeobox 5, 6
NFATC1	Nuclear factor of activated T cells, cytoplasmic, calcineurin dependent 1
NOTCH1	Notch1
ELN	Elastin

ventricular outflow tract. Because of the large number of genes with abnormal dosage in these conditions, identifying the causal genes for the cardiac features has proved difficult. Furthermore, the decreased penetrance of the CVMs suggests that genetic modifiers interact with dosage-sensitive genes on the same chromosome (in the case of trisomy 21) or other chromosomes to cause CVM. Thus, a threshold exists in both aneuploid and euploid populations for the number of genetic perturbations that can be tolerated before CVM results. For example, Creld1 and Hey2 were recently identified as potential modifier genes in trisomy 21.[9] Mice with mutant forms of these potential modifiers were intercrossed to the Ts65Dn mouse model of Down syndrome. Breeding loss-of-function alleles of either Creld1 or Hey2 onto the trisomic background causes a significant increase in the frequency of CVM. This finding supports a threshold hypothesis for additive effects of genetic modifiers in the sensitized trisomic population.

Submicroscopic chromosome deletions and duplications also underlie many genetic syndromes, and the term genomic disorder is used to refer to these conditions. Two classic genomic disorders, 22q11.2 deletion syndrome and Williams-Beuren syndrome (WBS), are discussed in further detail later.

UNDERSTANDING THE GENETIC BASIS OF SYNDROMIC CARDIOVASCULAR MALFORMATION CAN IDENTIFY IMPORTANT GENES FOR ISOLATED CARDIOVASCULAR MALFORMATION

WBS is a common genetic syndrome associated with CVM caused by deletion at 7q11.23, resulting in haploinsufficiency of multiple genes, including elastin (ELN). Supravalvar aortic stenosis (SVAS) is the classic cardiac finding in WBS, although other defects, including peripheral pulmonic stenosis, occur. After the description of WBS as a deletion at 7q11.23 in 1993,[10] Ewart and colleagues[11] showed close linkage of *ELN* and SVAS in 2 families. Deletions or point mutations limited to the *ELN* gene seem to result in nonsyndromic SVAS, whereas larger deletions spanning multiple genes lead to WBS. Studies in a mouse model with elastin deficiency have successfully corroborated the genetic findings with regard to SVAS and latent aortic disease.[12,13]

22q11.2 deletion syndrome provides a second example of a genomic disorder that led to the identification of a single gene causing CVM. CVMs occur in approximately 75% of patients with 22q11.2 deletion syndrome, with conotruncal defects predominating. After the identification of 22q11.2 deletion syndrome, significant effort was put into delineating the dosage-sensitive genes responsible for the CVMs using mouse development and genetics, ultimately identifying *Tbx1*.[14,15] Yagi and colleagues investigated *TBX1* mutations in families that had 22q11.2 deletion syndrome phenotype but no detectable deletion and found that *TBX1* mutations are responsible for many major phenotypes of the syndrome, including CVMs.[16] In much the same way that modifiers for the Ts65Dn mouse model of Down syndrome were identified, sonic hedgehog and retinoic acid developmental signaling pathways modify the phenotypes of a 22q11.2 deletion syndrome mouse model, suggesting that mice with reduced gene dosage are sensitized to these morphogens.[17] These disorders show that genes that cause CVMs may be associated with syndromic or isolated presentations. Comprehensive identification of dosage-sensitive candidate CVM genes and integration into an understanding of the genetic and developmental origins of CVM would facilitate the development of therapies to rescue the CVMs associated with both syndromic and isolated CVM.

BLURRING THE BOUNDARIES: SINGLE-GENE DEFECTS THAT CAN CAUSE BOTH SYNDROMIC AND ISOLATED CARDIOVASCULAR MALFORMATIONS

Genetic testing technologies have identified several genes that cause both syndromic and nonsyndromic CVMs (see **Tables 2** and **3**).[6] For example, CVMs, including aortic aneurysm, are reported in syndromic patients (ie, Marfan syndrome [MFS] and Loeys-Dietz syndrome [LDS]) with mutations affecting the transforming growth factor beta (TGFβ) pathway (*TGFB2, TGFBR1, TGFBR2, SMAD3, FBN1*) (see **Table 2**).[18,19] Nonsyndromic aortic disease is a frequently asymptomatic but potentially lethal disease characterized by cases of familial thoracic aortic aneurysm and dissection (FTAAD). This monogenic but genetically heterogeneous condition is primarily inherited as an autosomal dominant disorder with variable penetrance and expressivity. Mutations in *TGFB* genes have also been described in nonsyndromic patients with isolated CVM or aortic aneurysm (see **Table 3**).[19–22] These facts complicate the clinical approach to patients with CVMs and the choice of genetic testing. Furthermore, patients with mutations in *ACTA2*, a gene known to cause isolated FTAAD, can have a syndromic presentation[23] and pediatric patients with FTAAD frequently have subtle signs of a connective tissue disorder.[24] As the ability to identify genetic cause improves, boundaries between syndromic and nonsyndromic disease often become less distinct. Careful phenotyping and improved interpretation of genetic variation are important to better refine the understanding of the spectrum of clinical effects of specific genetic variation.

THE DEVELOPMENTAL BASIS FOR CARDIOVASCULAR MALFORMATIONS: GENES AND PATHWAYS REQUIRED FOR CRITICAL STAGES OF HEART FORMATION

Genetically engineered mice are extensively used in CVM research and have contributed greatly to an understanding of the genetic control and mechanistic basis of CVMs. Multiple cell types contribute to the development of a fully septated 4-chambered heart, including the first heart field and second heart field, cardiac neural crest

(NC), and epicardial and endocardial cell lineages (**Fig. 1**).[25] Both cardiac NC and endocardium-derived cushion mesenchyme are important precursors of the outflow tract (OFT) septa and semilunar valves.[26] At embryonic day 9.5 (E9.5), endocardium in the proximal OFT region gives rise to cushion mesenchyme via epithelial-mesenchymal transition (EMT) (see **Fig. 1**).[26,27] Neural crest (NC) cells enter the distal OFT (E10), proliferate, and eventually colonize the endocardial ridges of the proximal cushions.[28] NC cells undergo apoptosis (E11.5–E13.5), and are necessary for aortico-pulmonary septation and OFT alignment.[29] Endocardium-derived OFT cells also undergo proliferation but remain restricted to the endocardial ridges of the proximal OFT cushions (**Fig. 2**). Remodeling and fusion of the endocardial ridges of the proximal cushions results in the formation of fibrous OFT septum that undergoes differentiation (E13.5–E15.5) and eventually becomes a completely muscular structure (E16.5–E18.5) through a process called myocardialization.[27] Despite abundant contributions of NC to the OFT mesenchyme, few NC derivatives are present in the mature semilunar valves.[28] Although the precise role of NC cells and their interaction with endocardial EMT-derived OFT cells remain unclear, more recent studies have suggested that NC cells are also important for the remodeling of the semilunar valves.[28] Abnormal OFT cushion remodeling often results in semilunar valve thickening, defective OFT septation (persistent truncus arteriosus [PTA]), or alignment defects such as double-outlet right ventricle (DORV) and ventricular septal defect (VSD).[26] The signals and cellular events that mediate valve remodeling are poorly characterized, although apoptosis and alterations in extracellular matrix production have been described.[30,31] Similar developmental events are noted in atrioventricular (AV) cushion formation and remodeling except that the cardiac NC is absent in the AV cushions and both dorsal mesocardium and epicardium provide additional cushion components of the AV cushion mesenchymal complex (see **Fig. 2**).[32]

Developmental pathways acting independently or in combination contribute to heart development and have been reviewed recently.[6,33–35] For example, TGFβ and bone morphogenetic protein (BMP) family members play different roles during cardiac development (**Fig. 3**) (reviewed in Refs.[27,36]), and mutations in these genes result in distinct phenotypes.[36–39] In LDS, mutations in the TGFβ pathway genes cause

Key Developmental Stages	EMT	Neural Crest Entry	Cushion Remodeling	Leaflet Formation	Valve Maturation		Mature Leaflet	
E	8.5	9.5	10.5	11.5	12.5	13.5	14.5	16.5	18.5

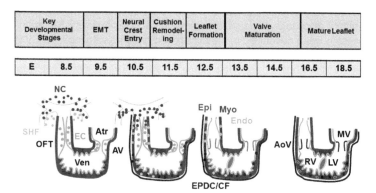

Fig. 1. Heart development. Endocardium (EC) (*aqua blue line*) forms the endocardial cushions (*green circles*) via cushion epithelial-mesenchymal transition (EMT) (E9.5). NC cells (*pink circles*) migrate into the outflow tract (OFT) during E10.5 to E12.5. Valve leaflets undergoing differentiation (*orange*) and maturation (*purple*) (E13.5–E18.5) are indicated. Only 1 semilunar valve is shown. AV, atrioventricular canal; LV, left ventricle; RV, right ventricle; SV, semilunar valves.

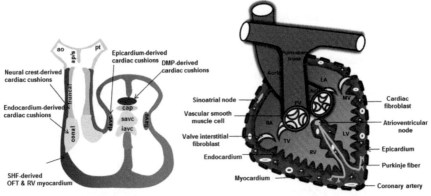

Fig. 2. Cardiac remodeling and septation. Myocardium, endocardium, cardiac fibroblasts, and epicardium are major cell types in the heart. (*Left*) Components of OFT and AV cushions are indicated. OFT contains well-demarcated conal (endocardium-derived) and truncal (NC-derived) cushions. AV cushion mesenchymal complex contains superior and inferior AV cushions (predominantly EC derived), right and left lateral AV cushions (rlavc, llavc) (with contributions from both epicardium and EC), mesenchymal cap (cap) and dorsal mesenchymal protrusion (dmp) (dorsal mesocardium derived). (*Right*) Fully septated 4-chambered heart. The valve annulus and vascular wall of the aorta and pulmonary trunk are predominantly composed of smooth muscle cells. Heart valves predominantly contain valve interstitial cells. Endocardium/endothelium is the innermost layer, whereas epicardium is the outermost layer. Both ventricular and atrial regions contain myocardium and cardiac fibroblasts along with coronary vasculature. Purkinje fiber and atrioventricular and sinoatrial nodes constitute the cardiac conduction system. AoV, aortic valve; LA, left atrium; MV, mitral valve; PV, pulmonary valve; RA, right atrium; TV, tricuspid valve.

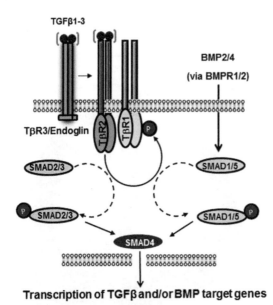

Transcription of TGFβ and/or BMP target genes

Fig. 3. The TGFβ signaling pathway. TGFβ binds to a common TGFβ receptor complex, and signals through phosphorylation of the canonical TGFβ-specific SMADs (ie, pSMAD2/3). The pSMAD2/3 forms a complex with SMAD4, which accumulates in the nucleus and can regulate target gene expression. SMAD4 also binds to BMP-specific SMADs (SMAD1/5/8), and therefore regulates BMP-target gene expression in heart development.

thoracic aortic aneurysm (TAA; see **Table 3**) and are also highly associated with BAV.[40] Paradoxically, increased levels of TGFβ1 are seen in these patients. Similar increases in TGFβ1 activity are also associated with BAV in Turner syndrome.[41] Overall, it remains unclear whether the loss of TGFB function and/or gain of TGFB function is the primary cause of CVM. In contrast, BMP signaling is required to induce differentiation of early cardiac progenitors, but BMP signaling is inhibited at later stages by Smad6a to permit chamber development mediated by Tbx2 and Tbx20. Importantly, the role of a particular signaling pathway can vary as development proceeds. For example, Wnt signals are critical for early cardiac precursor induction and proliferation, but later become inhibitory. Combinatorial interactions are the rule. Notch signaling interacts with both BMP and TGFβ pathways.[6,42] The cardiac transcription factor Nkx2.5 physically and functionally interacts with Gata4, Tbx5, and Mef2c, each of which forms additional unique and shared connections with other molecular, genetic, and signaling components.[6,34,35] Such signaling and transcriptional networks hint at the possibility that some CVMs may result from additive effects of multiple low-effect susceptibility alleles.

PHENOTYPIC HETEROGENEITY AND LOCUS HETEROGENEITY

Studies of gene-targeted mouse models indicate that loss of a single gene can result in a spectrum of CVMs (**Fig. 4; Tables 4** and **5** provide noncomprehensive examples). For example, the OFT malformations of the TGFβ2-deficient fetuses include DORV, PTA, abnormal morphology and thickening of aortic and/or pulmonary valves, aortic arch artery malformations (ie, interrupted aortic arch type A), double inlet left ventricle (DILV) and/or overriding of tricuspid valves orifice via a perimembranous inlet VSD,

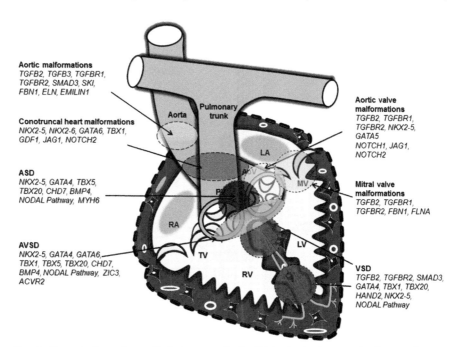

Aortic malformations
TGFB2, TGFB3, TGFBR1,
TGFBR2, SMAD3, SKI,
FBN1, ELN, EMILIN1

Conotruncal heart malformations
NKX2-5, NKX2-6, GATA6, TBX1,
GDF1, JAG1, NOTCH2

ASD
NKX2-5, GATA4, TBX5,
TBX20, CHD7, BMP4,
NODAL Pathway, MYH6

AVSD
NKX2-5, GATA4, GATA6,
TBX1, TBX5, TBX20, CHD7,
BMP4, NODAL Pathway, ZIC3,
ACVR2

Aortic valve malformations
TGFB2, TGFBR1,
TGFBR2, NKX2-5,
GATA5
NOTCH1, JAG1,
NOTCH2

Mitral valve malformations
TGFB2, TGFBR1,
TGFBR2, FBN1, FLNA

VSD
TGFB2, TGFBR2, SMAD3,
GATA4, TBX1, TBX20,
HAND2, NKX2-5,
NODAL Pathway

Aorta   Pulmonary trunk

LA

MV

RA   LV

TV

RV

Fig. 4. Phenotypic and genetic heterogeneity in CVMs. A single genetic abnormality can cause multiple types of CVMs. In addition, the same genetic abnormality can result in different CVMs. CVMs are indicated with colored circles.

Table 4
Phenotypic heterogeneity: the same genetic abnormality causes different heart defects

Gene	CVMs in Genetic Mouse Models
TGFB2	VSD, TAA, BAV
NKX2-5	VSD, AVSD, ASD
GATA4	ASD, VSD, AVSD
TBX1	AVSD, VSD
TBX20	VSD, AVSD, ASD
BMP4	VSD, AVSD, ASD
GATA6	VSD, AVSD, ASD
ZIC3	Heterotaxy, d-TGA, DORV, AVSD, other heterotaxy spectrum heart defects
JAG1	PS, ASD, TOF
GDF1	DORV, TOF, d-TGA
TBX5	ASD, VSD
Trisomy 21	ASD, VSD, PDA
45, X	BAV, HLHS, CoA
22q11.2 deletion	TOF, VSD, IAA type B

Abbreviations: BAV, bicuspid aortic valve; d-TGA, d-transposition of the great arteries; HLHS, hypoplastic left heart syndrome; IAA, interrupted aortic arch type A.

and abnormal morphology and thickening of tricuspid and mitral valves. Similarly, a range of CVM phenotypes is seen in mice that lack *Tbx1*, *Nkx2-5*, *Tbx20*, *Tbx5*, and *Gata4*.

Different CVM phenotypes are noted in patients with identical mutations, even among members of the same family (see **Table 4**). Null mutation in several genes can cause AVSD in mice, including *Nkx2-5*, *Gata4*, and *Tbx1*.[32] Additional examples are presented in **Fig. 4**. Developmental mechanisms that cause different CVMs in response to a mutation in a single gene remain incompletely understood.

MUTATIONS IN DEVELOPMENTAL PATHWAYS MAY RESULT IN LATENT DISEASE

There are numerous potential mechanisms through which genetic mutations could affect the complex differentiation and morphogenetic processes in heart

Table 5
Locus heterogeneity: the same CVM results from distinct genetic loci

CVM Type	Examples of Genetic Causes
BAV	TGFB signaling pathway single-gene mutations, aneuploidy (45,X)
VSD	TGFB and BMP signaling pathway single-gene mutations, aneuploidy (45,X; trisomy 21), 22q11.2 deletion
DORV	*GDF1, TBX1,* 22q11.2 deletion
AVSD	*ACVR2, NKX2-5, GATA4,* 22q11.2 deletion, aneuploidy (trisomy 21)
PS	*JAG1, NOTCH2*
TOF	*JAG1, NOTCH2,* 22q11.2 deletion
MVP	*TGFB2, FBN1, FLNA*
TAA	TGFB signaling pathway single-gene mutations, *MYH11, ACTA2, MYLK1, FBN1*
HCM	RASopathy gene mutations Sarcomeric gene mutation

development. Once developed, the cardiovascular system must undergo homeostasis to maintain function throughout life. This ability to repair and remodel following stress and injury uses many of the same mechanisms involved in the original development and remodeling of those tissues.[39] Failure of these processes can result in late-onset disease. Genes associated with CVMs (see **Fig. 4**)[36,39] are ideal candidates for these homeostatic, stress response, and repair processes. Improvement in outcomes requires a better understanding of mechanisms underlying CVMs and dysregulated homeostatic/repair processes.

There are many interesting examples of genes in which homozygous gene deletion in mice results in CVMs in embryos and latent cardiac disease in adult mice, including elastin, emilin 1, periostin, and fibrillin 1. Elastin null (Eln$^{-/-}$) mice die perinatally secondary to severe arterial obstruction reminiscent of SVAS,[12] whereas arteriopathy in the Eln$^{+/-}$ mouse manifests as systemic hypertension.[43] Juvenile Eln$^{+/-}$ mice show normal valve function, but progressive valve disease (predominantly aortic regurgitation) is identified in 17% of adult and 70% of aged adult Eln$^{+/-}$ mice by echocardiography.[13] Thus Eln$^{+/-}$ mice are a model of latent aortic valve disease and reduced elastin level leads to dysregulation in valve pathogenesis. Other good examples of mouse models of latent aortic disease include *Emilin1*, *Fibrillin-1*$^{+/C1039G}$, and *Fibrillin1*$^{mgR/mgR}$ (*Fbn1*$^{mgR/mgR}$), *Fibrillin-1*$^{+/C1039G}$ and *Fibrillin1*$^{mgR/mgR}$ being mouse models of MFS. The *Fbn1*$^{mgR/mgR}$ mice die spontaneously from rupture of the thoracic aorta between 2 and 4 months of age, and are useful in testing therapeutic strategies for aortic aneurysm. In contrast, *Fibrillin-1*$^{+/C1039G}$ mice, in which a point mutation seen in MFS has been made, represent a viable mouse model to study the development and progression of aortic aneurysm. The early manifestation of elastic fiber fragmentation and aberrant TGFβ signaling suggests that these processes are crucial intermediate factors that provide novel information for diagnosis and treatment of patients with aortic disease.[24,44]

DECREASED PENETRANCE, VARIABLE EXPRESSIVITY, AND COMPLEX INHERITANCE: LESSONS FROM MOUSE MODELS

Genetically engineered mice can serve as a useful example of modifying genetic influences that affect phenotype. A good example is the different phenotypes seen in *Tgfb2* null mice on mixed (129/Bl-Swiss) and inbred (C57BL/6) genetic backgrounds. The OFT malformations of the inbred null fetuses included DORV (100% cases), PTA (27.2% cases), and semilunar valve defects (100% cases). In addition, the null fetuses developed DILV and/or overriding of tricuspid valve orifice via a perimembranous inlet VSD (100% cases), and tricuspid/mitral valve defects (100%). Notably, the overall penetrance of the observed cardiac valve and septal defects was significantly higher in C57BL/6 inbred null fetuses compared with *Tgfb2* null fetuses on the mixed genetic background.[45] This difference is attributed to the differences in genetic modifiers between the strains.

EPIGENETIC FACTORS IN CARDIOVASCULAR MALFORMATION

An increasing recognition of epigenetic factors underlying CVMs has revealed an unanticipated breadth.[46] Epigenetics refers to functionally relevant changes to the genome that do not involve a change in the DNA sequence. DNA methylation and histone modification are major epigenetic mechanisms that alter chromatin remodeling and gene expression without altering the underlying genetic information.[5] A recent study by Pediatric Cardiac Genomics Consortium of the National Heart, Lung and Blood Institute identified de novo point mutations in several histone-modifying genes that collectively contribute to approximately 10% of severe CVM.[5,22] Refinements in technologies such as ChIP-seq (chromatin immunoprecipitation-sequencing) and systems biology approaches aid the understanding of global regulation and functional redundancies in cardiac transcription factors in CVMs.[34,35] MicroRNAs, a class of small noncoding RNAs, negatively regulate the expression of their target genes through posttranscriptional processes and also interact with epigenetic machinery.[47] Regulation of gene expression via mechanisms that affect epigenetic machinery identifies novel causes for CVMs.

FUTURE DEVELOPMENTS

The effect of gene variation on the assembly of distinct cardiac and extracardiac cell lineages during heart development is an important area that warrants future investigation. The relative importance and roles of different cell types in cardiac morphogenesis and remodeling remains to be fully understood. Defining gene function in specific cell types in mouse models at high resolution will enable predictions to be made about the phenotypic consequences of variants in humans that currently lack functional interpretation. Experiments that delineate fundamental differences/similarities in loss-of-function and gain-of-function genetic backgrounds in mice will provide insight into the consequences of gene dosage perturbation in humans and mechanisms of genetic disease. In addition, incorporation of new technologies such as NGS, gene expression profiling (ie, RNA sequencing), and gene editing CRISPR/Cas9-based methodologies to discover and validate novel genes involved in CVMs will significantly enhance the understanding of cardiac genetics and development.

SUMMARY

Cardiac development is a complex, multistep process under genetic regulation. A detailed understanding of the molecular basis of cardiac development is necessary to understand disease causation. Cardiovascular genetics is progressing at a rapid pace, leading to novel diagnostic genetic testing for CVMs. Recent efforts to integrate developmental studies from animal models with systems biology approaches offer significant promise for future CVM research. Understanding how genetic mutations affect the integration of multiple signal transduction pathways to cause CVM is an active area of research. The information gained from these developmental and genetic investigations should generate novel hypotheses for future experimentation and to provide diagnostic and therapeutic avenues for patients with CVM.

Best practices

What is the current practice?
Genetic Testing in Cardiovascular Malformations

- Genetic testing practices for congenital heart defects have yet to be standardized in many centers and testing is frequently underused.
- Guidelines for cardiac imaging and genetic testing for TAA and cardiomyopathy.
- A genetic diagnosis has important implications for patient management, screening recommendations for family members, and recurrence risk counseling.

Genetic Testing Options

- Chromosome analysis is the gold standard for diagnosis of aneuploidies and other large chromosomal abnormalities.
- CMA and fluorescence in situ hybridization (FISH) permit identification of microdeletion and duplication syndromes resulting from abnormalities too small to be detected by conventional chromosome analyses.
- NGS panels are the test of choice for some syndromic congenital heart defects, TAA, and cardiomyopathy.
- CMA and targeted NGS are nonredundant tests. Consulting a geneticist is important for establishing a differential, ordering the appropriate tests, and interpreting results.

Implications for Family Members

- First-degree relatives of patients with specific CVMs (ie, left ventricular outflow tract obstructive (LVOTO) defects, TAA) should undergo cardiac screening.
- Family-based risk assessment and recurrence risk information differ by type of cardiovascular malformation and should be provided to the family by a knowledgeable genetics professional.

What changes in current practice are likely to improve outcomes?

- Continued integration of genetic testing services into cardiovascular practice will improve diagnostic and prognostic accuracy and will support risk assessment and family planning initiatives.
- NGS technologies promise to greatly benefit patient diagnosis and gene discovery efforts.
- Appropriate cardiac screening and surveillance in at-risk relatives will identify latent disease.

Is there a clinical algorithm?

- An algorithm for congenital heart defects has been proposed recently.[6]
- Guidelines summarize genetic testing for syndromic and nonsyndromic TAA as well as cardiac screening in first-degree relatives.[48]

Major Recommendations

Genetic testing and referral decisions should be determined based on the nature of the cardiac defect.

A detailed pedigree should be obtained in all cases of CVM.

Chromosome analysis is recommended for patients with suspected aneuploidy.

Patients with multiple congenital anomalies, neurologic findings, developmental delay, and/or dysmorphic features should be referred for genetic evaluation.

CMA and/or FISH should be used in patients with conotruncal defects.

Patients with apparently nonsyndromic LVOTO, right ventricular outflow tract obstructive defects (RVOTO), AVSD, heterotaxy, or other complex defects should have CMA.

Patients with TAA should have a genetics evaluation and appropriate genetic testing.

Specific CVMs should trigger cardiac screening of first-degree relatives.

Rating for the Strength of the Evidence

C recommendation based on consensus, usual practice, expert opinion, disease-oriented evidence, and case series for studies of diagnosis, treatment, prevention, or screening

References

Pierpont ME, Basson CT, Benson DW Jr, et al. Genetic basis for congenital heart defects: current knowledge: a scientific statement from the American Heart Association Congenital Cardiac Defects Committee, Council on Cardiovascular Disease in the Young: endorsed by the American Academy of Pediatrics. Circulation 2007;115:3015–38.

Hiratzka LF, Bakris GL, Beckman JA, et al. 2010 ACCF/AHA/AATS/ACR/ASA/SCA/SCAI/SIR/STS/SVM guidelines for the diagnosis and management of patients with Thoracic Aortic Disease: a report of the American College of Cardiology Foundation/American Heart Association Task Force on Practice Guidelines, American Association for Thoracic Surgery, American College of Radiology, American Stroke Association, Society of Cardiovascular Anesthesiologists, Society for Cardiovascular Angiography and Interventions, Society of Interventional Radiology, Society of Thoracic Surgeons, and Society for Vascular Medicine. Circulation 2010;121(13):e266–369.

Cowan JR, Ware SM. Genetics and genetic testing in congenital heart disease. Clin Perinatol 2015;42:373–93.

Summary

Genetic evaluation and testing are increasingly important for CVMs. Improvements in genetic testing technologies have assisted gene discovery and helped to reshape standards of patient care. Risk assessment of family members and recurrence risk counseling are important components of management and care.

REFERENCES

1. Gillum RF. Epidemiology of congenital heart disease in the United States. Am Heart J 1994;127(4 Pt 1):919–27.
2. Chaoui R, Korner H, Bommer C, et al. Prenatal diagnosis of heart defects and associated chromosomal aberrations. Ultraschall Med 1999;20(5):177–84 [in German].
3. Tennstedt C, Chaoui R, Korner H, et al. Spectrum of congenital heart defects and extracardiac malformations associated with chromosomal abnormalities: results of a seven year necropsy study. Heart 1999;82(1):34–9.
4. Ferencz C, Boughman JA, Neill CA, et al. Congenital cardiovascular malformations: questions on inheritance. Baltimore-Washington Infant Study Group. J Am Coll Cardiol 1989;14(3):756–63.
5. Bruneau BG, Srivastava D. Congenital heart disease: entering a new era of human genetics. Circ Res 2014;114(4):598–9.
6. Cowan JR, Ware SM. Genetics and genetic testing in congenital heart disease. Clin Perinatol 2015;42(2):373–93, ix.
7. Lalani SR, Belmont JW. Genetic basis of congenital cardiovascular malformations. Eur J Med Genet 2014;57(8):402–13.

8. Oyen N, Poulsen G, Boyd HA, et al. Recurrence of congenital heart defects in families. Circulation 2009;120(4):295–301.
9. Li H, Cherry S, Klinedinst D, et al. Genetic modifiers predisposing to congenital heart disease in the sensitized Down syndrome population. Circ Cardiovasc Genet 2012;5(3):301–8.
10. Curran ME, Atkinson DL, Ewart AK, et al. The elastin gene is disrupted by a translocation associated with supravalvular aortic stenosis. Cell 1993;73(1):159–68.
11. Ewart AK, Jin W, Atkinson D, et al. Supravalvular aortic stenosis associated with a deletion disrupting the elastin gene. J Clin Invest 1994;93(3):1071–7.
12. Li DY, Brooke B, Davis EC, et al. Elastin is an essential determinant of arterial morphogenesis. Nature 1998;393(6682):276–80.
13. Hinton RB, Adelman-Brown J, Witt S, et al. Elastin haploinsufficiency results in progressive aortic valve malformation and latent valve disease in a mouse model. Circ Res 2010;107(4):549–57.
14. Lindsay EA, Vitelli F, Su H, et al. Tbx1 haploinsufficiency in the DiGeorge syndrome region causes aortic arch defects in mice. Nature 2001;410(6824):97–101.
15. Merscher S, Funke B, Epstein JA, et al. TBX1 is responsible for cardiovascular defects in velo-cardio-facial/DiGeorge syndrome. Cell 2001;104(4):619–29.
16. Yagi H, Furutani Y, Hamada H, et al. Role of TBX1 in human del22q11.2 syndrome. Lancet 2003;362(9393):1366–73.
17. Maynard TM, Gopalakrishna D, Meechan DW, et al. 22q11 gene dosage establishes an adaptive range for sonic hedgehog and retinoic acid signaling during early development. Hum Mol Genet 2013;22(2):300–12.
18. Braverman AC. Heritable thoracic aortic aneurysm disease: recognizing phenotypes, exploring genotypes. J Am Coll Cardiol 2015;65(13):1337–9.
19. Micha D, Guo DC, Hilhorst-Hofstee Y, et al. SMAD2 mutations are associated with arterial aneurysms and dissections. Hum Mutat 2015;36(12):1145–9.
20. Gago-Diaz M, Blanco-Verea A, Teixido-Tura G, et al. Whole exome sequencing for the identification of a new mutation in TGFB2 involved in a familial case of non-syndromic aortic disease. Clin Chim Acta 2014;437:88–92.
21. Matyas G, Naef P, Tollens M, et al. De novo mutation of the latency-associated peptide domain of TGFB3 in a patient with overgrowth and Loeys-Dietz syndrome features. Am J Med Genet A 2014;164A(8):2141–3.
22. Zaidi S, Choi M, Wakimoto H, et al. De novo mutations in histone-modifying genes in congenital heart disease. Nature 2013;498(7453):220–3.
23. Guo DC, Pannu H, Tran-Fadulu V, et al. Mutations in smooth muscle alpha-actin (ACTA2) lead to thoracic aortic aneurysms and dissections. Nat Genet 2007;39(12):1488–93.
24. Landis BJ, Ware SM, James J, et al. Clinical stratification of pediatric patients with idiopathic thoracic aortic aneurysm. J Pediatr 2015;167(1):131–7.
25. Kelly RG, Buckingham ME, Moorman AF. Heart fields and cardiac morphogenesis. Cold Spring Harb Perspect Med 2014;4(10):a015750.
26. Lin CJ, Lin CY, Chen CH, et al. Partitioning the heart: mechanisms of cardiac septation and valve development. Development 2012;139(18):3277–99.
27. Azhar M, Schultz JE, Grupp I, et al. Transforming growth factor beta in cardiovascular development and function. Cytokine Growth Factor Rev 2003;14(5):391–407.
28. Jain R, Engleka KA, Rentschler SL, et al. Cardiac neural crest orchestrates remodeling and functional maturation of mouse semilunar valves. J Clin Invest 2011;121(1):422–30.
29. Kirby ML, Gale TF, Stewart DE. Neural crest cells contribute to normal aorticopulmonary septation. Science 1983;220(4601):1059–61.

30. Markwald RR, Norris RA, Moreno-Rodriguez R, et al. Developmental basis of adult cardiovascular diseases: valvular heart diseases. Ann N Y Acad Sci 2010;1188:177–83.
31. Hinton RB Jr, Lincoln J, Deutsch GH, et al. Extracellular matrix remodeling and organization in developing and diseased aortic valves. Circ Res 2006;98(11):1431–8.
32. Briggs LE, Kakarla J, Wessels A. The pathogenesis of atrial and atrioventricular septal defects with special emphasis on the role of the dorsal mesenchymal protrusion. Differentiation 2012;84(1):117–30.
33. Rana MS, Christoffels VM, Moorman AF. A molecular and genetic outline of cardiac morphogenesis. Acta Physiol (Oxf) 2013;207(4):588–615.
34. Chong JJ, Forte E, Harvey RP. Developmental origins and lineage descendants of endogenous adult cardiac progenitor cells. Stem Cell Res 2014;13(3 Pt B):592–614.
35. Kathiriya IS, Nora EP, Bruneau BG. Investigating the transcriptional control of cardiovascular development. Circ Res 2015;116(4):700–14.
36. Arthur HM, Bamforth SD. TGFbeta signaling and congenital heart disease: insights from mouse studies. Birth Defects Res A Clin Mol Teratol 2011;91(6):423–34.
37. Hinck AP. Structural studies of the TGF-betas and their receptors - insights into evolution of the TGF-beta superfamily. FEBS Lett 2012;586(14):1860–70.
38. Akhurst RJ, Hata A. Targeting the TGFbeta signalling pathway in disease. Nat Rev Drug Discov 2012;11(10):790–811.
39. Doetschman T, Barnett JV, Runyan RB, et al. Transforming growth factor beta signaling in adult cardiovascular diseases and repair. Cell Tissue Res 2012;347(1):203–23.
40. Maccarrick G, Black JH III, Bowdin S, et al. Loeys-Dietz syndrome: a primer for diagnosis and management. Genet Med 2014;16(8):576–87.
41. Zhou J, Arepalli S, Cheng CM, et al. Perturbation of the transforming growth factor beta system in Turner syndrome. Beijing Da Xue Xue Bao 2012;44(5):720–4.
42. de la Pompa JL, Epstein JA. Coordinating tissue interactions: notch signaling in cardiac development and disease. Dev Cell 2012;22(2):244–54.
43. Carta L, Wagenseil JE, Knutsen RH, et al. Discrete contributions of elastic fiber components to arterial development and mechanical compliance. Arterioscler Thromb Vasc Biol 2009;29(12):2083–9.
44. Pierpont ME, Lacro RV. Children with thoracic aortic aneurysm: challenges in diagnosis and therapy. J Pediatr 2015;167(1):14–6.
45. Azhar M, Brown K, Gard C, et al. Transforming growth factor Beta2 is required for valve remodeling during heart development. Dev Dyn 2011;240(9):2127–41.
46. Chang CP, Bruneau BG. Epigenetics and cardiovascular development. Annu Rev Physiol 2012;74:41–68.
47. Kataoka M, Wang DZ. Non-coding RNAs including miRNAs and lncRNAs in cardiovascular biology and disease. Cells 2014;3(3):883–98.
48. Hiratzka LF, Bakris GL, Beckman JA, et al. 2010 ACCF/AHA/AATS/ACR/ASA/SCA/SCAI/SIR/STS/SVM guidelines for the diagnosis and management of patients with thoracic aortic disease: a report of the American College of Cardiology Foundation/American Heart Association Task Force on Practice Guidelines, American Association for Thoracic Surgery, American College of Radiology, American Stroke Association, Society of Cardiovascular Anesthesiologists, Society for Cardiovascular Angiography and Interventions, Society of Interventional Radiology, Society of Thoracic Surgeons, and Society for Vascular Medicine. Circulation 2010;121(13):e266–369.

Perinatal and Delivery Management of Infants with Congenital Heart Disease

Laura Sanapo, MD[a], Anita J. Moon-Grady, MD[b],
Mary T. Donofrio, MD[a,c],*

KEYWORDS

- Fetal echocardiography • Fetal cardiology • Congenital heart disease
- Neurodevelopment • Biophysical profile • Obstetric management
- Antenatal surveillance

KEY POINTS

- Prenatal diagnosis has improved neonatal outcomes of congenital heart disease (CHD) but perinatal morbidity and mortality are still significant in some cases.
- Fetal echocardiography can facilitate delivery and perinatal planning for infants with CHD.
- Antenatal surveillance of fetuses with CHD can identify prenatal progression of the lesion and decompensation, and may improve perinatal and postnatal outcomes.
- Successful perinatal management of neonates with a prenatal diagnosis of CHD requires close collaboration between obstetric, neonatal, and cardiology services.
- Delivery of infants prenatally diagnosed with CHD in most cases should not be scheduled before 39 weeks unless there is an obstetric indication or concern regarding fetal well-being.

Video content accompanies this article at http://www.perinatology.theclinics.com/

INTRODUCTION

Advances in prenatal imaging and increasing experience in fetal cardiology have improved the examination of the fetal cardiovascular system.[1] Fetal echocardiography

Disclosure: The authors have nothing to disclose.
[a] Division of Fetal and Transitional Medicine, Children's National Health System, 111 Michigan Avenue, Northwest, Suite M3-118, Washington, DC 20010, USA; [b] Fetal Cardiovascular Program, UCSF Benioff Children's Hospitals, University of California San Francisco, 550 16th Street, 5th Floor, Box 0544, San Francisco, CA 94158, USA; [c] Fetal Heart Program, Division of Cardiology, Children's National Health System, 111 Michigan Avenue, Northwest, Washington, DC 20010, USA
* Corresponding author. Fetal Heart Program, Division of Cardiology, Children's National Health System, 111 Michigan Avenue, Northwest, Washington, DC 20010.
E-mail address: MDonofri@childrensnational.org

Clin Perinatol 43 (2016) 55–71
http://dx.doi.org/10.1016/j.clp.2015.11.004
0095-5108/16/$ – see front matter © 2016 Elsevier Inc. All rights reserved.

is able to obtain precise details of cardiac structural and hemodynamic alterations in fetuses with congenital heart disease (CHD). Sequential examinations through gestation can predict the evolution of disease in utero and during the transition to postnatal circulation at delivery. This approach allows detailed prenatal counseling and enables planning to define perinatal management, selecting the fetuses at risk of postnatal hemodynamic instability who might require a specialized delivery plan.[2,3] The prenatal diagnosis and management of critical neonatal CHD has been shown to play an important role in improving the outcome of newborns with these conditions, allowing timely stabilization of the disease before cardiac surgery[4] and reducing the risk of perioperative morbidity,[4–9] including the risk of perioperative neurologic insults.[10] Despite evidence that fetal diagnosis has improved the outcome of some CHDs, critical forms may still be associated with significant morbidity and mortality caused by hemodynamic instability that occurs after birth, often shortly after separation from the placental circulation.[11] Therefore, prenatal assessment of the severity of the lesion and disease-specific delivery recommendations has been suggested to ensure the best care and avoid delays in treatment.[11–14] Perinatal management of neonates with a prenatal diagnosis of CHD requires a close collaboration between obstetric, neonatal, and cardiology services, and a well-delineated network with communication between the adult hospital and pediatric tertiary care center.[3]

This article reviews the most recent recommendations for the perinatal and delivery management of infants with a prenatal diagnosis of CHD.

FETAL ECHOCARDIOGRAPHY AND RISK OF HEMODYNAMIC INSTABILITY AT BIRTH

Most CHD is well tolerated in utero, does not present a risk of hemodynamic instability at birth or in the first days of life, and does not require specialized delivery care. However, some critical CHDs have an increased risk of hemodynamic instability after delivery and may require maintenance of patency of the fetal shunts and/or immediate intervention.[2] In order to identify the fetuses with CHD at risk of hemodynamic instability at birth, it is important to understand the physiology of the fetal circulation and the transition to the extrauterine circulation and how this process is compromised in newborns with a cardiac defect.

Fetal and Transitional Circulation

The fetal circulation is a highly efficient system that provides blood to the fetal body and the placenta. Fetal shunts allow the more highly oxygenated and nutrient-rich blood from the umbilical vein to be preferentially delivered to the left ventricle, therefore entering the systemic circulation. The remainder of the umbilical vein blood mixes with less oxygenated blood from the fetal body and passes to the right heart, and via the ductus arteriosus is directed into the descending aorta supplying the lower body and the placenta.[15] The fetoplacental circulation is characterized by low resistance, whereas the circulation to the fetal lungs is limited by high resistance. At delivery, multiple important changes occur. Cord clamping interrupts the low-resistance placental circulation, whereas initiation of respiration decreases the pulmonary vascular resistance and increases pulmonary blood flow and ultimately the blood volume returning to the left atrium through the pulmonary veins. Consequently, the left atrial pressure increases and functional closure of the foramen ovale occurs. With the closure of the ductus venosus (within the first week of life) and the ductus arteriosus (usually within 12–72 hours),[16] the fetal circulation transitions to the postnatal circulation in series.[17]

In specific cases of CHD, the presence of in utero cardiac shunting permits redistribution of blood flow to maintain cardiac output and adequate oxygen delivery to the fetal body to maintain a normal fetoplacental circulation. For this reason, most CHDs are well tolerated in utero,[17] although the altered circulatory pattern may impair systemic oxygenation and affect fetal growth and brain develop-ment.[18–21] The risk of hemodynamic instability after birth depends on 3 factors: (1) the type of CHD, including whether the defect is shunt dependent; (2) whether there is cardiac dysfunction either from a primary cardiomyopathy, structural anomaly leading to an excessive pressure or volume load to the heart, or a cardiac rhythm abnormality; and (3) whether there is an associated abnormality of the res-piratory system.

Models of Risk Assessment of Hemodynamic Instability at Birth

Several postnatal risk stratification protocols for babies diagnosed in utero with CHD have been proposed[11,12,14] and more recently summarized as part of the American Heart Association Statement on Fetal Cardiology[2] (**Table 1**). The risk of potential compromise at birth is most often determined prenatally by the fetal cardiologist, tak-ing into account the specific CHD as well as patient-specific findings noted on fetal echocardiogram (**Table 2**). A recent evaluation of a risk assessment protocol applied prospectively to a patient population at the Children's National Health System showed high accuracy with a sensitivity ranging from 0.83 to 0.99 for prediction of postnatal care and need for specialized intervention at birth.[12]

CHDs can be divided into 3 main categories, according to the predicted risk of he-modynamic instability at birth: (1) CHD without risk of hemodynamic instability during or immediately after delivery, or in the neonatal period; (2) CHD with minimal risk of hemodynamic instability; and (3) CHD with high risk of instability.

Congenital heart disease without predicted risk of hemodynamic instability at birth

This group includes left-to-right shunt lesions such as ventricular septal defects, atrial septal defects, atrioventricular septal defects, and mild valve abnormalities. Left-to-right shunt lesions most often become hemodynamically unstable weeks after birth when the decrease in the pulmonary vascular resistance causes significant left-to-right shunting and associated pulmonary overcirculation.[15] Similarly, infants prenatally diagnosed with a mild isolated valve abnormality and normal cardiac function are usu-ally stable after birth. These conditions do not require specialized care in the delivery room, and babies often can be delivered at local hospitals and be evaluated either in the nursery or as an outpatient.[12,22]

Congenital heart disease with minimal risk of hemodynamic instability at birth

This group mainly includes CHDs that depend on the patency of the ductus arteriosus for maintenance of the systemic or pulmonary circulation after birth. The ductus arteriosus does not generally close immediately at birth, but after 12 to 72 hours,[16] and therefore these babies are not expected to be compromised in the delivery room or immediate perinatal period.[12,13] In these cases, babies may be delivered at a location that can institute therapy with prostaglandin E1 for maintenance of ductal patency. After initial stabilization, transport of the newborn to the tertiary care cardiac center for anticipated intervention and/or sur-gery should be arranged.

The prediction of the need for patency of ductus arteriosus after birth may be diffi-cult but there are several criteria available (see **Table 2**). In case of pulmonary outflow tract obstruction, such as critical pulmonary stenosis or atresia, severe tricuspid valve stenosis or atresia without or with a small ventricular septal defect, or severe tetralogy of Fallot (TOF), the following findings have been shown to be fairly reliable predictors of

Table 1
Type of CHD and delivery recommendations

Definition	Example CHD	Delivery Recommendations	DR Recommendations
CHD in which palliative care is planned	CHD with severe/fatal chromosome abnormality or multisystem disease	Arrange for family support/palliative care services Normal delivery at local hospital	—
CHD without predicted risk of hemodynamic instability in the DR of first days of life	VSD, AVSD, mild TOF	Arrange cardiology consultation or outpatient evaluation Normal delivery at local hospital	Routine DR care Neonatal evaluation
CHD with minimal risk of hemodynamic instability in DR requiring postnatal catheterization/surgery	Ductal-dependent lesions, including HLHS, critical coarctation, severe AS, IAA, PA/IVS, severe TOF	Consider planned induction, usually near term Delivery at hospital with neonatologist and accessible cardiology consultation	Neonatologist in DR Routine DR care, initiate PGE if indicated Transport for catheterization/surgery
CHD with likely hemodynamic instability in DR requiring immediate specialty care for stabilization	d-TGA with concerning atrial septum primum (it is reasonable to consider all d-TGA fetuses without an ASD at risk) Uncontrolled arrhythmias CHB with heart failure	Planned induction at 38–39 wk; consider CS if necessary to coordinate services Delivery at hospital that can execute rapid care, including necessary stabilizing/lifesaving procedures	Neonatologist and cardiac specialist in DR, including all necessary equipment Plan for intervention as indicated by diagnosis Plan for urgent transport if indicated
CHD with expected hemodynamic instability with placental separation requiring immediate catheterization/surgery in DR to improve chance of survival	HLHS/severely RFO or IAS d-TGA/severely RFO or IAS and abnormal DA Obstructed TAPVR Ebstein anomaly with hydrops TOF with APV and severe airway obstruction Uncontrolled arrhythmias with hydrops CHB with low ventricular rate, EFE, and/or hydrops	CS in cardiac facility with necessary specialists in the DR usually at 38–39 wk	Specialized cardiac care team in DR Plan for intervention as indicated by diagnosis; may include catheterization, surgery, or ECMO

Abbreviations: APV, absent pulmonary valve; AS, aortic stenosis; ASD, atrial septal defect; AVSD, atrioventricular septal defect; CHB, complete heart block; CS, cesarean section; DA, ductus arteriosus; DR, delivery room; d-TGA, d-transposition of the great arteries; ECMO, extracorporeal membrane oxygenation; EFE, endocardial fibroelastosis; HLHS, hypoplastic left heart syndrome; IAA, interrupted aortic arch; IAS, intact atrial septum; PA/IVS, pulmonary atresia/intact ventricular septum; PGE, prostaglandin; RFO, restrictive foramen ovale; TAPVR, total anomalous pulmonary venous return; TOF, tetralogy of Fallot; VSD, ventricular septal defect.
Source: American Heart Association, Inc.

Table 2
Current recommendations for fetal predictors for delivery planning

CHD	Fetal Echocardiographic Finding	Delivery Recommendation
Ductal-dependent lesions	Ductal-dependent pulmonary circulation: 　Aorta to pulmonary flow in the DA 　Reversed orientation of the DA Ductal-dependent systemic circulation: 　Left-to-right atrial flow across the foramen ovale	No specialized care in the DR Initiation of prostaglandin E1
HLHS with RFO or IAS	Ratio of pulmonary vein forward to reversed velocity-time integral <3 Maternal hyperoxygenation in third trimester with no change in fetal branch pulmonary artery pulsatility index	Plan for possible urgent intervention to decompress left atrium (catheterization balloon or stent; surgery)
d-TGA	Reported FO findings predictive of restriction: 　Angle of septum primum <30° to the atrial septum 　Bowing of septum primum into the left atrium >50% 　Lack of normal swinging motion of septum primum 　Hypermobile septum primum (all fetuses with d-TGA and concerning septum primum should be considered at risk) Abnormal DA findings: 　Small (low z score) 　Accelerated forward, bidirectional, or reversed diastolic flow	Plan for urgent balloon atrial septostomy, on site if possible in the DR or ICU Initiation of prostaglandin E1 Consider therapy for pulmonary hypertension with abnormal DA flow
TOF with APV	Lung finding suggestive of lobar emphysema (fluid trapping) on MRI	Specialized ventilation Consider ECMO
Ebstein anomaly	Hydrops fetalis Uncontrolled arrhythmia	Consider early delivery with measures to decrease pulmonary resistance, treat arrhythmias, and support cardiac output
TAPVR, obstructed	Decompressing vein below the diaphragm Accelerated flow in decompressing vein	Consider ECMO
Tachyarrhythmias	Rapid heart rate Decreased heart function Pericardial effusion/hydrops fetalis	Consider early delivery if appropriate gestational age Urgent cardioversion or medical therapy in DR if possible
CHB	Decreasing CVP score (to <7) Very low ventricular rate Decreased heart function/EFE Hydrops fetalis	Consider early delivery Consider medical chronotrope or temporary pacing in DR if possible

Abbreviations: CHB, complete heart block; CVP, cardiovascular profile; d-TGA, transposition of the great arteries; DA, ductus arteriosus; ECMO, extracorporeal membrane oxygenation; EFE, endocardial fibroelastosis; FO, foramen ovale; HLHS, hypoplastic left heart syndrome; IAS, intact atrial septum; ICU, intensive care unit; MRI, magnetic resonance imaging; RFO, restrictive foramen ovale; TAPVR, total anomalous pulmonary venous return; TOF with APV, Tetralogy of Fallot with absent pulmonary valve.
Source: American Heart Association, Inc.

the necessity of patency of the ductus arteriosus or significant cyanosis and need for neonatal intervention to improve pulmonary blood flow after birth:

- Reversed flow in the ductus arteriosus, described as flow from the aorta to the pulmonary artery through the ductus (**Fig. 1**, Video 1)[23,24]
- Reversed orientation of the ductus arteriosus, defined as the angle of junction between the ductus arteriosus and the aorta being less than 90°[25]
- Pulmonary valve z score less than −3 measured after 16 weeks of gestation (in cases of TOF)[26]

In cases of obstruction to the systemic circulation, inadequacy of the left heart to maintain systemic output after birth can be predicted based on the following:

- Reversed flow across the foramen ovale, defined as flow directed from the left atrium to the right atrium (**Fig. 2**)[23,27]
- Systolic flow reversal in the distal transverse aortic arch, implying perfusion of the aortic arch via the ductus arteriosus (**Fig. 3**, Video 2)[23,27]

Congenital heart disease with high risk of hemodynamic instability at birth

This group includes cardiac defects that require immediate stabilization after birth with intervention in the immediate perinatal period. Fetuses with these conditions should be delivered at a hospital with neonatology and pediatric cardiology preferably on site, with rapid access to an interventional cardiac catheterization service and cardiac surgery. Examples of CHD in this category include hypoplastic left heart syndrome (HLHS) with a restrictive or closed foramen ovale, d-transposition of the great arteries (d-TGA), uncontrolled arrhythmias, complete heart block, TOF with absent pulmonary valve and concern for airway obstruction or with hydrops, severe Ebstein anomaly with hydrops, and obstructed total anomalous pulmonary venous return.

Fetal echocardiographic findings that have been shown to be predictive of the need for intervention to open the foramen ovale in cases of HLHS and d-TGA have been reported (see **Table 2**). In HLHS, the presence of the following findings increases the likelihood of need for intervention to open the atrial septum at birth:

- A ratio of forward pulmonary vein flow to reversed flow less than 3 (where the pulmonary flow is expressed as velocity-time integral) (**Fig. 4**)[5]
- Lack of vasoreactivity in the fetal branch of the pulmonary artery during the maternal hyperoxygenation testing performed in the third trimester[28]

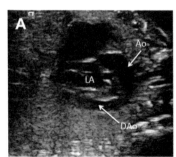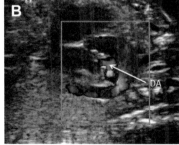

Fig. 1. Fetus with TOF. (*A*) Sagittal two-dimensional imaging of the aortic/ductal arches. (*B*) Color Doppler shows reversed flow (*red*) in the ductus arteriosus. Ao, aorta; DA, ductus arteriosus; DAo, descending aorta; LA, left atrium.

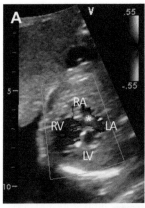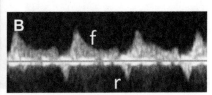

Fig. 2. Fetus with hypoplastic left heart syndrome (HLHS). (A) Axial 4-chamber view. Color Doppler shows reversed flow (*red*) across the foramen ovale. (B) Pulmonary vein flow with a velocity-time integral forward/reversed flow ratio greater than 5 indicating a nonrestrictive atrial septum. The asterisk indicates the foramen ovale. f, forward flow; LV, left ventricle; r, reversed flow; RA, right atrium; RV, right ventricle.

In fetuses with d-TGA, specific echocardiographic features of the septum primum have been shown to have a high specificity to predict the need for atrial septostomy, although specificity is not adequate[12]:

- Angle of septum primum less than 30° to the atrial septum[29]
- Bowing of the septum primum into the left atrium greater than 50% (**Fig. 5**)[29]
- Lack of normal swinging motion of septum primum[29]
- Hypermobility of septum primum (Video 3)[30]

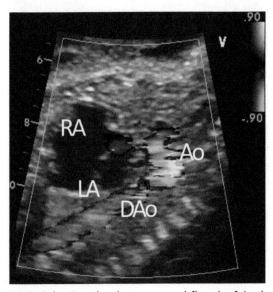

Fig. 3. Fetus with HLHS. Color Doppler shows reversed flow (*red*) in the transverse aortic arch.

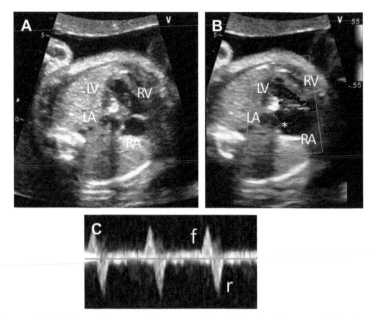

Fig. 4. Fetus with HLHS and intact atrial septum. (*A*) Axial 4-chamber view. (*B*) Color Doppler shows no flow across the foramen ovale. (*C*) Pulmonary vein flow with a velocity-time integral forward/reversed flow ratio less than 3. The asterisk indicates the foramen ovale.

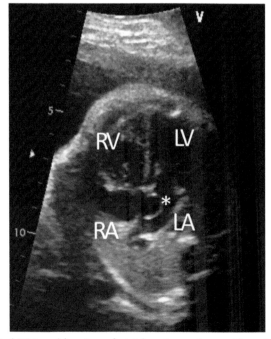

Fig. 5. Fetus with d-TGA and bowing of atrial septum primum. The asterisk indicates the atrial septum.

Given that the predictive value of these findings with regard to the need for urgent atrial septostomy in d-TGA is still limited, it is reasonable to consider all fetuses with d-TGA to be at risk of hemodynamic instability at birth and it is therefore recommended that all fetuses with d-TGA be delivered at a hospital with rapid access to a pediatric cardiologist able to perform a septostomy if needed.

At present there are limited data available to guide decisions regarding delivery management of complex rare diseases that are thought to be at risk of intrauterine demise and poor neonatal outcome because of pulmonary comorbidity, heart failure, and/or compromised cardiac output, such as TOF with absent pulmonary valve complex and severe Ebstein anomaly. However, because rapid deterioration in the perinatal period can be seen with these defects,[31] delivery in a setting that affords immediate access to specialized teams including neonatology, pediatric cardiology, and cardiothoracic surgery is probably prudent if there is any antenatal evidence of fetal compromise (effusions, hydrops, poor growth, nonreassuring fetal monitoring).

ANTENATAL FETAL SURVEILLANCE AFTER A DIAGNOSIS OF CONGENITAL HEART DISEASE

There may be a role for increased antenatal surveillance of a fetus with CHD. Goals of increased monitoring through the pregnancy may include evaluation for progression of the severity of the lesion in utero (ie, from non–ductal dependent to ductal dependent) and the early recognition of fetal compromise, including impairment of the fetal growth, evidence of fetal hypoxemia with altered umbilical and/or cerebral Doppler blood flow, or the development of fetal hydrops (as a manifestation of fetal congestive heart failure). Findings on serial assessment may require adjustment of the plans for perinatal and delivery management in order to improve perinatal and postnatal outcome.

Cardiotocography and Biophysical Profile

Computerized cardiotocography (CTG) and biophysical profile are tests used to identify fetuses at risk of intrauterine hypoxia and acidosis[32] and they are currently used for the fetal surveillance in high-risk pregnancies with the aim of selecting fetuses at risk of poor perinatal outcome. Recommendations regarding frequency and timing have been defined for specific obstetric complications such as advanced maternal age, diabetes, hypertension, and previous stillbirth, or specific fetal conditions such as intrauterine growth restriction and multiple gestations.[33] No guidelines are available that support this testing in fetuses with isolated CHD. Nevertheless, it is prudent to consider their use in the CHD population, especially when additional comorbidities exist or the cardiac defect puts the fetus at risk for heart failure or significant arrhythmias.

Cardiovascular Profile Score

The cardiovascular profile (CVP) score may be used to assess the risk of congestive heart failure in fetuses with a diagnosis of CHD.[34] It consists of 5 parameters: edema, effusions, or overt hydrops fetalis; heart size; cardiac function; and Doppler findings of the ductus venosus and umbilical veins and umbilical artery. Any variables may be rated from 0 to 2 with a final score ranging from a maximum of 10 to a minimum of 0 (**Table 3**).

Table 3
The cardiovascular profile score

Category	2 Points	1 Point	0 Point
Hydrops	None	Ascites or pericardial or pleural effusion	Skin edema
Heart size (HA/CA)	>0.2 and ≤0.35	0.35–0.5	<0.2 or >0.5
Cardiac function	Normal MV and TV, biphasic diastolic filling, LV or RV SFs >0.28	Holosystolic TR or LV or RV SFs <0.28	Holosystolic MR or TR dP/dt <400, monophasic diastolic filling
Arterial umbilical Doppler	Normal	AEDV	REDV
Venous Doppler	Normal	DV atrial reversal	UV pulsations

Abbreviations: AEDV, absent end-diastolic velocity; DV, ductus venosus; HA/CA, heart to chest area ratio; LV, left ventricle; MR, mitral valve regurgitation; MV, mitral valve; REDV, reversed end-diastolic velocity; RV, right ventricle; SF, ventricular shortening fraction; TR dP/dt, change in pressure over time of TR jet; TR, tricuspid valve regurgitation; TV, tricuspid valve; UV, umbilical vein.

From Wieczorek A, Hernandez-Robles J, Ewing L, et al. Prediction of outcome of fetal congenital heart disease using a cardiovascular profile score. Ultrasound Obstet Gynecol 2008;31:285; with permission.

The use of the CVP score has been evaluated in CHD and fetal rhythm abnormalities,[35–37] with a score less than or equal to 7 correlating with a higher risk of perinatal compromise or death. Among the 5 parameters, the presence of hydrops fetalis and severe cardiomegaly, defined as heart/chest area ratio greater than 0.5, have showed the most statistically significant association with mortality. The presence of hydrops or CVP less than 7 may represent an indication for urgent delivery and planning for potential immediate postnatal intervention.

DELIVERY PLANNING FOR NEONATES PRENATALLY DIAGNOSED WITH CONGENITAL HEART DISEASE

Delivery planning should take into account 3 main factors: (1) the risk of hemodynamic instability at birth, (2) the resources of the region, (3) the presence of obstetric complications.

Location of Delivery and Transportation of the Newborn

Most newborns with CHD do not need any specialized care in the perinatal period and recommendations are made to deliver at the local hospital and be followed as outpatients.[2] However, if the presence of a specialized cardiac team after delivery is anticipated (see **Table 1**), the location of delivery should take into account these special needs. Determination of the site of delivery may depend on the availability of a pediatric cardiac unit in close proximity. In some regions where the number of specialized cardiac centers is limited, strategies have been developed to safely plan the delivery and perinatal management of infants prenatally diagnosed with CHD.[14,22] These plans include either creation of highly specialized neonatal units locally or maternal-fetal transport with delivery nearer to a cardiac center in patients determined to be at high risk of hemodynamic instability. In order to improve the neonatal outcome of the infants with CHD associated with hemodynamic instability with placental separation and avoid transportation of critically ill newborns, some freestanding children's hospitals have planned deliveries in their facilities to accommodate these particularly high-risk patients, thus minimizing time to lifesaving intervention.[11,38]

Timing of Delivery

Recent studies have shown that infants prenatally diagnosed with critical forms of CHD tend to be delivered earlier than neonates in whom the diagnosis of CHD is made after birth.[10,39,40] This finding is particularly worrisome given that otherwise healthy neonates born at 37 to 38 weeks have increased risk of worse outcomes compared with those born at later term (39–40 weeks).[41] This finding has also been observed in babies with CHD. Studies have shown that babies with CHD have longer postoperative lengths of stay and higher mortality if delivered before 39 weeks.[40,42,43] Therefore, in the absence of fetal or maternal indications for earlier delivery, the potential advantages of an elective delivery of fetuses with CHD early should be carefully considered.

In addition to an increased mortality, there is growing evidence that the decision about timing of delivery of infants with CHD should also consider the potential effect of the gestational age at birth on the neurologic outcome. It has been shown that fetuses with critical CHDs, such as d-TGA or single-ventricle physiology, have delays in brain maturation that manifest as alteration of brain growth, brain metabolism, and the microstructure of the white matter of the pyramidal tract[44–47] and that suggest that brain development may lag by as much as 4 weeks in term neonates with CHD before heart surgery. Given these findings, it has been suggested that planning for the delivery of babies with CHD near or at full term may improve brain development and decrease susceptibility to injury postnatally[46]; however, further studies are needed to establish whether this will translate to improvement in long-term neurologic outcome.

Planning of the delivery of babies with CHD is also affected by the overall risk of preterm birth (occurring in 12.8% of all US births).[48] To date, although there are effective predictors of preterm birth before 34 weeks, such as cervicovaginal fetal fibronectin and cervical length based on ultrasonography evaluations, there is no way to identify the exact timing of the delivery among women with risk factors or symptoms of preterm labor.[49,50] For these reasons, close communication between the obstetrician and the pediatric cardiologist is necessary if spontaneous preterm birth seems likely.

Mode of Delivery

Data from retrospective studies show that prenatal diagnosis of a major CHD, such as HLHS, d-TGA, double-outlet right ventricle, or TOF, increases the likelihood for planned delivery and cesarean section. In fetuses with CHD, the mode of delivery has not been shown to affect the Apgar score, presurgical and postsurgical morbidity including the risk of hemodynamic instability, metabolic acidosis, and end-organ dysfunction, the length of hospitalization, or survival to surgery or discharge.[51,52] Two retrospective studies have concluded that labor is safe for fetuses with CHD in most cases,[53,54] but the impact on the long-term functional and neurodevelopmental outcomes is largely unknown.

Fetal Surveillance During Labor

The decision to perform a vaginal delivery in women with a prenatal diagnosis of fetal CHD opens a debate regarding how to monitor these fetuses during labor with the aim of promptly identifying and intervening for those at risk of hypoxemia and acidosis in order to minimize risk of hypoxic ischemic encephalopathy and adverse long-term neurologic outcome.

The use of CTG to record the fetal heart rate and the uterine contractile activity can stratify the risk of intrapartum hypoxia and neonatal acidosis,[55,56] but this test in practice has low positive predictive value for neonatal hypoxia and acidosis.[57] The introduction of continuous CTG in labor has not been shown to decrease the incidence of cerebral palsy or infant death among low-risk or high-risk pregnancies but has been associated with a decrease in the incidence of neonatal seizures. However, it is also associated with a higher percentage of cesarean and instrumental vaginal deliveries.[57]

The fetal heart rate is determined by the interaction between the cardiovascular center in the medulla oblongata, the vagus nerve, and the heart. It has been hypothesized that fetal anomalies involving the central nervous system or the heart may alter the fetal heart rate patterns without correlating with a hypoxic or acidotic state.[58] The few retrospective studies evaluating the use of CTG in labor of fetuses with CHD[53,58,59] have shown that these fetuses show a higher percentage of nonreassuring fetal heart rate tracings, but no characteristic fetal heart rate patterns have been related to specific heart defects. As with normal fetuses, the use of continuous CTG in labor for fetuses with CHD has been associated with an increased rate of emergent cesarean delivery.[58] In addition, CTG is limited in the assessment of the heart rate in fetuses with significant arrhythmias. To overcome these limitations, the fetal electrocardiogram, performed with scalp electrode, has been proposed in labor to monitor fetuses with a prenatal diagnosis of congenital heart block. Despite encouraging results, the only available data are based on case reports.[60,61]

Other types of fetal surveillance during labor, such as abdominal fetal electrocardiogram, pulse oximetry, and fetal scalp blood sampling for estimation of lactate, may serve as tools to select those fetuses with nonreassuring fetal heart rate tracings suggesting a risk of hypoxemia and acidosis; however, there are no data to support their routine use in fetuses with CHD.[62] Given the lack of data, the CTG remains the main tool for routine surveillance during labor for fetuses with CHD, with the interpretation of the tracings presently based on the classification systems proposed for all pregnancies.[55,56]

SUMMARY

The prenatal diagnosis of severe CHD is associated with improvement in preoperative condition, with a reduction in morbidity, including neonatal hypoxemia, need for invasive respiratory support, and metabolic acidosis, and an increased survival in select defects, including HLHS and d-TGA. Furthermore, detection of CHD in utero allows better parental counseling and delivery planning, especially when the need for urgent postnatal intervention is anticipated based on available predictive models. Perinatal management should be tailored to the specific needs of the mother and fetus, and should include decisions regarding location, timing, and mode of delivery that in general minimize the risk of early or operative delivery. In selected cases, there may be compelling maternal or fetal indications for earlier delivery, including a variety of obstetric indications, such as spontaneous onset of labor, maternal comorbidities, pregnancy complications, or nonreassuring results of fetal testing. Collaboration between obstetric and pediatric specialty services and careful attention to perinatal management and delivery planning after a prenatal diagnosis of CHD is made can improve the perinatal status of newborns with potential for improvement in both survival and long-term functional and neurodevelopmental outcome.

Best practices

What is the current practice?

CHD recognized before delivery

Objective: to minimize perinatal morbidity and mortality for both infant and mother, optimize infant status before surgical intervention, and improve short-term and long-term outcomes

What changes in current practice are likely to improve outcomes?

Prenatal diagnosis has the potential to confer improved survival and long-term outcome, specifically a neurodevelopmental advantage, if certain modifiable risk factors can be addressed during delivery planning

Where: triage of delivery to appropriate facility/level of care based on prediction of newborn hemodynamic status at birth

When: delivery as close to term as possible with avoidance of iatrogenic late preterm and early term delivery

How: avoidance of routine early induction of labor and of operative delivery in cases lacking clear obstetric indication

Major recommendations

- Perinatal management should emphasize maternal-fetal health and both short-term and long-term outcomes
- Most CHDs, such as shunt lesions or mild valve abnormality, with normal cardiac function may be delivered without anticipation of specialized delivery room care
- Delivery planning in a specialized center may be beneficial for certain high-risk lesions
- Vaginal delivery after spontaneous-onset labor is probably best for mother and baby in most cases; iatrogenic late-term and early term delivery should be discouraged
- Cardiotocography should be considered as a method of surveillance in labor for fetuses with heart malformations and the interpretation of the tracing is based on the same classification systems proposed for normal fetuses

---

SUPPLEMENTARY DATA

Supplementary data related to this article can be found at http://dx.doi.org/10.1016/j.clp.2015.11.004.

REFERENCES

1. Allan LD, Sharland GK, Milburn A, et al. Prospective diagnosis of 1,006 consecutive cases of congenital heart disease in the fetus. J Am Coll Cardiol 1994;23:1452–8.
2. Donofrio MT, Moon-Grady AJ, Hornberger LK, et al, American Heart Association Adults With Congenital Heart Disease Joint Committee of the Council on Cardiovascular Disease in the Young and Council on Clinical Cardiology, Council on Cardiovascular Surgery and Anesthesia, and Council on Cardiovascular and Stroke Nursing. Diagnosis and treatment of fetal cardiac disease: a scientific statement from the American Heart Association. Circulation 2014;129:2183–242.
3. Brown KL, Sullivan ID. Prenatal detection for major congenital heart disease: a key process measure for congenital heart networks. Heart 2014;100:359–60.

4. Tworetzky W, McElhinney DB, Reddy VM, et al. Improved surgical outcome after fetal diagnosis of hypoplastic left heart syndrome. Circulation 2001;103:1269–73.

5. Divanović A, Hor K, Cnota J, et al. Prediction and perinatal management of severely restrictive atrial septum in fetuses with critical left heart obstruction: clinical experience using pulmonary venous Doppler analysis. J Thorac Cardiovasc Surg 2011;141:988–94.

6. Tzifa A, Barker C, Tibby SM, et al. Prenatal diagnosis of pulmonary atresia: impact on clinical presentation and early outcome. Arch Dis Child Fetal Neonatal Ed 2007;92:F199–203.

7. Franklin O, Burch M, Manning N, et al. Prenatal diagnosis of coarctation of the aorta improves survival and reduces morbidity. Heart 2002;87:67–9.

8. Eapen RS, Rowland DG, Franklin WH. Effect of prenatal diagnosis of critical left heart obstruction on perinatal morbidity and mortality. Am J Perinatol 1998;15:237–42.

9. Kumar RK, Newburger JW, Gauvreau K, et al. Comparison of outcome when hypoplastic left heart syndrome and transposition of the great arteries are diagnosed prenatally versus when diagnosis of these two conditions is made only postnatally. Am J Cardiol 1999;83:1649–53.

10. Kipps AK, Feuille C, Azakie A, et al. Prenatal diagnosis of hypoplastic left heart syndrome in current era. Am J Cardiol 2011;108:421–7.

11. Donofrio MT, Levy RJ, Schuette JJ, et al. Specialized delivery room planning for fetuses with critical congenital heart disease. Am J Cardiol 2013;111:737–47.

12. Donofrio MT, Skurow-Todd K, Berger JT, et al. Risk-stratified postnatal care of newborns with congenital heart disease determined by fetal echocardiography. J Am Soc Echocardiogr 2015;28(11):1339–49.

13. Johnson BA, Ades A. Delivery room and early postnatal management of neonates who have prenatally diagnosed congenital heart disease. Clin Perinatol 2005;32:921–46.

14. Berkley EM, Goens MB, Karr S, et al. Utility of fetal echocardiography in postnatal management of infants with prenatally diagnosed congenital heart disease. Prenat Diagn 2009;29:654–8.

15. Rudolph AM. The fetal circulation and postnatal adaptation. In: Rudolph AM, editor. Congenital diseases of the heart: clinical-physiological considerations. Armonk (NY): Futura Publishing Company; 2001. p. 3–44.

16. Lim MK, Hanretty K, Houston AB, et al. Intermittent ductal patency in healthy newborn infants: demonstration by colour Doppler flow mapping. Arch Dis Child 1992;67:1217–8.

17. Friedman AH, Fahey JT. The transition from fetal to neonatal circulation: normal responses and implications for infants with heart disease. Semin Perinatol 1993;17:106–21.

18. Rosenthal GL. Patterns of prenatal growth among infants with cardiovascular malformations: possible fetal hemodynamic effects. Am J Epidemiol 1996;143:505–13.

19. Limperopoulos C, Tworetzky W, McElhinney DB, et al. Brain volume and metabolism in fetuses with congenital heart disease: evaluation with quantitative magnetic resonance imaging and spectroscopy. Circulation 2010;121:26–33.

20. Donofrio MT, Duplessis AJ, Limperopoulos C. Impact of congenital heart disease on fetal brain development and injury. Curr Opin Pediatr 2011;23:502–11.

21. Manzar S, Nair AK, Pai MG, et al. Head size at birth in neonates with transposition of great arteries and hypoplastic left heart syndrome. Saudi Med J 2005;26:453–6.

22. Anagnostou K, Messenger L, Yates R, et al. Outcome of infants with prenatally diagnosed congenital heart disease delivered outside specialist paediatric cardiac centres. Arch Dis Child Fetal Neonatal Ed 2013;98:F218–21.

23. Berning RA, Silverman NH, Villegas M, et al. Reversed shunting across the ductus arteriosus or atrial septum in utero heralds severe congenital heart disease. J Am Coll Cardiol 1996;27:481–6.

24. Quartermain MD, Glatz AC, Goldberg DJ, et al. Pulmonary outflow tract obstruction in fetuses with complex congenital heart disease: predicting the need for neonatal intervention. Ultrasound Obstet Gynecol 2013;41:47–53.

25. Hinton R, Michelfelder E. Significance of reverse orientation of the ductus arteriosus in neonates with pulmonary outflow tract obstruction for early intervention. Am J Cardiol 2006;97:716–9.

26. Arya B, Levasseur SM, Woldu K, et al. Fetal echocardiographic measurements and the need for neonatal surgical intervention in tetralogy of Fallot. Pediatr Cardiol 2014;35:810–6.

27. Mäkikallio K, McElhinney DB, Levine JC, et al. Fetal aortic valve stenosis and the evolution of hypoplastic left heart syndrome: patient selection for fetal intervention. Circulation 2006;113:1401–5.

28. Szwast A, Tian Z, McCann M, et al. Vasoreactive response to maternal hyperoxygenation in the fetus with hypoplastic left heart syndrome. Circ Cardiovasc Imaging 2010;3:172–8.

29. Jouannic JM, Gavard L, Fermont L, et al. Sensitivity and specificity of prenatal features of physiological shunts to predict neonatal clinical status in transposition of the great arteries. Circulation 2004;110:1743–6.

30. Punn R, Silverman NH. Fetal predictors of urgent balloon atrial septostomy in neonates with complete transposition. J Am Soc Echocardiogr 2011;24: 425–30.

31. Freud LR, Escobar-Diaz MC, Kalish BT, et al. Outcomes and predictors of perinatal mortality in fetuses with Ebstein anomaly or tricuspid valve dysplasia in the current era: a multi-center study. Circulation 2015;132(6):481–9.

32. Manning FA, Harman CR, Morrison I, et al. Fetal assessment based on fetal biophysical profile scoring. IV. An analysis of perinatal morbidity and mortality. Am J Obstet Gynecol 1990;162:703–9.

33. ACOG practice bulletin. Antepartum fetal surveillance. Number 9, October 1999 (replaces technical bulletin number 188, January 1994). Clinical management guidelines for obstetrician-gynecologists. Int J Gynaecol Obstet 2000;68:175–85.

34. Falkensammer CB, Paul J, Huhta JC. Fetal congestive heart failure: correlation of Tei-index and cardiovascular-score. J Perinat Med 2001;29:390–8.

35. Wieczorek A, Hernandez-Robles J, Ewing L, et al. Prediction of outcome of fetal congenital heart disease using a cardiovascular profile score. Ultrasound Obstet Gynecol 2008;31:284–8.

36. Huhta JC. Right ventricular function in the human fetus. J Perinat Med 2001;29: 381–9.

37. Donofrio MT, Gullquist SD, Mehta ID, et al. Congenital complete heart block: fetal management protocol, review of the literature, and report of the smallest successful pacemaker implantation. J Perinatol 2004;24:112–7.

38. Howell LJ. The Garbose Family Special Delivery Unit: a new paradigm for maternal-fetal and neonatal care. Semin Pediatr Surg 2013;22:3–9.

39. Levey A, Glickstein JS, Kleinman CS, et al. The impact of prenatal diagnosis of complex congenital heart disease on neonatal outcomes. Pediatr Cardiol 2010; 31:587–97.

40. Costello JM, Polito A, Brown DW, et al. Birth before 39 weeks' gestation is associated with worse outcomes in neonates with heart disease. Pediatrics 2010;126:277–84.

41. Cheng YW, Nicholson JM, Nakagawa S, et al. Perinatal outcomes in low-risk term pregnancies: do they differ by week of gestation? Am J Obstet Gynecol 2008;199:370.e1–7.

42. Cnota JF, Gupta R, Michelfelder EC, et al. Congenital heart disease infant death rates decrease as gestational age advances from 34 to 40 weeks. J Pediatr 2011;159:761–5.

43. Costello JM, Pasquali SK, Jacobs JP, et al. Gestational age at birth and outcomes after neonatal cardiac surgery: an analysis of the society of thoracic surgeons congenital heart surgery database. Circulation 2014;129:2511–7.

44. Miller SP, McQuillen PS, Hamrick S, et al. Abnormal brain development in newborns with congenital heart disease. N Engl J Med 2007;357:1928–38.

45. Partridge SC, Vigneron DB, Charlton NN, et al. Pyramidal tract maturation after brain injury in newborns with heart disease. Ann Neurol 2006;59:640–51.

46. Licht DJ, Shera DM, Clancy RR, et al. Brain maturation is delayed in infants with complex congenital heart defects. J Thorac Cardiovasc Surg 2009;137:529–36.

47. Clouchoux C, du Plessis AJ, Bouyssi-Kobar M, et al. Delayed cortical development in fetuses with complex congenital heart disease. Cereb Cortex 2013;23:2932–43.

48. Martin JA, Hamilton BE, Sutton PD, et al, Centers for Disease Control and Prevention National Center for Health Statistics National Vital Statistics System. Births: final data for 2006. Natl Vital Stat Rep 2009;57:1–104.

49. Honest H, Forbes CA, Durée KH, et al. Screening to prevent spontaneous preterm birth: systematic reviews of accuracy and effectiveness literature with economic modelling. Health Technol Assess 2009;13:1–627.

50. Lockwood CJ. Predicting premature delivery–no easy task. N Engl J Med 2002;346:282–4.

51. Peterson AL, Quartermain MD, Ades A, et al. Impact of mode of delivery on markers of perinatal hemodynamics in infants with hypoplastic left heart syndrome. J Pediatr 2011;159:64–9.

52. Trento LU, Pruetz JD, Chang RK, et al. Prenatal diagnosis of congenital heart disease: impact of mode of delivery on neonatal outcome. Prenat Diagn 2012;32:1250–5.

53. Walsh CA, MacTiernan A, Farrell S, et al. Mode of delivery in pregnancies complicated by major fetal congenital heart disease: a retrospective cohort study. J Perinatol 2014;34:901–5.

54. Reis PM, Punch MR, Bove EL, et al. Obstetric management of 219 infants with hypoplastic left heart syndrome. Am J Obstet Gynecol 1998;179:1150–4.

55. American College of Obstetricians and Gynecologists. ACOG practice bulletin No. 106: intrapartum fetal heart rate monitoring: nomenclature, interpretation, and general management principles. Obstet Gynecol 2009;114:192–202.

56. Parer JT, Ikeda T, King TL. The 2008 National Institute of Child Health and Human Development report on fetal heart rate monitoring. Obstet Gynecol 2009;114:136–8.

57. Alfirevic Z, Devane D, Gyte GML. Continuous cardiotocography (CTG) as a form of electronic fetal monitoring (EFM) for fetal assessment during labour. Cochrane Database Syst Rev 2013;(5):CD006066.

58. Ueda K, Ikeda T, Iwanaga N, et al. Intrapartum fetal heart rate monitoring in cases of congenital heart disease. Am J Obstet Gynecol 2009;201:64.e1–6.

59. Morikawa M, Endo D, Yamada T, et al. Electronic fetal heart rate monitoring in five fetuses with Ebstein's anomaly. J Obstet Gynaecol Res 2014;40:424–8.
60. Katz AR, Ross PJ, Bekheit-Saad S. Utilization of fetal scalp pH and direct fetal electrocardiogram in the intrapartum management of congenital complete heart block in an adolescent primigravida. J Adolesc Health Care 1980;1:152–4.
61. Friedman DM, Zervoudakis I, Buyon JP. Perinatal monitoring of fetal well-being in the presence of congenital heart block. Am J Perinatol 1998;15:669–73.
62. East CE, Leader LR, Sheehan P, et al. Intrapartum fetal scalp lactate sampling for fetal assessment in the presence of a non-reassuring fetal heart rate trace. Cochrane Database Syst Rev 2015;(5):CD006174.

Screening for Critical Congenital Heart Disease

Matthew E. Oster, MD, MPH[a,b,]*, Lazaros Kochilas, MD, MSCR[a,b]

KEYWORDS

- Newborn screening • Critical congenital heart disease • Pulse oximetry

KEY POINTS

- Critical congenital heart disease (CCHD) screening with pulse oximetry can detect many cases of CCHD before a child becomes symptomatic.
- An infant who fails CCHD screening warrants a thorough evaluation, not only for CCHD, but also for other causes of hypoxemia.
- An infant who passes CCHD screening may still have CCHD, as the sensitivity of pulse oximetry is poor for certain types of CCHD. A negative CCHD screen does not rule out the presence of disease.

INTRODUCTION

Screening for critical congenital heart disease (CCHD) using pulse oximetry was first proposed in the early 2000s.[1] Since that time, screening for CCHD has become common in most developed countries around the world, with CCHD being added to the United States Recommended Uniform Screening Panel (RUSP) in 2011.[2] In the United States, nearly all newborns are now screened for CCHD using pulse oximetry. This article reviews some of the history of screening for CCHD, the recommended approach to screening, considerations for screening in special settings such as the neonatal intensive care unit (NICU), and, most importantly, the limitations of existing screening practices.

WHAT IS CRITICAL CONGENITAL HEART DISEASE SCREENING?

The goal of any public health screening program is to identify disease in an asymptomatic individual. To that end, physicians have been screening children for CCHD for years. In many cases, a child with CCHD has been detected either by routine antenatal

Disclosures: None.
[a] Children's Healthcare of Atlanta, Atlanta, GA, USA; [b] Emory University School of Medicine, Atlanta, GA, USA
* Corresponding author. Sibley Heart Center Cardiology, Children's Healthcare of Atlanta, 2835 Brandywine Road, Suite 300, Atlanta, GA 30341.
E-mail address: osterm@kidsheart.com

Clin Perinatol 43 (2016) 73–80
http://dx.doi.org/10.1016/j.clp.2015.11.005
0095-5108/16/$ – see front matter © 2016 Elsevier Inc. All rights reserved.

ultrasound or the newborn physical examination; technically, these are both common screening tests, not only for CCHD, but for a number of other important conditions as well. However, due to either the limitations of antenatal ultrasound[3] or the lack of findings on physical examination,[4] until recently, up to 30% of children with CCHD were being discharged to home from the nursery with undiagnosed CCHD.[5,6]

With pulse oximetry, however, it is possible to detect low levels of oxygen saturation in newborns who otherwise appear well and before any overt signs of cyanosis or heart disease are present on examination.[4] Typically, clinically detectable cyanosis requires a concentration of at least 5 g/dL of deoxygenated hemoglobin, and this level of hypoxemia may not be seen in the first few hours for a newborn even in the presence of a cyanotic heart lesion. This is in part because the high affinity of fetal hemoglobin and partially because of the existence of fetal pathways that can mask the ultimate physiology of even the most severe congenital heart diseases. If pulse oximetry detects either a low oxygen saturation level or a notable difference between the upper and lower extremities, the health care provider will be alerted to the possibility of an underlying CCHD and can undertake an appropriate evaluation. There are many types of CCHD that can be detected by pulse oximetry based on their underlying physiology, as hypoxemia may result from restriction of effective pulmonary blood flow, mandatory recirculation in the pulmonary or systemic compartment, impediment of the pulmonary venous return toward the systemic circulation, or at least mixing of the systemic arterial and venous blood flow at some level.

Table 1 outlines the 12 most common types of CCHD that are surveilled by the US Centers for Disease Control and Prevention (CDC) and are associated with abnormal oxygen saturations. However, other less common or less severe defects can also be detected as long as their physiology includes any of the elements described previously. These defects range in their birth prevalence, their likelihood of being detected prenatally, and in their degree of hypoxemia during the neonatal transition (ie, their likelihood of being detected via pulse oximetry). Today, many types of CCHD such as hypoplastic left heart syndrome can often be detected by routine fetal ultrasonography or newborn physical examination. But several types of CCHD, such as total anomalous pulmonary venous return, can escape both of these modalities, and are thus ideal targets for screening with pulse oximetry.[7]

Table 1
Selected targets of critical congenital heart disease screening using pulse oximetry

		Lower Birth Prevalence (<1 per 10,000 US Births)	Higher Birth Prevalence (>1.5 per 10,000 US Births)
Higher sensitivity of pulse oximetry	Higher prenatal detection rate	Pulmonary atresia Tricuspid atresia Truncus arteriosus	HLHS
	Lower prenatal detection rate	TAPVR	d-TGA
Lower sensitivity of pulse oximetry	Higher prenatal detection rate	Double outlet right ventricle	—
	Lower prenatal detection rate	Ebstein anomaly Interrupted aortic arch Single ventricle complex	Coarctation of the aorta TOF

Abbreviations: d-TGA, d-Transposition of the Great Arteries; HLHS, Hypoplastic left heart syndrome; TAPVR, Total anomalous pulmonary venous return; TOF, Tetralogy of Fallot.
Adapted from Ailes EC, Gilboa SM, Honein MA, et al. Estimated number of infants detected and missed by critical congenital heart defect screening. Pediatrics 2015;135(6):1000–8.

TECHNIQUE FOR CRITICAL CONGENITAL HEART DISEASE SCREENING

A general protocol for implementing CCHD screening in a well-baby nursery was proposed in 2011 shortly before CCHD screening was added to the United States RUSP.[2] Modeled after a protocol that had been demonstrated to identify CCHD in Sweden,[8] this protocol has been endorsed by the American Academy of Pediatrics (AAP), American Heart Association (AHA), and American College of Cardiology (ACC). There are several important elements of this protocol (**Fig. 1**) to consider:

- Setting. This protocol was intended for use only in the well-baby nursery on a child who is asymptomatic. There are no published guidelines for screening in the NICU or other settings.
- Timing. The protocol recommends screening after 24 hours of age. Earlier screening can be performed, but there may be notable alterations in the sensitivity (some types of CCHD may not have yet developed hypoxemia) and specificity (many newborns without CCHD will still have low oxygen saturation levels in the

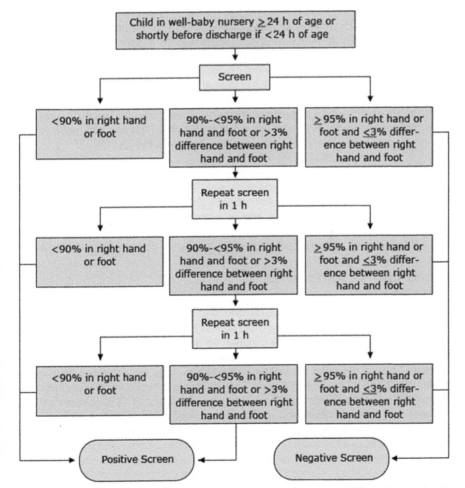

Fig. 1. CCHD screening algorithm endorsed by the AAP, AHA, and ACC. (*From* Centers for Disease Control and Prevention. Congenital heart defects: information for health care providers. Available at: http://www.cdc.gov/ncbddd/heartdefects/hcp.html. Accessed December 17, 2015.)

first 24 hours of life). There are no guidelines as to how late a child can be screened, but screening should be performed prior to discharge from the hospital.

- Anatomic location. Two separate sites—the right hand (typically preductal) and either foot (always postductal)—are needed to allow measurement of oxygen saturation in both a preductal and postductal location. This can be performed either simultaneously or in a relatively rapid succession by moving the probe from one extremity to the other.
- Repeat measurement. The purpose of repeating measurements is to decrease the false-positive rate (ie, to increase the specificity of screening). This should be done within a relatively short time frame (about 1 hour), and the child should be observed for the development of symptoms. If at any point a child develops symptoms, further evaluation should proceed accordingly.
- Equipment. Only US Food and Drug Administration (FDA)-approved pulse oximeters should be used.[9] Although pulse oximetry screening has been shown overall to be cost-effective, using disposable probes (instead of reusable probes) can have dramatic effects on increasing costs.[10,11]

Although the algorithm described previously is the most commonly used algorithm and is recommended by the AAP, AHA, and ACC, some states or hospitals are using modified versions of this algorithm. For example, in New Jersey, public health officials preferred to strive for a higher sensitivity at the sacrifice of a lower specificity. Thus, by the New Jersey algorithm, a child must have a saturation of at least 95% in both the right hand and either foot instead of only either one. In Tennessee, health officials aimed to simplify the algorithm in an attempt to reduce time, costs, and errors. Considering the fact that in only very rare instances should the right arm saturation be less than the foot saturation from a physiologic standpoint, the Tennessee algorithm first tests the foot only. If this level is at least 97%, the right arm saturation is assumed to also be high, and no further testing is necessary. If the level in the foot is less than 90%, then the child fails screening. But if the level in the foot is 90% to 96%, the right arm is tested, and the algorithm in **Fig. 1** is then followed. Unfortunately, data are limited to determine which algorithm is best by means of sensitivity, specificity, cost, and ease of use. Because algorithms in different settings are typically driven by the local conditions, it is prudent for a nursery to follow the CCHD screening guidelines set forth by the local state department of health, if any.

INTERPRETATION OF SCREENING RESULTS
The Positive Screen

The child who has a positive screen (ie, has failed screening) warrants further evaluation to determine the cause of hypoxemia. Although the goal of screening is to identify children with CCHD, many of these children will have some other etiology of hypoxemia such as sepsis, pneumonia, or persistent pulmonary hypertension of the newborn. Thus, a thorough evaluation of hypoxemia may be warranted beyond the workup for CCHD.[12] The type of evaluation should be prioritized as clinically indicated and available at a particular institution. If a cause other than CCHD is identified and addressed (ie, there is resolution of the hypoxemia), a full cardiac evaluation may not be needed; this is an important consideration for nurseries in remote areas that would otherwise have to transfer a child in order to obtain a pediatric echocardiogram. However, in the absence of an identifiable cause of hypoxemia, echocardiogram prior to discharge to home is standard of care. Given the complexities of some cases of CCHD, it is preferred that this echocardiogram be performed and interpreted by individuals trained specifically in pediatric echocardiography. The role of telemedicine to guide the performance of such a study by an individual without specific pediatric echocardiographic expertise and/or the performance of a limited echocardiogram to rule out critical abnormalities remains to be identified.

The Negative Screen

It is important to realize that a child who has a negative screen (ie, has passed screening) may still have significant heart disease.[13] First, even in the setting of an appropriately followed protocol, the sensitivity of CCHD screening remains poor for select defects, notably coarctation of the aorta. Coarctation of the aorta is the CCHD most commonly missed in the first 24 hours of life, with approximately 870 of the 1420 annual cases in the United States not detected by prenatal diagnosis or standard clinical means in the first 24 hours of life.[7] Of these, only 315 cases are expected to be detected via pulse oximetry, yielding a sensitivity of only 36%. With currently available technology, CCHD screening with pulse oximetry is not designed to detect heart defects that do not typically have hypoxemia. In the case of coarctation of the aorta, the diagnosis can possibly be detected by pulse oximetry via the difference between pre- and postductal oxygen saturations. However, this differential cyanosis may be present only within a short window during neonatal transitioning when the ductus arteriosus is still patent and in the presence of coarctation that allows desaturated blood flow to the lower part of the body. Newer technologies that are based on the analysis of the pulse oximetry signal to detect changes in peripheral perfusion are still being investigated as possible tools to detect occult coarctation of the aorta.[14]

Second, there are many types of heart disease that may require surgery, but do not typically have hypoxemia during early neonatal life. Atrioventricular canal defect, l-transposition of the great arteries, atrial septal defect, and ventricular septal defect are but a few examples. Given the low sensitivity of pulse oximetry for certain types of CCHD and the lack of hypoxemia in other significant CHD, clinicians should not consider significant heart disease to be ruled out by a negative screen with pulse oximetry. Rather, clinicians should suspect CHD in any child who has evidence of shortness of breath, poor feeding, poor femoral pulses, pathologic murmur, or other signs or symptoms of CHD. For details on clinical approach to evaluate infants with suspected CHD, see: Jaeggi E, Annika Öhman A. Fetal and Neonatal Arrhythmias, in this issue.

SPECIAL SETTINGS
Neonatal Intensive Care Unit

As stated previously, CCHD screening was intended for asymptomatic newborns in the well-baby nursery. Yet, many states have legislation that mandates screening of all newborns. This poses a challenge for some children, particularly those in a NICU. The AAP has provided some guidance on this issue.[15] Any infant who has had a complete postnatal echocardiogram does not need to subsequently have CCHD screening performed. Any infant who is on oxygen supplementation should first be weaned from oxygen prior to CCHD screening, even if this means a delay in the screening (provided that the infant is being monitored in the NICU while on oxygen). In the event that an infant cannot be weaned from oxygen, an echocardiogram is warranted prior to discharge from the hospital. In all other infants, screening should be performed per the regular guidelines, keeping in mind that there may be a higher false positive rate in the NICU as compared to the well-baby nursery.[16]

High Altitude

At higher elevations, infants will have lower oxygen saturations at baseline,[17] resulting in a greater false-positive rate if the algorithm in **Fig. 1** is used. Modified algorithms have been tried in the setting of high altitude.[17] Hospitals in such areas should refer to their state health department's guidance for screening in these settings.

Home Births

In many home births, waiting until 24 hours of age is not always feasible, resulting in a greater false-positive rate if screening is performed early. Modified algorithms have been tried in the setting of home births,[18] but further research is needed in these areas. Any infant with a low oxygen level requires a thorough evaluation and possible transfer to appropriate care.

LIMITATIONS OF SCREENING

Beyond the limitations of the test itself mentioned previously, the biggest limitation of CCHD screening in practice has been human error in the failure to follow the specified protocol, whatever protocol that may be. In a study in Minnesota, approximately 29% of all infants who had to be retested were cases of misinterpretation of the algorithm.[19] Use of electronic applications or data collection can help alleviate some of these problems.[20] Furthermore, appropriate education of all staff and providers is a key component of any successful screening program; such training information is available from the AAP,[15] CDC,[21] and Children's National Medical Center.[22]

SUMMARY

CCHD can lead to significant morbidity and mortality if not detected in a timely fashion. Although traditional CCHD screening methods of prenatal ultrasound and postnatal physical examination can identify the majority of cases of CCHD, many children are still undiagnosed at 24 hours of age. Screening for CCHD using pulse oximetry can help narrow this diagnostic gap. Children who fail CCHD screening with pulse oximetry should have a thorough evaluation to determine the presence of not only CCHD, but also other potential causes of hypoxemia. But, CCHD screening with pulse oximetry is not a perfect test; many children with CCHD, particularly those with coarctation of the aorta, will still be missed.

Best practices

What is the current practice?

- CCHD

Best Practice/Guideline/Care Path Objective(s)

- To detect cases of CCHD prior to the onset of symptoms

Is there a clinical algorithm?

- The most common algorithm is the one endorsed by the AAP, AHA, and ACC, but there are other modified versions of this algorithm in use.

Summary statement

- In the infant who fails CCHD screening, clinicians should evaluate for causes of hypoxemia, including CCHD; in the infant who passes CCHD screening, clinicians should realize that CCHD has not been ruled out.

REFERENCES

1. Hoke TR, Donohue PK, Bawa PK, et al. Oxygen saturation as a screening test for critical congenital heart disease: a preliminary study. Pediatr Cardiol 2002;23(4): 403–9.
2. Kemper AR, Mahle WT, Martin GR, et al. Strategies for implementing screening for critical congenital heart disease. Pediatrics 2011;128(5):e1259–67.
3. Pinto NM, Keenan HT, Minich LL, et al. Barriers to prenatal detection of congenital heart disease: a population-based study. Ultrasound Obstet Gynecol 2012;40(4): 418–25.
4. Hokanson J. Pulse oximetry screening for unrecognized congenital heart disease in neonates. Neonatal Today 2010;5(12):1–6.
5. Oster ME, Lee KA, Honein MA, et al. Temporal trends in survival among infants with critical congenital heart defects. Pediatrics 2013;131(5):e1502–8.
6. Dawson AL, Cassell CH, Riehle-Colarusso T, et al. Factors associated with late detection of critical congenital heart disease in newborns. Pediatrics 2013; 132(3):e604–11.
7. Ailes EC, Gilboa SM, Honein MA, et al. Estimated number of infants detected and missed by critical congenital heart defect screening. Pediatrics 2015;135(6): 1000–8.
8. de-Wahl Granelli A, Wennergren M, Sandberg K, et al. Impact of pulse oximetry screening on the detection of duct dependent congenital heart disease: a Swedish prospective screening study in 39,821 newborns. BMJ 2009;338:a3037.
9. Pulse oximeters—premarket notification submissions: guidance for industry and food and drug administration staff. 2015. Available at: http://www.fda.gov/RegulatoryInformation/Guidances/ucm341718.htm. Accessed August 10, 2015.
10. Peterson C, Grosse SD, Oster ME, et al. Cost-effectiveness of routine screening for critical congenital heart disease in U.S. newborns. Pediatrics 2013;132(3):e595–603.
11. Reeder MR, Kim J, Nance A, et al. Evaluating cost and resource use associated with pulse oximetry screening for critical congenital heart disease: empiric estimates and sources of variation. Birth Defects Res A Clin Mol Teratol 2015; 103(11):962–71.
12. Singh A, Rasiah SV, Ewer AK. The impact of routine predischarge pulse oximetry screening in a regional neonatal unit. Arch Dis Child Fetal Neonatal Ed 2014; 99(4):F297–302.
13. Oster ME, Colarusso T, Glidewell J. Screening for critical congenital heart disease: a matter of sensitivity. Pediatr Cardiol 2013;34(1):203–4.
14. Granelli A, Ostman-Smith I. Noninvasive peripheral perfusion index as a possible tool for screening for critical left heart obstruction. Acta Paediatr 2007;96(10): 1455–9.
15. Newborn screening for CCHD: answers and resources for primary care pediatricians. Available at: https://www.aap.org/en-us/advocacy-and-policy/aap-health-initiatives/PEHDIC/Pages/Newborn-Screening-for-CCHD.aspx. Accessed August 9, 2015.
16. Manja V, Mathew B, Carrion V, et al. Critical congenital heart disease screening by pulse oximetry in a neonatal intensive care unit. J Perinatol 2015;35(1):67–71.
17. Ravert P, Detwiler TL, Dickinson JK. Mean oxygen saturation in well neonates at altitudes between 4498 and 8150 feet. Adv Neonatal Care 2011;11(6):412–7.
18. Narayen IC, Blom NA, Verhart MS, et al. Adapted protocol for pulse oximetry screening for congenital heart defects in a country with homebirths. Eur J Pediatr 2015;174(1):129–32.

19. Kochilas LK, Lohr JL, Bruhn E, et al. Implementation of critical congenital heart disease screening in Minnesota. Pediatrics 2013;132(3):e587–94.
20. Oster ME, Kuo K, Mahle WT. Quality improvement in screening for critical congenital heart disease. J Am Coll Cardiol 2013;61(10):E475.
21. Information for healthcare providers. Available at: http://www.cdc.gov/ncbddd/heartdefects/hcp.html. Accessed August 10, 2015.
22. Congenital heart disease screening program toolkit. Available at: http://www.babysfirsttest.org/sites/default/files/CCHD%20Toolkit.pdf. Accessed August 10, 2015.

Recognition of Undiagnosed Neonatal Heart Disease

David Teitel, MD

KEYWORDS

- Aortic transposition • Left-to-right shunt • Cyanosis • Left heart obstructive lesions
- Foramen ovale • Pulmonary hypertension of the newborn • Hypoperfusion
- Right-to-left shunt

KEY POINTS

- Symptomatic congenital heart disease usually presents in early infancy and may present as 1 of 3 clinical presentations: cyanosis, hypoperfusion, or respiratory distress/failure to thrive (without hypoperfusion).
- Cyanotic heart disease can be subdivided into lesions with decreased pulmonary blood flow and those with the aorta receiving blood from the venous ventricle (aortic transposition in which the circulations are mostly separated).
- Hypoperfusion is caused either by obstruction to the inflow or outflow of the left ventricle or by the inability of the left ventricle to deliver an adequate systemic blood flow in the absence of obstruction.
- Respiratory distress/failure to thrive caused by congenital cardiac defects has the common pathophysiological problem of a left-to-right shunt causing excessive pulmonary blood flow, with or without an associated right-to-left shunt.
- The initial evaluation of the newborn with symptomatic heart disease should be directed at defining the presenting pathophysiologic process, and the initial management should be similarly focused.

INTRODUCTION

Heart defects are the most common congenital malformation. In the general population, the incidence is about 7 to 10 per 1000 live births (excluding bicuspid aortic valve and hemodynamically insignificant lesions such as very small secundum atrial and muscular ventricular septal defects [VSDs]), and the incidence is much higher in

Disclosure: None.
Pediatric Heart Center, UCSF Benioff Children's Hospital San Francisco, UCSF, 550 16th Street, Mission Hall, 5th Floor, 5733, San Francisco, CA 94143-0544, USA
E-mail address: david.teitel@ucsf.edu

Clin Perinatol 43 (2016) 81–98
http://dx.doi.org/10.1016/j.clp.2015.11.006   perinatology.theclinics.com

stillborn infants and abortuses.[1,2] About 60% of newborns with heart defects require an intervention, either surgery or catheter-based, at some time in their lives. About half of those require intervention in the first year of life, and two-thirds of this latter group (20% of all heart defects) are critical, defined as a defect that requires an intervention within the first month of life or serious morbidity or mortality is likely. At the current birth rate in the United States, this means that there are approximately 40,000 infants born each year with congenital heart disease and that approximately 8000 require diagnosis and intervention in the newborn period to avoid severe injury or death. Thus, early recognition of symptomatic heart disease is essential to prevent morbidity in the many infants born with critical heart disease each year.[3–5]

The following sections elucidate the physiology, presentation, and general approach to the treatment of symptomatic heart disease in the newborn.

CONGENITAL HEART DEFECTS

The number of distinct congenital heart defects is sufficiently large that pediatric cardiologists with more than 30 years' experience still see congenital heart defects that they have never seen before. Thus, it is necessary to take a logical approach to understanding congenital heart disease rather than an approach in which the various lesions are memorized. Moreover, treatment of cardiac defects in the newborn requires a physiology-based approach, to ameliorate the cardiovascular derangements that are caused by the transition from the fetal to newborn circulation. It is noteworthy that, because of the presence of 3 interconnected circulations in the fetus (the systemic, pulmonary, and placental circulation, connected by the ductus venosus, the ductus arteriosus, and the foramen ovale), even the most complex cardiac defect rarely causes symptoms in the fetus. Birth is associated with abolition of the placental circulation and functional closure of the ductus arteriosus and foramen ovale, leading to 2 circulations in series, both requiring normal vascular connections and biventricular function for hemodynamic stability and adequate oxygen uptake and delivery. Thus, it is not surprising that symptomatic heart disease frequently occurs in the newborn period.

The most effective and logical approach is to consider the physiologic consequences of congenital heart defects that cause symptoms in the newborn. Using this approach, heart defects can be separated into 3 symptomatic modes of presentation.[6] They are

1. Cyanosis (decreased arterial oxygen saturation causing central cyanosis, which impairs systemic oxygen delivery)
2. Hypoperfusion (decreased systemic perfusion of either the upper or the lower body circulation or both)
3. Respiratory distress/failure to thrive (visible distress or subclinical, leading to poor growth; this is in the presence of normal perfusion)

Within each of the 3 modes of presentation, there are 2 pathophysiologic processes that may cause that presentation. These modes of presentation are

1. Cyanosis
   a. Decreased pulmonary blood flow
   b. Separated systemic and pulmonary circulations (variants of d-transposition of the great arteries in which the aorta is malposed over the systemic venous [SV] ventricle)
2. Hypoperfusion
   a. Left-sided obstruction

   b. Inadequate systemic blood flow without obstruction (myopathic heart or a he-
      modynamic steal)
3. Respiratory distress/failure to thrive (with normal perfusion)
   a. Increased pulmonary blood flow with only a left-to-right shunt
   b. Increased pulmonary blood flow with a dominant left-to-right shunt and an
      associated right-to-left shunt

Cyanosis

Cyanosis is the most important sign to elicit when evaluating the newborn for the presence of symptomatic heart disease. The newborn who presents with cyanosis without
significant respiratory distress almost always has structural congenital heart disease.
Moreover, because it is the most common manifestation of symptomatic congenital
heart disease, can be diagnosed with careful visual inspection alone, and may be
associated with critically decreased oxygen delivery leading to severe morbidity or
death within hours or days of life, it is essential to be able to quickly and accurately
identify its presence.[3,4]

Differential diagnosis of neonatal cyanosis

Cyanosis in the newborn may be caused by lung disease, cyanotic congenital heart
defects, or pulmonary hypertension of the newborn (PPHN). The pathophysiologic
mechanisms in each group are different. Lung disease causes cyanosis because there
is impaired oxygen transfer at the alveolar-capillary level. Heart disease causes
cyanosis because either there is inadequate pulmonary blood flow, which leads to a
right-to-left shunt of deoxygenated blood to the body, or the fully oxygenated blood
is not available to the systemic circulation (these mechanisms are discussed in greater
detail later), whereas PPHN may be caused by a combination of these processes. It is
often initiated by lung diseases such as meconium aspiration leading to impaired oxygen transfer, and the alveolar hypoxia causes failure of pulmonary resistance to fall,
which in turn causes right-to-left shunting of deoxygenated venous blood via the foramen ovale or ductus arteriosus to the systemic arterial (SA) circulation (**Fig. 1**).

   Determining the underlying cause of cyanosis can be a major diagnostic challenge.
Adding to the challenge is the fact that around 50% of infants with critical heart disease do not have murmurs (whereas around 20%–30% of infants with normal hearts
do have heart murmurs), and the electrocardiogram is normal in most newborns with
cyanotic heart disease.

   There are 3 key points to remember when considering the cause of cyanosis in the
newborn:

First: the presence of respiratory distress Infants with lung disease have abnormal
lung mechanics so that they are usually much more distressed than most infants
with cyanotic heart disease. Infants with PPHN may or may not have severe respiratory distress depending on its cause.

Second: the difference in cyanosis between the upper and lower body Recall that, in
the normal fetus, blood flow to the upper body is supplied entirely by the left ventricle,
and blood flow to the lower body is mostly supplied by the right ventricle, via the ductus arteriosus. Immediately at birth, the ductus is still patent, but blood flow across the
ductus in the normal newborn reverses because pulmonary vascular resistance decreases dramatically. Thus, blood flow to both the upper and the lower body is supplied immediately and entirely by the left ventricle and is fully oxygenated. In infants
with only lung disease (that is, without associated pulmonary hypertension), the

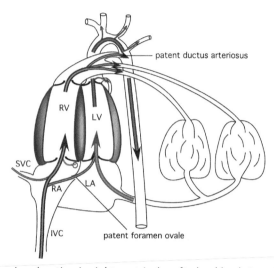

Fig. 1. PPHN. Excessive elevation in right ventricular afterload leads to a right-to-left shunt at the foramen ovale, and pulmonary vascular resistance above systemic levels leads to a right-to-left shunt across the ductus arteriosus. Thus, upper body saturation is abnormally low and lower body saturation is further decreased. IVC, inferior vena cava; LA, left atrium; LV, left ventricle; RA, right atrium; RV, right ventricle; SVC, superior vena cava.

oxygen saturation is always decreased equally in the upper and lower body (**Table 1**). In infants with PPHN, upper body pulse oximetry may be decreased due to a right-to-left shunt across the foramen ovale and/or associated lung disease, but oxygen saturation in the lower body may be even lower, because of a persistent right-to-left shunt across the ductus arteriosus (see **Fig. 1**). In cyanotic heart disease caused by decreased pulmonary blood flow (see later discussion), the pressure in the pulmonary artery must be lower than that in the aorta, so that the ductus can only shunt left to right; thus, like infants with lung disease, oxygen saturation is always decreased equally in the upper and lower body. In cyanotic infants with separated circulations

Table 1		
Oxygen saturations and responses to 100% oxygen in patients with cyanosis due to various pathophysiologic processes		
Pathophysiology	**Upper Body Saturation/Po$_2$**	**Lower Body Saturation/Po$_2$**
Lung disease (*without* pulmonary hypertension)	Decreased saturation, Po$_2$ increases greatly in 100% O$_2$	*Always same* saturation and Po$_2$ response as upper body
Pulmonary hypertension (with or without lung disease)	Normal or decreased saturation, Po$_2$ increases greatly in 100% O$_2$	Same saturation and Po$_2$ as upper body *or lower*
Cyanotic heart disease due to decreased pulmonary blood flow	Decreased saturation with small increase in Po$_2$ in 100% O$_2$	*Always same* saturation and Po$_2$ response as upper body
Cyanotic heart disease due to aortic transposition	Decreased saturation with small increase in Po$_2$ in 100% O$_2$	Same saturation and Po$_2$ as upper body *or higher*

(transposition variants, see later discussion), the ductus may shunt right to left, but if so, the lower body saturation would be higher, because it is the left ventricle, not the right, that is connected to the pulmonary artery. If a patient is cyanotic and has a higher lower body saturation, the great arteries are transposed.

Third: the response to oxygen Infants with lung disease have decreased alveolar oxygen concentration and often an increased alveolar-arteriolar gradient, whereas those with heart disease do not. Thus, increasing the inspired oxygen concentration will have a far greater effect on infants with lung abnormality alone than in those with cyanotic heart disease. The response in PPHN is variable and often intermediate, depending on the extent of the right-to-left foraminal shunt; this can be demonstrated by administering high concentrations of inspired oxygen to the infant (sometimes called the hyperoxia test) and checking upper body arterial blood oxygen levels (see **Table 1**). Rarely will an infant with cyanotic heart disease have an increase in arterial oxygen concentration more than 150 mm Hg when exposed to 100% oxygen. If oxygen saturation by pulse oximetry does not increase more than 95%, then arterial blood gas measurements are not necessary.

Congenital heart defects causing cyanosis
Either infants with cyanotic heart disease have inadequate blood flow through the pulmonary vascular bed that is decreased (decreased pulmonary blood flow) or the amount is normal, or even increased, but SV blood, which is poorly oxygenated, is preferentially directed across the aortic valve to the body. The latter anatomy creates relatively separated systemic and pulmonary circulations. There are many variants of this, as noted in later discussion, but they all have, in common, d-transposition of the aorta over the SV ventricle. It is of great value to consider these 2 pathophysiologic processes causing cyanosis separately, because lesions within each category tend to have similar presentations and therapeutic approaches.

Decreased pulmonary blood flow The neurohormonal mechanisms that control the cardiovascular system are directed toward maintaining a normal or increased amount of systemic blood flow in order to maintain adequate oxygen delivery. Because systemic blood flow is normal or increased, SV return must be as well. In congenital heart defects with decreased pulmonary blood flow, some of that SV return does not enter the pulmonary circulation but rather is shunted right to left, back into the systemic circulation. The amount of poorly oxygenated (desaturated) blood that is shunted right to left determines how cyanotic the patient is. If half of the desaturated blood (presume that it is 50% saturated because the SA saturation is decreased) is shunted to the aorta and mixes with the other half, which entered the lung and thus is fully saturated, then the half that is 50% saturated mixes with the half that is 100% saturated, and the resultant SA saturation is 75%. Any saturation level less than about 85% in a newborn with a normal hemoglobin concentration leads the infant to have central cyanosis, visible by looking at the infant's tongue, gums, or buccal mucosa.

Most congenital heart defects with decreased pulmonary blood flow have obstruction either to the inflow of blood to the right ventricle or to the outflow of blood from it. A much smaller number of lesions are associated not with obstruction but with insufficiency of either the tricuspid or pulmonary valve. The most common of these is Ebstein anomaly,[7] in which inferior displacement of the septal leaflet of the tricuspid valve causes severe tricuspid insufficiency. All of these lesions can be considered sequentially, along lines of blood flow (**Table 2**). In each, pulmonary arterial pressure must be lower than systemic, so that any shunt across the ductus arteriosus must be left to right.

Table 2
Common defects causing cyanosis due to decreased pulmonary blood flow

Anatomic Level	Structural Defect
Tricuspid valve	*Unguarded tricuspid valve* Tricuspid valve hypoplasia (usually with hypoplastic right ventricle and pulmonary atresia) Tricuspid valve atresia *Ebstein anomaly*
Right ventricle	Hypoplastic right ventricle (usually with pulmonary atresia and intact ventricular septum) Tetralogy of Fallot (subpulmonic stenosis with VSD)
Pulmonary valve	Pulmonary stenosis with intact ventricular septum Pulmonary atresia with intact ventricular septum Pulmonary stenosis or atresia with VSD ($\pm$ single ventricle, malposed aorta, or aortopulmonary collateral vessels) *Absent pulmonary valve syndrome*
Pulmonary artery	Supravalvar pulmonary artery stenosis Branch pulmonary artery stenosis

Those lesions presented in italics are primarily associated with valve insufficiency rather than obstruction to blood flow.

The association of anterior malalignment of the outlet ventricular septum, a VSD, and outlet (infundibular) obstruction leading to a right-to-left shunt across the VSD is called tetralogy of Fallot and is one of the most common forms of cyanotic congenital heart disease (**Fig. 2**). If the obstruction to the right ventricular outflow tract is severe in utero, the pulmonary arteries are also hypoplastic,[8] leading to an early presentation of cyanosis as the ductus begins to close.

Aortic transposition over the venous ventricle (separated systemic and pulmonary circulations) The second group of lesions associated with cyanosis in the newborn and infant can be considered together as defects in which the aorta is anteriorly

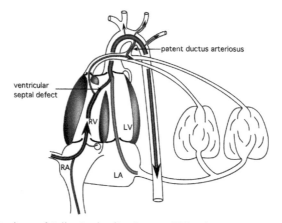

Fig. 2. Severe tetralogy of Fallot in the first hours of life. There is severe obstruction of the right ventricular outflow tract so that only a small amount of SV blood crosses the pulmonary valve to the pulmonary circulation. The majority crosses the VSD to the left ventricle and aorta and is not oxygenated. The ductus arteriosus is still open, allowing an adequate amount of blood flow to the lungs via a left-to-right ductal shunt. As it closes, pulmonary blood flow decreases, and cyanosis becomes apparent.

and rightward displaced, committed to the SV ventricle (usually, but not always, this is the right ventricle). SV rather than pulmonary venous (PV) blood preferentially flows across the aortic valve to the body via the ascending aorta. Pulmonary blood flow may be normal, increased, or decreased in this group of lesions, depending on the associated lesions; in most cases, it is either normal or increased. Each lesion is considered a physiologic variant of transposition of the great arteries, although it is best to consider only the aortic malposition as essential because the pulmonary artery may remain on the right side of the ventricular septum (double outlet of the right ventricle of the transposition type, or Taussig-Bing anomaly[9]; **Box 1**).

The classic and most common lesion in this group is d-transposition of the great arteries with intact ventricular septum, also called simple d-transposition of the great arteries (**Fig. 3**).

D-transposition of the aorta can be associated with almost any other defect of the heart or great vessels. The patient may have an associated atrial septal defect, but more commonly, the patient has an associated ventricular septal defect (VSD). The various associated lesions are presented in **Box 1**.

Distinguishing "decreased pulmonary blood flow" lesions from "separated circulations (aortic transposition)" There are two ways to help distinguish decreased pulmonary blood flow from cyanosis caused by d-transposition of the aorta: differential pulse oximetry and the timing of cyanosis.

Differential pulse oximetry Briefly, every patient with decreased pulmonary blood flow has the same pulse oximetry level in the upper and lower body, whereas patients with aortic transposition can have higher pulse oximetry readings in the lower body if the ductus arteriosus is still patent.

Timing of cyanosis The earlier and more severe the cyanosis, the more likely the newborn has d-transposition of the aorta rather than decreased pulmonary blood flow because, in d-transposition of the aorta, the aorta remains committed to the SV ventricle, causing significant, often intense, cyanosis, immediately after birth. This is in contrast to the infant with decreased pulmonary blood flow. The ductus arteriosus is usually widely patent at birth. The ductus arteriosus maintains normal or increased pulmonary blood flow initially. Mixing of the relatively high amount of PV return with the normal amount of SV return leads to either mild or no visible cyanosis. As the ductus arteriosus begins to close in the first few hours of life, pulmonary blood flow gradually decreases and cyanosis becomes apparent. Because the ductus may close

---

Box 1
Defects associated with aortic transposition, along lines of blood flow

Transposition complexes, that is, aorta malposed over venous ventricle ±:

Atrial septal defect

Ventricular septal defect

Subaortic stenosis (only in presence of double-outlet right ventricle: Taussig-Bing anomaly)

Subpulmonary and/or pulmonary valve stenosis (usually with VSD)

Pulmonary artery transposed or not (double outlet right ventricle – Taussig-Bing anomaly)

Patent ductus arteriosus

Aortic arch interruption/coarctation (interruption occurs only with Taussig-Bing anomaly)

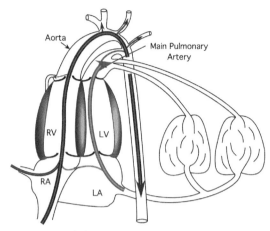

Fig. 3. Simple d-transposition of the great arteries. In this common lesion, the pulmonary artery is also malposed, over the left ventricle. The ductus remains open in the immediate postnatal period, but the right ventricle ejects very desaturated blood out the aortic valve. In the absence of a large atrial communication, the infant is severely cyanotic immediately at birth.

more slowly in some infants and because visible cyanosis requires pulse oximetry levels much lower than normal, usually around 85%, routine pulse oximetry screening[10] has allowed for the early diagnosis of many of these patients who had previously been discharged as being normal infants.

Initial management for cyanotic heart disease Infants with cyanosis due to suspected congenital heart disease can almost always be stabilized by giving prostaglandin E1 (PGE$_1$) to maintain ductal patency as long as there is an adequate atrial communication. The ductus arteriosus maintains a significant shunt of blood from the aorta to the pulmonary artery. Because various mechanisms maintain normal systemic blood flow, pulmonary blood flow is elevated. In the case of decreased pulmonary blood flow, this maintains an adequate SA oxygen saturation, as noted above. It is very rare that these infants have an inadequate atrial communication because the flow across the foramen ovale is increased in utero, usually causing a secundum atrial septal defect, which then maintains a right-to-left atrial shunt after birth, decompressing the right atrium. In the case of aortic transposition, the left-to-right ductal increases left atrial blood volume and pressure, causing a left-to-right atrial shunt, which in turn affords more highly oxygenated blood to the aorta. Some infants with d-transposition of the great arteries have a small atrial communication, and the increased left atrial pressure closes the flap of the foramen ovale (see **Fig. 3**), causing respiratory distress in addition to cyanosis, and these infants can rapidly decompensate. In such infants, a balloon atrial septostomy must be performed as quickly as possible to allow oxygenated blood to cross the atrial septum to enter the systemic circulation.

Hypoperfusion

Systemic hypoperfusion is the second most common presentation of the newborn with symptomatic heart disease and represents the most common cause of mortality. Unlike cyanosis, hypoperfusion is often caused by noncardiac diseases, particularly sepsis, so that heart disease is not always considered in a timely manner. This finding is particularly true when no murmur is present because many clinicians consider that its absence excludes congenital heart disease. Unfortunately, some of the most common and lethal forms of cardiac disease that present in the newborn and infant are not associated with murmurs.

Pathophysiologic processes

As with cyanosis, hypoperfusion on a cardiac basis can be divided into 2 pathophysiologic mechanisms, which may overlap in an individual patient. Hypoperfusion may be caused by left-sided obstruction (either obstruction to filling of the left of the heart, or obstruction to outflow from it) or it may result from left ventricular dysfunction or a hemodynamic steal; that is, the left ventricle is incapable of delivering adequate systemic blood flow without obstruction. Decreased left ventricular function is a common cause of hypoperfusion from noncardiac causes, but only left ventricular dysfunction caused by congenital heart disease is discussed in this section.

Congenital heart defects causing hypoperfusion

Left-sided obstruction The left side of the heart may be obstructed at its inflow or outflow (**Table 3**). Many inflow lesions are associated with secondary outflow lesions because the reduced blood flow into the left heart structures in the fetus causes left-sided hypoplasia.

A very common form of inflow disease is hypoplastic left heart syndrome. When the mitral valve is critically obstructed, there is severe hypoplasia of the left ventricle, often with secondary aortic valve atresia. Hypoplastic left heart syndrome usually presents within the first hours or days of life, as the ductus arteriosus begins to close. Systemic blood flow is entirely dependent on ductal size; therefore, as it begins to constrict, blood flow to the body decreases and signs of hypoperfusion manifest. The infant shows the typical signs of cardiovascular collapse with poor pulses, hypotension, tachycardia, tachypnea, pallor with poor capillary refill, and cool extremities. Metabolic acidosis with elevated lactate levels are present, and the downward spiral, as the right ventricle starts to fail as well, is rapid. Death usually occurs within the first few days of life if untreated.

Coarctation of the aorta is also a very common cause of left-sided obstruction, and it is extremely important to consider throughout the neonatal period. It is an easily correctable lesion, but diagnosis is often delayed, leading to cardiovascular collapse, which may in turn cause severe neurologic injury or death.

Table 3
Common defects causing hypoperfusion due to left heart obstruction

Anatomic Level	Structural Defect
Pulmonary veins	Total anomalous PV connection with obstruction
Left atrium	Cor triatriatum Supravalvar mitral web/ring
Mitral valve	Atresia Stenosis ($\pm$ parachute mitral valve)
Left ventricle	Hypoplastic left heart syndrome Subaortic stenosis
Aortic valve	Atresia (part of hypoplastic left heart syndrome) Stenosis
Aorta	Supravalvar aortic stenosis Aortic arch hypoplasia Aortic arch interruption Coarctation of the aorta

One reason for the delay in diagnosis is that, unlike hypoplastic left heart syndrome, infants with coarctation usually go home from the hospital without symptoms or signs of heart disease, not only because the ductus arteriosus assists in blood supply to the lower body but also because the way that it closes delays the development of obstruction. Coarctation occurs in the region of the aorta across from the ductus arteriosus, at the distal end of the aortic isthmus (**Fig. 4**). Ductal closure begins in the middle of the ductus and progresses toward the ends, which may leave the aortic side, or ductal ampulla, relatively large for some time. As it is opposed the area of the coarctation, the obstruction is minimized. Thus, many infants even with a severe coarctation of the aorta present with symptoms of hypoperfusion at about 7 to 14 days of age (this is not true of infants who have ductal tissue surrounding the area of coarctation; as the ductus begins to constrict the area constricts as well, leading to a very early presentation of hypoperfusion). However, decreased pulses usually can be appreciated well before this time, which makes it essential for the clinician to carefully evaluate upper and lower body pulses to exclude coarctation of the aorta at birth and through the first month of life, and to consider obstructive heart disease when an infant presents with hypoperfusion during that time period. Routine pulse oximetry screening improves the likelihood of early diagnosis of infants with coarctation of the aorta but only if the ductus is adequately patent at the time of screening, which is often not the case. If performed on the lower extremity while the ductus is reasonably large, a right-to-left ductal shunt will be reflected by decreased saturations. Unfortunately, the ductus arteriosus usually constricts very quickly so that most newborns with coarctation of the aorta will not have this finding at routine screening.

Hypoperfusion without obstruction Ventricular dysfunction without obstruction presents similarly to the obstructed heart and may be difficult to differentiate on clinical examination (**Table 4**). It is more commonly caused by nonstructural processes that impair cardiac function, such as arrhythmias, myocardial infections, metabolic or hematologic derangements, or systemic infections. Rarely, but importantly, hypoperfusion without obstruction may be the presentation of structural congenital

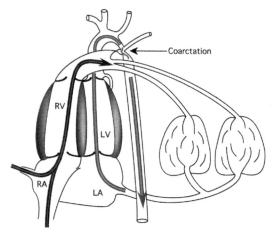

Fig. 4. Although there is a discrete and prominent posterior shelf that will eventually lead to severe aortic coarctation, the presence of a ductal ampulla in the first few days or weeks of life during closure of the midportion of the ductus arteriosus mitigates the severity of the obstruction.

Table 4
Categories of disease processes causing hypoperfusion due to ventricular dysfunction without obstruction, and examples

Category	Causes
Primary	Cardiomyopathies (dilated, hypertrophic, restrictive)
Vascular	Arteriovenous malformations such as vein of Galen malformation
Arrhythmic	Bradycardia (eg, congenital complete heart block) or tachycardia (eg, supraventricular tachycardia)
Ischemic	Embolic, structural coronary abnormalities
Infectious	Myocarditis, sepsis
Hematologic	Anemia, polycythemia
Metabolic	Decreased oxygen, calcium, magnesium, glucose, carnitine, glucocorticoids, thyroxin
Infiltrative	Malignancies, storage diseases

The primary cardiovascular causes are separated from the others by a thick line.

cardiovascular disease. Hypoperfusion without obstruction occurs when the cardiac muscle does not form correctly, such as in a congenital cardiomyopathies, when there is impaired myocardial blood flow, such as in atresia an ostium of a coronary artery, or when blood from the left ventricle flows directly, in an obligatory manner, away from the systemic vascular bed (a hemodynamic steal). The most common and dramatic of the lesions is the vein of Galen aneurysm,[11] or other cerebral arteriovenous malformations. The diagnosis of a cerebral arteriovenous malformation is obvious if the clinician auscultates the head for bruits, which, if it is a regular part of the examination, will not be forgotten.

Initial management for hypoperfusion due to congenital cardiac disease

The therapeutic approach to the infant with hypoperfusion and possible obstruction must be rapid and directed at the central problems: respiratory distress and decreased systemic blood flow. Respiratory distress is addressed by sedating and mechanically ventilating the infant. Sedation decreases oxygen demand by decreasing heart rate and catecholamine stimulation, while mechanical ventilation improves oxygenation and ventilation, and eliminates the metabolic demand of breathing (up to 50% of oxygen consumption in the distressed infant). Maintenance of a neutral thermal environment also aids in the decrease in oxygen consumption.

Improvement in systemic blood flow is the next consideration. Before surgical or transcatheter relief of the obstruction of the lesion itself, infusion of PGE_1 is essential: it will relieve the obstruction at the ductus arteriosus and should be begun in all patients who have a presumptive diagnosis of left heart obstruction. The potential benefits of PGE_1 infusion in every patient with presumptive obstruction far outweigh the potential risks, as long as the clinician is aware of and rapidly responds to the respiratory depression and vasodilatory effects of the drug. Volume infusion and inotropic support may be beneficial, but should be used with caution. For example, if obstruction is present, extra volume can be detrimental, further overloading the right atrium. This obstruction can be rapidly determined clinically by evaluating the size of the liver. If left ventricular dysfunction is suspected, the inotropic agent should also have vasodilatory actions (eg, milrinone) so that blood is not further directed toward the malformation or across the regurgitant valve. Maximizing ventricular function and minimizing organ injury should include reversal of any metabolic derangement that is present (such as metabolic acidosis or hypocalcemia). Rapid treatment of other possible diagnoses (such as sepsis or hypoadrenalism) should also be undertaken, but that is beyond the scope of this review.

Respiratory Distress/Failure to Thrive

Newborns and infants with excessive pulmonary blood flow present with respiratory distress and/or failure to thrive without overt cyanosis. This presentation is the least common of symptomatic heart disease in the neonatal period but the most common in the subsequent months. Although the mechanism of the respiratory distress is not certain, it is associated with excessive pulmonary blood flow, and almost always only if pulmonary arterial pressures are increased (for example, young infants with an atrial septal defect and a large left-to-right shunt have normal pulmonary arterial pressures and are rarely symptomatic, only so if they have concomitant chronic lung disease). Respiratory distress usually manifests during the period of the physiologic anemia of infancy (about 6 weeks of age), when cardiac output, and thus pulmonary blood flow, is highest.

Often, the respiratory distress is subtle so that the primary sign of excessive pulmonary blood flow is failure to thrive. Because a large component of oxygen consumption in the infant is related to breathing, any increase in work of breathing may redirect oxygen consumption from anabolic processes. The work of breathing added to the work of feeding and absorption may cause a large increase in energy expenditure for the infant, manifesting as sweating with feeding and shortened feeding. Decrease in intake in combination with an increase in demand commonly leads to failure to thrive in these infants; this is called "high output heart failure," because the heart is failing to meet the metabolic demands of the body for growth despite a higher than normal cardiac output.

In the absence of a heart murmur, the diagnosis of this type of heart disease also is often missed until a serendipitous event, such as a wheezing episode, leads to a chest radiograph or pulse oximetry, which alerts the clinician that the problem may be cardiac.

Pathophysiologic processes (and other considerations)

There is a very diverse group of congenital cardiac malformations that, despite their differences, have a common pathophysiologic endpoint of increased pulmonary blood flow. The lesions can be divided into 2 hemodynamic groups, those lesions in which there is only a left-to-right shunt and those that have a large left-to-right shunt, but, in addition, have a right-to-left shunt, so that the SA saturation is somewhat decreased. The latter group has bidirectional shunting with increased pulmonary blood flow. Such lesions are often mislabeled as forms of cyanotic heart disease, but this label does not take into account the pathophysiology, which determines both the symptoms and the therapeutic approach. This point is illustrated in **Fig. 5**.

Fig. 5A represents a patient with a VSD, in which there is markedly elevated pulmonary blood flow, while the SA blood is fully saturated. This shunt is purely left to right. **Fig. 5B** represents a patient with truncus arteriosus, in which the aorta and pulmonary arteries arise together from a common truncal valve, overriding both ventricles. Because SV and PV blood mix in the outlet of the ventricles, some SV blood enters the aorta so that SA saturation is lower than PV saturation. However, pulmonary vascular resistance is much lower than systemic vascular resistance, so that far more of the mixed blood goes into the pulmonary artery. The combined blood is highly saturated; the patient suffers not from cyanosis but from excessive pulmonary blood flow. The following calculation illustrates this point:

- If pulmonary blood flow is 3 times systemic and if SV is 50% and PV is 100%, then SA will be 87.5%, assuming that the systemic and PV returns fully mixed

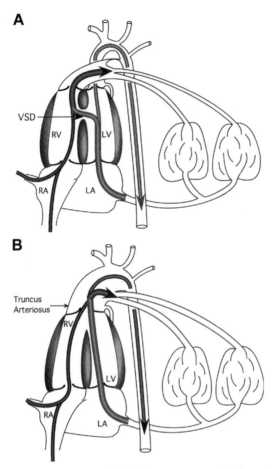

Fig. 5. (*A*) Patient with a VSD in which all of the SV return goes out the pulmonary valve. It is joined by a large amount of PV return because pulmonary vascular resistance is lower than systemic vascular resistance, so that there is a large amount of pulmonary blood flow. Note that no SV blood crosses the VSD to the aorta, so that SA blood is fully saturated. This is a pure left-to-right shunt. (*B*) Patient with truncus arteriosus, in which the aorta and pulmonary arteries arise together from a common truncal valve, overriding both ventricles. SV and PV blood mix in the outlet of the ventricles, so that some SV enters the aorta. Thus, SA saturation is lower than PV saturation. However, pulmonary vascular resistance is much lower than systemic vascular resistance, so that far more of the mixed blood goes into the pulmonary artery.

in the ventricles. In fact, because the aortic outflow is angled anteriorly, the same direction as the left ventricle, PV blood is preferentially directed toward the aorta rather than the pulmonary arteries, and SA is usually in the low 90s, well above the level whereby a clinician can perceive cyanosis.

Congenital heart defects causing respiratory distress/failure to thrive
Left-to-right shunt alone As with the other hemodynamic categories, left-to-right shunts are best considered along lines of blood flow (**Table 5**).

Table 5	
Common defects causing pure left-to-right shunts	
Anatomic Level	**Structural Defect**
Atrial septum	Secundum atrial septal defect
	Primum atrial septal defect
	Sinus venosus atrial septal defect
Atrioventricular septum	*Complete atrioventricular septal defect*
	Partial atrioventricular septal defect
Ventricular septum	*Inlet VSD*
	Perimembranous VSD
	Muscular VSD (may cause symptoms if a large midmuscular defect is present)
	Outlet VSD
Truncal/aortopulmonary septum	*Aortopulmonary window*
	Anomalous origin of the right pulmonary artery from the ascending aorta
Arterial communication	Patent ductus arteriosus (may cause symptoms if very large or premature infant)
	Arteriovenous malformation
Venous communication	Partial anomalous PV connection

Defects in italics may present in infancy.

VSDs are the most common causes of left-to-right shunts. There are many different types of VSDs,[12] but, in the absence of malalignment of the outlet septum or other causes of obstruction of one or the other outflow, the presentation depends on the size of the defect, the downstream resistance, and systemic blood flow (see **Fig. 5**A). Newborns with VSD and no other problems are rarely symptomatic in the first days or weeks of life, but usually present around 6 weeks to 3 months of age with respiratory distress and failure to thrive. As noted above, defects in the atrial septum rarely present with symptoms in early infancy likely because the normal pulmonary arterial pressures minimize the production of interstitial fluid. Conversely, large defects at the arterial level (ie, aortopulmonary window) may present at a very early age because diastolic as well as systolic pulmonary arterial pressures are elevated. Obligatory shunts such as a vein of Galen malformation may present soon after birth.[11]

Bidirectional shunting with excessive pulmonary blood flow Infants in whom there is a right-to-left shunt of SV blood out the aorta will have a decrease in SA saturation, but if at the same time pulmonary blood flow is increased significantly, the resultant SA oxygen saturation will only be mildly decreased. It will neither be clinically appreciable nor metabolically significant. Thus, these infants present similarly to those with a pure left-to-right shunt, not like those infants with cyanotic heart disease. The defects are considered along lines of blood flow in **Table 6**.

Truncus arteriosus is a relatively common bidirectional shunting lesion that is highly associated with chromosome 22q11 microdeletion, particularly when there is a right aortic arch or an interruption of the arch.[13] The newborn with truncus arteriosus occasionally does present with clinical cyanosis, but this would only be apparent in the first hours of life, until pulmonary vascular resistance drops to normal newborn levels. A large left-to-right shunt that develops rapidly and the elevated systolic and diastolic pulmonary arterial pressures lead to production of a large amount of interstitial fluid. Therefore, these infants present very early, within days or weeks of life, with respiratory distress and failure to thrive, not with symptomatic cyanosis.

Table 6	
Common defects causing bidirectional (but dominant left-to-right) shunts	
Anatomic Level	**Structural Defect**
Atrial septum	Common atrium (usually left atrial isomerism)
Atrioventricular septum	Complete atrioventricular septal defect with common ventricle (usually left atrial isomerism)
Ventricular septum	Single ventricle physiology: 1. Double inlet left ventricle (usually L-malposed aorta) and unobstructed outflow tracts 2. Atrioventricular valve atresia/stenosis (mitral or tricuspid) with large VSD and unobstructed outflow tracts
Truncal/aortopulmonary septum	Truncus arteriosus
Arterial communication	Truncus arteriosus
Venous communication	Total anomalous PV connection without obstruction

All defects often present in infancy.

Initial management of respiratory distress/failure to thrive lesions The medical management of all patients with symptomatic excessive pulmonary blood flow is similar. It should be directed at minimizing respiratory symptoms and maximizing growth. To minimize respiratory symptoms, therapy should attempt to either decrease absolute pulmonary blood flow or remove interstitial fluid. To maximize growth, therapy should attempt to maximize caloric intake.

Pulmonary blood flow depends on the relative resistances of the pulmonary and systemic beds as well as on the absolute amount of systemic blood flow. Therefore, to decrease pulmonary blood flow, strategies can be directed at minimizing systemic blood flow, decreasing systemic vascular resistance, or increasing pulmonary vascular resistance. To minimize absolute systemic blood flow while maintaining systemic oxygen delivery, the clinician should ensure that blood hemoglobin content is maximized, because systemic oxygen content is increased with increasing hemoglobin. Systemic vascular resistance can be decreased by a variety of agents, but most commonly, an ACE inhibitor is used. Unfortunately, in most infants, systemic resistance is already quite low, and in those in high-output heart failure, it may even be even lower. Thus, this therapeutic approach is often of little benefit. Increasing pulmonary vascular resistance can be accomplished by either increasing hematocrit greater than 55%, increasing P_{CO_2}, or decreasing F_{IO_2}, although these manipulations are rarely implemented unless the patient is very symptomatic (often requiring mechanical ventilation) and cannot undergo surgery because of an active infection or other comorbidity.

Decreasing interstitial fluid in the lungs is a mainstay in the treatment of these infants. Diuretics are commonly used. They can significantly decrease the work of breathing, allowing the infant to both feed better and direct those calories toward growth. Care needs to be given toward maintaining normal hydration status, particularly when the infant has decreased intake or vomiting and diarrhea, preventing electrolyte disturbances.

The second mainstay of treatment of these infants is ensuring adequate caloric intake. Because of the increased oxygen consumption associated with the respiratory distress and associated catecholamine stimulation of the high output state, this is not an easy goal. Increasing caloric density, as tolerated, is routinely used, and antireflux therapy is common. Occasionally, nasogastric or g-tube feeding is required, particularly when the infant is premature, or is in uncontrollable failure and needs to grow before repair or palliative surgery is considered.

Cardiovascular Examination

The cardiovascular examination should be performed systematically, evaluating for the presence of symptomatic heart disease at each step, considering whether the infant has cyanosis, hypoperfusion, or respiratory distress. It is useful to assess the newborn first generally and then specifically, the latter from the distal body to proximally, evaluating the heart itself, including the presence of murmurs, last. Murmurs are not specific for symptomatic heart disease, and focusing on them first without consideration of the specific lesions that may be present will often be misleading.

The newborn should be observed unclothed and in a neutral thermal environment. Vital signs including pulse oximetry of the lower extremity and, if this is decreased, of the upper extremity as well, should first be noted. Plotting the older infant on a growth chart should be done at the same time.

The first sign to assess on general observation is central cyanosis, and thus, is important to observe the gums, tongue, and buccal mucosa, all of which have little vasoconstrictor tone. Next, the respiratory status should be closely evaluated. Respiratory rate and effort should be determined, and the presence of subcostal and intercostal retractions as well as grunting should be considered. Auscultation over the nose for grunting can be helpful.

Following the general evaluation, the peripheral examination should be undertaken, by evaluation of the pulses in the lower and upper extremities, capillary refill time, skin color, and temperature. If the infant has good pedal pulses, it is not necessary to feel for femoral pulses. This method is the best for excluding significant coarctation of the aorta (at the time of the examination only; later obstruction can occur, as noted above).

By this time, the clinician will already know whether the newborn has symptomatic heart disease. The remainder of the examination is to determine its severity, the pathophysiologic process, and possibly the specific diagnosis if there are pathognomonic findings. All of this is of secondary importance to the diagnosis of symptomatic heart disease, which on its own should lead to the appropriate intervention.

Following examination of the periphery, the abdomen can be evaluated. Percussion of the right and left upper abdomen and of the lower ribs will determine the location and size of the liver as well as the presence of splenomegaly. Liver sidedness is very important in the cardiovascular examination because many patients with complex disease have situs abnormalities such as situs ambiguous (right atrial isomerism, or asplenia, or left atrial isomerism, or polysplenia) or situs inversus. The size of the liver is also a good index of SV pressure and is particularly important when the patient is hypoperfused. Hepatomegaly in a patient with hypoperfusion indicates elevated venous pressures and suggests that fluid resuscitation may be contraindicated.

Auscultation of the lungs is performed to determine the presence of rales or rhonchi, particularly in the patient with hypoperfusion, indicating alveolar edema, or respiratory distress. It is wise at the same time to auscultate over the anterior fontanel and the liver, for bruits, which would indicate the presence of an arteriovenous malformation.

Last is the evaluation of the heart. Palpation is first performed. The precordium is felt over the parasternal and subxiphoid regions to determine whether there is right ventricular hypertension or a thrill secondary to a left-to-right shunt across a VSD. The former is most important, particularly in a cyanotic infant. The absence of a right ventricular impulse indicates that the patient neither has d-transposition of the aorta nor right ventricular outflow obstruction (such as tetralogy of Fallot) but must have inflow obstruction, either tricuspid atresia or pulmonary atresia with intact ventricular septum. Unlike an older infant or child, even the normal newborn has a palpable right ventricular impulse because the right ventricle is thick and pumps under somewhat high pressures, and the sternum is thin and compliant. Palpation of the apical impulse is often difficult because of the increased right ventricular impulse. Last, a thrill should be sought in the suprasternal notch, indicative of left ventricular obstruction. Next is auscultation of the heart. S1 is rarely abnormal. The location and loudness of S2 should be determined, to locate aortic valve position and to estimate pulmonary blood flow and pulmonary arterial diastolic pressures. The latter is difficult because splitting is often not appreciated due to the normally fast newborn heart rate. Auscultation for extra heart sounds is important, particularly if a specific diagnosis is being entertained. For example, if an infant presents with mildly decreased saturations and is tachypneic, auscultation of a systolic ejection click is highly supportive of the diagnosis of truncus arteriosus. Similarly, auscultation of a systolic ejection click in a patient with a suprasternal notch thrill indicates that the aortic outflow obstruction is at the valvar level. Last, auscultation for murmurs should be performed. Because symptomatic heart disease is most important to diagnose in the immediate newborn period, murmurs are considered only as they related to the specific pathophysiology being considered. For example, the presence of to-and-fro pulmonary outflow murmurs in an infant with severe respiratory distress indicates that the diagnosis is tetralogy of Fallot with absent pulmonary valve. A to-and-fro murmur in the tricuspid region in a severely cyanotic infant supports the diagnosis of Ebstein anomaly. It is important to reiterate that many normal newborns have murmurs (often of physiologic peripheral pulmonary artery stenosis or of a closing ductus arteriosus), and many infants with critical congenital heart disease do not.

Following the cardiovascular examination, the clinician will know whether the newborn has symptomatic heart disease. She or he will know the mode of presentation and, with the history and simple ancillary tests (particularly a chest radiograph and electrocardiogram), the likely pathophysiologic process, and possibly even the specific diagnosis. With that information, the initiation of acute therapy can be undertaken immediately. Subsequent evaluation by the cardiologist will arrive at a specific diagnosis and plan of care. However, the most important intervention in the infant with symptomatic congenital heart disease is performed by the first physicians involved. With careful cardiovascular evaluation and consideration of the pathophysiologic processes, most of these infants can be rapidly stabilized and transferred over for definitive care by those physicians, with the infant being in stable cardiovascular and metabolic states.

REFERENCES

1. Hoffman JI, Kaplan S, Liberthson RR. Prevalence of congenital heart disease. Am Heart J 2004;147(3):425–39.
2. Hoffman JI, Kaplan S. The incidence of congenital heart disease. J Am Coll Cardiol 2002;39(12):1890–900.
3. Chang RK, Gurvitz M, Rodriguez S. Missed diagnosis of critical congenital heart disease. Arch Pediatr Adolesc Med 2008;162(10):969–74.
4. Liberman RF, Getz KD, Lin AE, et al. Delayed diagnosis of critical congenital heart defects: trends and associated factors. Pediatrics 2014;134(2): e373–81.
5. Wren C, Reinhardt Z, Khawaja K. Twenty-year trends in diagnosis of life-threatening neonatal cardiovascular malformations. Arch Dis Child Fetal Neonatal Ed 2008;93(1):F33–5.

6. Artman M, Mahony L, Teitel DF. Neonatal cardiology. 2nd edition. New York: McGraw-Hill Medical; 2010.

7. Shinkawa T, Polimenakos AC, Gomez-Fifer CA, et al. Management and long-term outcome of neonatal Ebstein anomaly. J Thorac Cardiovasc Surg 2010;139(2): 354–8.

8. Hornberger LK, Sanders SP, Sahn DJ, et al. In utero pulmonary artery and aortic growth and potential for progression of pulmonary outflow tract obstruction in tetralogy of Fallot. J Am Coll Cardiol 1995;25(3):739–45.

9. Konstantinov IE. Taussig-Bing anomaly: from original description to the current era. Tex Heart Inst J 2009;36(6):580–5.

10. Mahle WT, Newburger JW, Matherne GP, et al. Role of pulse oximetry in examining newborns for congenital heart disease: a scientific statement from the American Heart Association and American Academy of Pediatrics. Circulation 2009; 120(5):447–58.

11. Khullar D, Andeejani AM, Bulsara KR. Evolution of treatment options for vein of Galen malformations. J Neurosurg Pediatr 2010;6(5):444–51.

12. Anderson RH, Lenox CC, Zuberbuhler JR. The morphology of ventricular septal defects. Perspect Pediatr Pathol 1984;8(3):235–68.

13. Butto F, Lucas RV Jr, Edwards JE. Persistent truncus arteriosus: pathologic anatomy in 54 cases. Pediatr Cardiol 1986;7(2):95–101.

Fetal and Neonatal Arrhythmias

Edgar Jaeggi, MD, FRCPC*, Annika Öhman, MD

KEYWORDS

- Arrhythmia • Fetal • Pediatric • Tachycardia • Bradycardia • Diagnosis

KEY POINTS

- Arrhythmias may present as an irregularity of the cardiac rhythm, as slow or fast heart rate, or as a combination of irregular rhythm and abnormal rate.
- The identification of the underlying arrhythmia mechanism and hemodynamic impact is critical because the management and prognosis differ among the various disorders.
- The most common arrhythmia is an irregular heart rhythm caused by premature atrial contractions (PACs). Isolated PACs are usually benign and self-resolving.
- Dysrhythmias presenting with sustained slow or fast heart rates are uncommon but potentially life threatening because of the hemodynamic consequences and the underlying cause. Antiarrhythmic treatment to control the tachycardia is often key to ensuring a good outcome.

INTRODUCTION

Understanding the normal rhythm is essential for diagnosing any dysrhythmia. This article reviews the normal electrophysiology and then addresses the mechanisms, features, management, and outcomes of the common fetal and neonatal rhythm disorders.

NORMAL IMPULSE GENERATION AND PROPAGATION

The main function of the heart is to pump blood throughout the body to allow a sufficient supply of oxygen and nutrients to the tissues while removing toxic wastes. Cardiac output, the volume of ejected blood per minute, is equal to the stroke volume of each ventricle in a single heart beat times the heart rate. The normal heart rate ranges between 120 and 160 beats/min (bpm) in the mid to late gestational fetus and between

Disclosures: None.
Labatt Family Heart Centre, Hospital for Sick Children, University of Toronto, 555 University Avenue, Toronto, Ontario M5G 1X8, Canada
* Corresponding author.
E-mail address: edgar.jaeggi@sickkids.ca

Clin Perinatol 43 (2016) 99–112
http://dx.doi.org/10.1016/j.clp.2015.11.007
0095-5108/16/$ – see front matter © 2016 Elsevier Inc. All rights reserved.

100 and 150 bpm in the newborn. Heart rate is usually controlled by the sinoatrial (SA) nodal cells. These cells are capable of spontaneously depolarizing and thus acting as a pacemaker. The electrical impulse from the SA node is then propagated across the atria, the atrioventricular (AV) node, and the His-Purkinje system throughout the ventricles, allowing the sequential depolarization of the atrial and ventricular myocardium with each heartbeat. The cardiac mechanical actions, contraction of myocytes in systole, and relaxation in diastole are then orchestrated by rapid cyclic changes in their transmembrane action potentials and ion currents with each heartbeat. Following depolarization, the conducted impulse is prevented from immediately reactivating the conduction system and myocardium by refractoriness of the tissue that just has been activated. The heart must then await a new electrical impulse from the SA node to initiate the next heartbeat.

METHODS OF PERINATAL CARDIAC RHYTHM ASSESSMENT

The electrocardiogram (ECG) is the main diagnostic tool after birth to record the electrical activity of the heart. The normal ECG entails a sinus P wave with a P-wave axis between 0 and +90° (positive P wave in lead II) that precedes each QRS complex within a regular, normal PR interval. The neonatal cardiac rhythm is typically regular and the rate within the normal range for patient age. Because noninvasive fetal electrocardiography is available at a few centers only, the antenatal rhythm evaluation is primarily based on the chronology of atrial and ventricular systolic mechanical events that are recorded by echocardiography. M-mode imaging is useful to simultaneously record the atrial and ventricular systolic wall motions.[1] Similarly, simultaneous pulse wave Doppler evaluation of the mitral inflow and aortic outflow (mitral valve/aorta) or, preferably, the superior vena cava (SVC) and the ascending aorta (SVC/aorta Doppler) is used to examine the sequence and time relationship of blood flow events that are secondary to atrial and ventricular contractions.[2] The beginning of the mitral A wave and the retrograde SVC a wave reflect the onset of atrial systole, whereas the onset of aortic forward flow marks the beginning of ventricular systole. The diagnosis of a normal fetal cardiac rhythm is based on the documentation of a regular atrial and ventricular rhythm with a normal rate for gestational age (**Fig. 1**A).[3] Each atrial event is followed by a ventricular event within a normal AV time interval, which confirms normal 1:1 AV conduction.[4] Although echocardiography provides useful information on mechanical systolic events, it does not inform on the morphology, duration, and amplitude of electrical events. Hence, it is not possible to confirm repolarization abnormalities like long QT syndrome (LQTS) solely by echocardiography.

MECHANISMS OF ARRHYTHMIAS

Arrhythmias may present as an irregular cardiac rhythm, as a slow or fast heart rate, or as a combination of abnormal rhythm and rate. The contributing causes can be broadly divided into abnormalities in the generation and the propagation of electrical impulses. These disturbances result from critical alterations in electrical activity and may occur in every region of the heart.

Abnormal Impulse Generation

Cardiac cells in the atria, AV node, and His-Purkinje system can spontaneously depolarize and manifest automaticity outside the SA node. They are called latent pacemakers because they are physiologically suppressed by the faster sinus rate. Rhythm disorders whose origin is the SA node include a sinus node that fires at an unusually fast or slow rate. Ectopic cardiac rhythms occur when the dominant

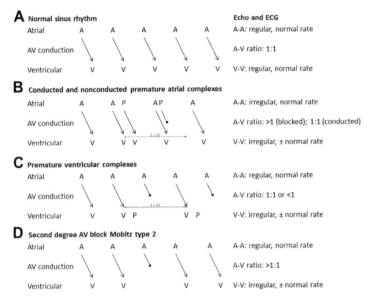

Fig. 1. (*A–D*) The sequence of electrical activation and impulse propagation of (*A*) the normal sinus rhythm compared with (*B–D*) the main disorders of an irregular heart rhythm. →, nonconducted atrial beat; A, normal atrial event; Echo, echocardiography; P, premature atrial or ventricular complex; V, normal ventricular event.

pacemaker shifts from the SA node to a latent pacemaker, either when the sinus rate decreases to less than the intrinsic rate of the secondary pacemaker (atrial or junctional escape rhythm) or the intrinsic rate of a secondary pacemaker increases to more than the normal sinus rate (atrial ectopic tachycardia, junctional ectopic tachycardia, ventricular tachycardia [VT]), or the sinus beat fails to conduct across the AV node, leaving a secondary junctional or ventricular pacemaker free to fire at its slower intrinsic rhythm.

Abnormal Impulse Propagation

Reentry is the propagation of an impulse through myocardial tissue already activated by the same impulse in a circular movement. Reentry is the underlying mechanism of most types of perinatal tachyarrhythmia, including atrial flutter (AF) and AV reentrant tachycardia (AVRT). AF is sustained by a macroreentrant circuit that is confined to the atria. AVRT, the most common mechanism of a fast heart rate in the young, is a reentrant circuit that uses the AV node to conduct from the atria to the ventricles and a fast-conducting accessory pathway to propagate the ventricular impulse back to the atria. On the other side, nonconduction of the impulse occurs when it arrives in nonexcitable tissue, either because it is still refractory after a recent depolarization (eg, blocked premature atrial contraction [PAC]) or because of abnormal tissue (eg, heart block).

CONSEQUENCES OF ARRHYTHMIAS

Compared with adults, the fetal and neonatal heart beats significantly faster, is structurally and functionally immature, and performs close to the maximum of the ventricular function curve. Because of the limited pump reserve of immature hearts, any significant change in heart rate leads to a decline in cardiac output, impaired cardiac filling, and venous congestion, the severity of which depends on arrhythmia characteristics and myocardial properties. As a general rule, the more abnormal the heart rate and the younger the age, the less likely it is that a significant arrhythmia will be well tolerated by the fetus and infant. Rhythm disorders that manifest with enduring slow (complete heart block) or fast (AVRT) heart rates represent the main cardiac causes of fetal hydrops, prematurity, and perinatal death. To provide optimal care on any new arrhythmia diagnosis it is therefore essential to first discern the mechanism and the hemodynamic impact of the rhythm disorder and then to decide on the need of treatment, if this option is available.

ASSESSMENT OF ARRHYTHMIAS

Although arrhythmias have diverse causes, most abnormalities can be deducted by the experienced investigator. **Box 1** presents a stepwise approach that can be used to diagnose and differentiate most fetal arrhythmias and that may also be used for neonatal patients.

Box 1
Stepwise approach to the assessment of fetal rhythm abnormalities

Atrial (A) rate and rhythm (A-A):

Absent – slow – normal – fast

Regular – irregular – regular-irregular (eg, atrial bigeminy)

Ventricular (V) rate and rhythm (V-V):

Slow – normal – fast

Regular – irregular – regular-irregular (eg, ventricular bigeminy)

Ratio of atrial and ventricular events:

Normal 1:1 (equal A and V)

Greater than 1:1 (more A than V)

Less than 1:1 (more V and A)

Relationship and timing of atrial and ventricular events:

Normal AV time – prolonged AV time – A-V dissociation

Arrhythmia pattern:

Duration: brief (<10%) – intermittent (10%–50%) – sustained (>50%) – incessant (100%)

Onset/termination: sudden or gradual; triggered by other event (ie, PAC)

Health state:

Effusions, heart size and function, AV valve regurgitation; fetal movements; ↓ or ↑ amniotic fluid

Structural heart disease and other associations:

Heart block: anti-Ro antibodies; left isomerism; congenital corrected transposition

Supraventricular tachycardia: Ebstein anomaly

Sinus tachycardia: Graves disease; beta-mimetic therapy; myocarditis

Sinus bradycardia, 2:1 AV block, VT: LQTS; anti-Ro antibodies

---

ARRHYTHMIAS PRESENTING WITH AN IRREGULAR RHYTHM

Probably the most frequent presentation of an irregular rhythm disorder is coincidental during a routine assessment of an otherwise asymptomatic patient. The main differential diagnosis of the underlying mechanisms includes (**Fig. 1B–D**):

- PAC
- Premature ventricular contractions (PVCs)
- Second-degree AV block

Premature Atrial Contractions

PACs account for most patients with an irregular heartbeat at any age. ECG criteria of PACs include the documentation of premature P waves with abnormal P-wave axes and with an AV conduction that may be normal, aberrant (bundle branch block), or blocked. By echocardiography, a PAC is detected by a shorter than normal atrial (A-A) interval (see **Fig. 1B**). If the AV conduction is normal, the premature atrial event is followed by a timely related premature ventricular event. If the PAC is premature enough to fail conduction across the refractory AV node, no ventricular event is observed, which manifests as a skipped heartbeat. The true fetal incidence of PACs is unknown but the arrhythmia seems to be common. In healthy newborns, PACs were documented in 51% over a 24-hour ECG surveillance study.[5] At least after birth, isolated PACs may be considered a finding within the normal range unless they are associated with other conditions, such as electrolyte abnormalities, myocarditis, or tachyarrhythmia. Before birth, PACs have been associated with less than a 1% risk of fetal tachycardia, although a higher risk has been suggested for atrial bigeminy and couplets.[6,7] PACs are usually spontaneously resolving and no medical treatment is warranted.

Premature Ventricular Contractions

PVCs are uncommon observations during fetal life. In healthy newborns, PVCs were documented in 18% by 24-hour ECG.[5] The ECG diagnosis is based on a premature QRS complex that is not preceded by a P wave. Moreover, the QRS morphology of the PVC differs from normally conducted ventricular beats. By echocardiography, the PVC is not preceded by an atrial beat, whereas the atrial intervals are usually normal and regular (see **Fig. 1C**).

Isolated atrial and ventricular ectopy are typically benign and self-limited, and no treatment is required.[5] Fetal heart rate should be monitored weekly or every other week by an obstetrician or midwife until the PACs or PVCs have resolved. In addition, recently published American Heart Association (AHA) guidelines also recommend fetal echocardiography to assess the cardiac structure and function and to determine the mechanism of the arrhythmia if the fetus presents with frequent ectopic beats, if there is any question about the mechanism, or if the ectopic beats persist beyond 1 to 2 weeks.[6]

An irregular rhythm can also be caused by second-degree AV block, which is characterized by failure of AV conduction of some, but not all, atrial activity to the ventricles (see **Fig. 1D**). The atrial rate is normal and the ventricular rate depends on the number of conducted atrial impulses. In Mobitz type I or Wenckebach-type AV block, the nonconducted atrial event is preceded by progressive PR/AV lengthening. In Mobitz type II, the AV conduction is either normal or blocked. Type II is considered serious because the site of the conduction block is below the AV node. Second-degree fetal AV block has been associated with antibody-mediated conduction disease and may benefit from antiinflammatory treatment to prevent progression to complete heart block (CHB).[8]

ARRHYTHMIAS PRESENTING WITH A SLOW HEART RATE

Fetal bradycardia is defined by a heart rate less than 110 bpm; in the newborn it is a resting heart rate less than 100 bpm on a surface ECG. Occasional, brief sinus bradycardia is a benign physiologic response whereby the rate of the SA node is slower than normal for age. Of more concern is bradycardia that is prolonged or persistent, which should trigger a more detailed assessment for the cause. The main mechanisms of perinatal bradycardia include (**Fig. 2**):

- Sinus bradycardia
- CHB
- Functional AV block: nonconducted atrial bigeminy and 2:1 AV block

Sinus Bradycardia

Sinus bradycardia is defined as a rhythm that originates from the SA node but in which the rate is slow for age (see **Fig. 2**A). A subsidiary pacemaker (ie, in the lower atrium) may become the dominant pacemaker if the rate of the SA node decreases to less than that of the secondary pacemaker. By echocardiography, fetal sinus or atrial bradycardia resembles that of a normal rhythm with the only difference that the atrial and ventricular rates are slow for gestational age, usually in the range between 80 and 110 bpm. Sinus bradycardia per se is well tolerated but may be secondary to fetal distress, sinus node dysfunction (anti-Ro antibody related, left isomerism), and LQTS (KCNQ1 mutations).[9–12]

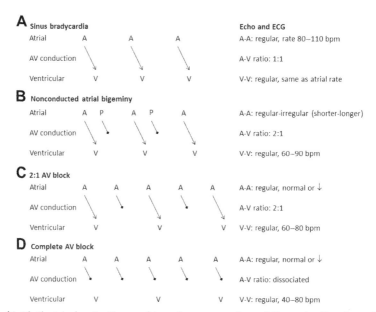

Fig. 2. (*A–D*) Electrical activation and impulse propagation of the main disorders of a slow heart rate. P, premature atrial complex.

The perinatal management of sinus bradycardia depends on the underlying cause and may include no treatment, antiinflammatory medication for myocarditis (anti-Ro antibodies, parvovirus), premature delivery (fetal distress), and postnatal therapy with β-blocker with or without pacing (LQTS).

Complete Heart Block

CHB is defined as a complete failure of the normal propagation of atrial impulses to the ventricles (see **Fig. 2D**). It is the most common congenital conduction abnormality and accounts for about 40% of all major arrhythmias before birth. The typical fetal echo-cardiogram shows a regular normal atrial rhythm and rate, whereas the ventricles beat independently at a much slower rate of between 40 and 80 bpm. On the ECG, the QRS morphology of congenital CHB is usually narrow complex, which means that the ventricular escape rhythm is junctional (**Fig. 3.**). In about half of fetal cases with CHB, it is associated with major structural heart disease, most importantly left atrial isomerism, which carries a very high risk of in-utero demise.[13,14] In the absence of structural heart disease, congenital CHB is strongly linked to the fetal transplacental passage of anti-Ro antibodies, which are prevalent in about 2% of pregnant women.[15] In 1% to 5% of exposed fetuses, the maternal antibodies lead to complications, including CHB, sinus bradycardia, myocarditis, endocardial fibroelastosis, and/or dilated cardiomyopathy. Although isolated fetal CHB is often tolerated, at the severe end of the disease spectrum it results in low cardiac output, fetal hydrops, and death. Risk factors associated with perinatal death include fetal hydrops, endocardial fibroe-lastosis, myocarditis, and bradycardia less than 50 to 55 bpm.[16,17]

There is currently no consensus about the indications of prenatal therapy for isolated CHB. There is no treatment available to reverse CHB.[18] However, dexamethasone, intravenous immune globulin (IVIG), β-adrenergic medication, and postnatal pacing have been used to prevent or treat more severe immune-mediated myocardial inflam-mation, to augment cardiac output and to improve the chances of survival.[19,20] In contrast, possible treatment-related adverse events that may preclude the routine use of high-dose steroids include fetal growth restriction, oligohydramnios, and maternal mood/behavioral changes.[17,19] Chronic prenatal steroid therapy for CHB

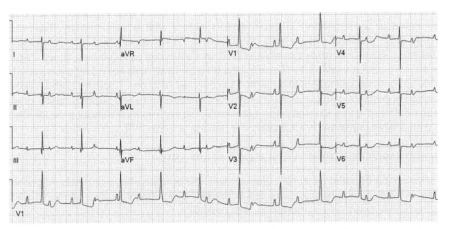

Fig. 3. ECG recording of a newborn with immune-mediated congenital CHB. The atrial rate is 135 bpm, the narrow complex ventricular rate is 105 bpm, and there is complete AV disso-ciation. The baby has no immediate indication for a permanent pacemaker implantation.

had no obvious impact on neurocognitive function at school age.[21] In our institution, maternal dexamethasone (8 mg/d for 2 weeks; 4 mg/d to 28 weeks; 2 mg/d to birth) is routinely used to treat immune-mediated cardiac disease from the time of diagnosis to birth.[22] Maternal IVIG (1 g/kg every 2–3 weeks) is added if we detect signs of endocardial fibroelastosis and ventricular dysfunction. In contrast, idiopathic isolated CHB (not associated with maternal anti-Ro antibodies) can be managed without antiinflammatory medication. If the average fetal heart rate is less than 50 bpm, we also use transplacental salbutamol (usually 10 mg 3 times a day orally) and postnatal isoprenaline infusion to maintain an adequate ventricular output until the neonatal implantation of a permanent pacemaker system. Current American College of Cardiology/AHA guidelines[23] recommend permanent pacing for CHB in children for the following class 1 indications: (1) symptomatic bradycardia, ventricular dysfunction, or low cardiac output; (2) wide-complex QRS escape rhythm; and (3) infants with ventricular rate less than 55 bpm or with congenital heart disease and a ventricular rate less than 70 bpm. During the past decade, the neonatal survival rate of isolated congenital CHB was 95% at our center, which is improved compared with predominantly untreated patient cohorts reported by us and others.[16,17,19,24] Most patients with isolated congenital CHB require permanent pacing during childhood and most commonly during the first month of life.[25]

Functional Atrioventricular Block

Functional AV block may occur when the AV node is refractory not excitable; that is, following recent depolarization or because of QT prolongation. In nonconducted atrial bigeminy (see **Fig. 2**B), every second atrial impulse occurs prematurely enough to fail conduction by the physiologically refractory AV junction. By echocardiography, the interatrial intervals are irregular but in a regular pattern alternating between a shorter (A-PAC [time interval between sinus beat to premature atrial beat]) and a longer (PAC-A [time interval between premature to normal beat]) atrial interval. If each PAC is nonconducted and each SA beat (A) is forwarded to the ventricles, the ventricular rate will be half of that of the averaged atrial rate, which is in the range between 60 and 90 bpm in fetuses. Nonconducted atrial bigeminy is a possible cause of fetal bradycardia and may last for days to weeks. Blocked PACs are benign, well tolerated, and resolve spontaneously. Weekly assessment by an obstetrician is recommended until resolution of the PACs is documented.

Atrial bigeminy should not be confused with 2:1 AV block (see **Fig. 2**D), which may be related to a congenital QT prolongation. Unlike with atrial bigeminy, the atrial rhythm in 2:1 AV block seems fairly constant and 1:1 AV conduction recurs at slower atrial rates. Similar to other possible LQTS manifestations (unexplained sinus bradycardia, VT), patients with 2:1 AV block (and their families) should undergo a complete work-up for the possibility of an inherited ion channel disorder. Because of the predisposition of patients with LQTS for VT-related cardiac arrests and sudden death, postnatal treatment with a long-acting β-blocker (ie, nadolol) with or without a pacemaker or implantable cardioverter-defibrillator is usually required.[9,10]

ARRHYTHMIAS PRESENTING WITH A FAST HEART RATE

The detection of a fast heart rate greater than 180 bpm in a fetus or newborn constitutes a medical emergency because it carries a significant risk of hemodynamic compromise, heart failure, morbidity, and mortality.

Possible mechanisms include (**Fig. 4**):

- Supraventricular tachycardia (SVT), including AVRT, atrial ectopic tachycardia (AET), and permanent junctional reciprocating tachycardia (PJRT)

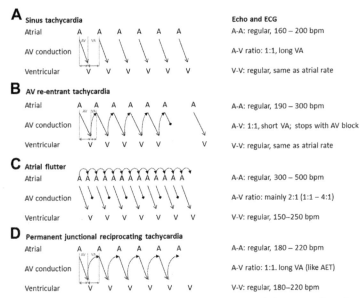

Fig. 4. (*A–D*) Electrical activation and impulse propagation of the main disorders of a fast heart rate. Long VA indicates that the tachycardia VA interval is longer than the AV interval, which is the case in sinus tachycardia, permanent junctional reciprocating tachycardia, and atrial ectopic tachycardia (not shown). The VA interval is shorter than the AV interval in AVRT (short VA or short RP tachycardia). ⋯, reentrant pathway; →, nonconducted atrial event; V, ventricular event.

- AF
- Sinus tachycardia
- Rare: VT

Atrioventricular Reentrant Tachycardia and Atrial Flutter

AVRT and AF account for 90% of the fetal and neonatal tachyarrhythmias.[26] Both arrhythmias are readily distinguished by echocardiography and electrocardiography.

Atrioventricular Reentrant Tachycardia

AVRT commonly manifests as an intermittent or persistent tachycardia between 190 and 300 bpm. It can occur any time after the first trimester. The usual reentrant circuit involves the AV node for anterograde conduction (AV) and a fast retrograde ventriculo-atrial (VA) conducting accessory pathway. AVRT starts suddenly with a PAC and terminates with AV block. Most hearts are structurally normal, but Ebstein anomaly of the tricuspid valve is a known association with accessory pathways. By fetal echocardiography, the tachycardia has a short VA pattern because the atrial contraction occurs closely after the ventricular contraction (see **Fig. 4**B). Because of the almost simultaneous atrial and ventricular contraction the AV valves are closed during atrial systole and there is pronounced a-wave flow reversal in the precordial veins and the ductus venosus. On the tachycardia ECG (**Fig. 5**), a retrograde P wave is seen immediately following QRS (short RP tachycardia). The QRS morphology is typically regular and narrow complex unless there is rate-related bundle branch block. A delta wave is

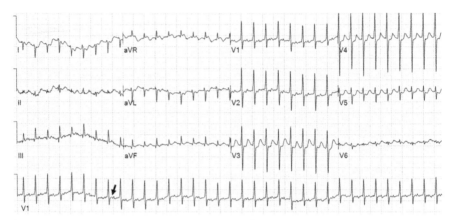

Fig. 5. Neonatal AVRT with a ventricular rate of 265 bpm. P waves are seen in the ST segment in leads III and V1 (*arrow*). The short RP interval is typical for this arrhythmia.

seen if there is anterograde pathway conduction during sinus rhythm (Wolff-Parkinson-White syndrome).

Close observation without drug therapy may be a safe approach for fetuses with infrequent, brief SVT episodes, because heart failure rarely develops unless the arrhythmia is very fast and/or becomes more persistent. In contrast, fetuses with incessant tachyarrhythmia tend to develop heart failure with hydrops if left in tachycardia. Fetal hydrops, cardiovascular collapse, and death are strongly associated with incessant AVRT but even intermittent tachycardia may have serious consequences.[27] In retrospective studies, 40% of fetuses with AVRT presented with hydrops and this was associated with a perinatal mortality between 21% and 27%. In contrast, the rate of perinatal mortality was less than 5% for those cases without hydrops.[26,27] Rapid pharmacologic cardioversion to a normal sinus rhythm is therefore most pressing for hydropic fetuses with incessant tachyarrhythmia. Moreover, fetal hydrops resolves over time once the cardiac rhythm is normalized by antiarrhythmic therapy. Possible medications to treat fetal SVT until birth include maternal digoxin, flecainide, or sotalol either alone or in combination, whereas amiodarone and direct fetal therapy are usually reserved for treatment-resistant, poorly tolerated tachycardia. Newborns in sinus rhythm may not require postnatal antiarrhythmic treatment but close observation for 2- 3 days and thereafter for SVT recurrence is advised. Neonatal incessant AVRT warrants acute cardioversion by vagal stimulation (facial immersion in iced water or ice pack), rapid intravenous bolus injection over 1 to 2 seconds of the short-acting adenosine immediately followed by a rapid saline flush, transesophageal atrial overdrive pacing, and/or additional antiarrhythmic medication, whereas electrical cardioversion is rarely required. Prophylactic antiarrhythmic treatment (ie, with propranolol) is then often used to prevent SVT recurrence during the first 6 to 12 months of life or longer. In our experience, AVRT associated with manifest pathway conduction during sinus rhythm (Wolff-Parkinson-White syndrome) is more likely to persist and to require long-term postnatal antiarrhythmic treatment.[28]

Atrial Flutter

AF is sustained by a circular macroreentrant pathway within the atrial wall, whereas the AV node is not part of the reentry circuit (see **Fig. 4**C). Atrial rates range between 300 and 500 bpm, which is commonly associated with 2:1 AV conduction and ventricular rates between 150 to 250 bpm.[29] Normal or near-normal ventricular rates are observed in AF with slower 3:1 or 4:1 AV conduction.

ECG diagnosis of AF is straightforward with saw-tooth flutter waves that are best seen in leads II, III, and aVF (**Fig. 6**). In the absence of structural heart disease, AF is almost exclusively observed in babies during the third trimester or at birth. AF is usually tolerated and fetal hydrops and death are uncommon. Sotalol or digoxin is the first-line medication to treat fetal AF.[26] The treatment aim is either to suppress the arrhythmia or, if this is not achieved, to slow the ventricular rate to a more normal heart rate. If AF persists to birth, sinus rhythm can be restored by transesophageal overdrive pacing or synchronized electrical cardioversion. Neonatal recurrence of AF is unusual and long-term treatment is rarely required.

Other

Other tachyarrhythmia mechanisms are less common and may be difficult to differentiate from each other without ECG. Before birth, sinus tachycardia, PJRT, and AET present similarly as long VA tachycardia with heart rates less than 220 bpm. Sinus tachycardia is usually 20 to 30 bpm slower than AET and PJRT and characterized by atrial rates of less than 200 bpm, normal 1:1 AV conduction, and some variability of the fetal heart rate (see **Fig. 4A**). Sinus tachycardia greater than 200 bpm is occasionally seen in critically ill babies. A variety of fetal and maternal conditions may be responsible for sustained sinus tachycardia, including distress, anemia, and infections. The importance of sinus tachycardia is recognizing and treating the underlying cause. PJRT is an AV reentry tachycardia with a fairly slow retrograde conducting accessory pathway, which explains the long VA pattern (see **Fig. 4D**). The typical ECG pattern is that of an incessant tachycardia with long RP intervals and inverted P waves in the inferior leads II, III, and aVF. Spontaneous resolution of PJRT is unusual. Definitive treatment of PJRT is possible with radiofrequency ablation of the pathway in later life.

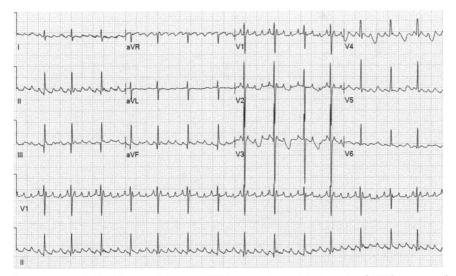

Fig. 6. Neonatal AF with an atrial rate of 460 bpm and a ventricular rate of 115 bpm caused by 4:1 AV conduction. Saw-tooth flutter waves are best seen in leads II, aVF, and V1.

Atrial Ectopic Tachycardia

AET (**Fig. 7**) arises from an ectopic focus within the atria and is most commonly sustained. During AET, intermittent changes in tachycardia rate with warming up and cooling down may be observed. Although AET is usually 1:1, conduction delay with AV block may be seen. Short-term antiarrhythmic treatment is often required but AET usually resolves before 6 months of life.

Ventricular Tachycardia

VT is a rare arrhythmia in babies. The fetal echocardiogram shows a tachycardia less than 200 bpm that is often incessant on presentation. The ventricular rate is higher than the atrial rate and there is no clear relation between ventricular and atrial events (AV dissociation). The postnatal definition of VT is that of a ventricular rate that is greater than or equal to 120 bpm or 25% faster than the normal sinus rate. The term accelerated ventricular rate is used if the ventricular rate is less than 120 bpm. The characteristic ECG of VT shows QRS widening with a bundle branch block pattern as well as AV dissociation. VT needs to be differentiated from other rare mechanisms in infants that also produce wide QRS tachycardia, including SVT/AF with bundle branch block and SVT with anterograde conduction across an accessory pathway. If the QRS in the tachycardia is wide, then the diagnosis of VT is more likely.

When evaluating a fetus or newborn for VT, possible causes include viral and anti-Ro antibody-mediated myocarditis; cardiac tumors; structural heart disease; hereditary cardiomyopathy, including LQTS; and electrolyte imbalance. In the absence of an identifiable predisposing condition, perinatal VT is often a benign finding (idiopathic VT). Treatment and prognosis depend on the VT mechanism and pattern, the hemodynamic impact, and associated conditions. Before birth, short-term maternal intravenous magnesium has been recommended as first-line medication for VT greater than 200 bpm.[6] Other treatments to acutely control VT may include intravenous lidocaine, oral β-blocker, and mexiletine. In the absence of LQTS, amiodarone, flecainide, or sotalol may also be useful.

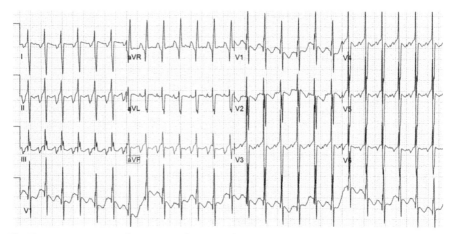

Fig. 7. Incessant AET with a ventricular rate of 190 bpm. The RP interval is prolonged and there are deeply inverted P waves in leads I, II, and III.

SUMMARY

Clinically relevant rhythm disorders are not common but may be associated with significant morbidity and mortality. Precise diagnosis is required before treatment is considered. AVRT is the most common type of SVT in fetuses and neonates. Antiarrhythmic treatment up to 12 months may be needed to prevent recurrence. CHB is the most common cause of persistent slow heart rate. Most survivors to birth require postnatal ventricular pacing.

REFERENCES

1. Jaeggi E, Fouron JC, Fournier A, et al. Ventriculo-atrial time interval measured on M mode echocardiography: a determining element in diagnosis, treatment, and prognosis of fetal supraventricular tachycardia. Heart 1998;79(6):582–7.
2. Fouron JC. Fetal arrhythmias: the Saint-Justine Hospital experience. Prenat Diagn 2004;24(13):1068–80.
3. Mitchell JL, Cuneo BF, Etheridge SP, et al. Fetal heart rate predictors of long QT syndrome. Circulation 2012;126(23):2688–95.
4. Nii M, Hamilton RM, Fenwick L, et al. Assessment of fetal atrioventricular time intervals by tissue Doppler and pulse Doppler echocardiography: normal values and correlation with fetal electrocardiography. Heart 2006;92(12):1831–7.
5. Nagashima M, Matsushima M, Ogawa A, et al. Cardiac arrhythmias in healthy children revealed by 24-hour ambulatory ECG monitoring. Pediatr Cardiol 1987;8(2):103–8.
6. Donofrio MT, Moon-Grady AJ, Hornberger LK, et al. Diagnosis and treatment of fetal cardiac disease: a scientific statement from the American Heart Association. Circulation 2014;129(21):2183–242.
7. Sonesson SE, Eliasson H, Conner P, et al. Doppler echocardiographic isovolumetric time intervals in diagnosis of fetal blocked atrial bigeminy and 2:1 atrioventricular block. Ultrasound Obstet Gynecol 2014;44(2):171–5.
8. Raboisson MJ, Fouron JC, Sonesson SE, et al. Fetal Doppler echocardiographic diagnosis and successful steroid therapy of Luciani-Wenckebach phenomenon and endocardial fibroelastosis related to maternal anti-Ro and anti-La antibodies. J Am Soc Echocardiogr 2005;18(4):375–80.
9. Horigome H, Nagashima M, Sumitomo N, et al. Clinical characteristics and genetic background of congenital long-QT syndrome diagnosed in fetal, neonatal, and infantile life: a nationwide questionnaire survey in Japan. Circ Arrhythm Electrophysiol 2010;3(1):10–7.
10. Cuneo BF, Etheridge SP, Horigome H, et al. Arrhythmia phenotype during fetal life suggests long-QT syndrome genotype: risk stratification of perinatal long-QT syndrome. Circ Arrhythm Electrophysiol 2013;6(5):946–51.
11. Chockalingam P, Jaeggi ET, Rammeloo LA, et al. Persistent fetal sinus bradycardia associated with maternal anti-SSA/Ro and anti-SSB/La antibodies. J Rheumatol 2011;38(12):2682–5.
12. Lin JH, Chang CI, Wang JK, et al. Intrauterine diagnosis of heterotaxy syndrome. Am Heart J 2002;143(6):1002–8.
13. Berg C, Geipel A, Kohl T, et al. Atrioventricular block detected in fetal life: associated anomalies and potential prognostic markers. Ultrasound Obstet Gynecol 2005;26(1):4–15.
14. Jaeggi ET, Hornberger LK, Smallhorn JF, et al. Prenatal diagnosis of complete atrioventricular block associated with structural heart disease: combined

experience of two tertiary care centers and review of the literature. Ultrasound Obstet Gynecol 2005;26(1):16–21.

15. Jaeggi E, Laskin C, Hamilton R, et al. The importance of the level of maternal anti-Ro/SSA antibodies as a prognostic marker of the development of cardiac neonatal lupus erythematosus a prospective study of 186 antibody-exposed fetuses and infants. J Am Coll Cardiol 2010;55(24):2778–84.

16. Izmirly PM, Saxena A, Kim MY, et al. Maternal and fetal factors associated with mortality and morbidity in a multi-racial/ethnic registry of anti-SSA/Ro-associated cardiac neonatal lupus. Circulation 2011;124(18):1927–35.

17. Eliasson H, Sonesson SE, Sharland G, et al. Isolated atrioventricular block in the fetus: a retrospective, multinational, multicenter study of 175 patients. Circulation 2011;124(18):1919–26.

18. Saleeb S, Copel J, Friedman D, et al. Comparison of treatment with fluorinated glucocorticoids to the natural history of autoantibody-associated congenital heart block: retrospective review of the research registry for neonatal lupus. Arthritis Rheum 1999;42(11):2335–45.

19. Jaeggi ET, Fouron JC, Silverman ED, et al. Transplacental fetal treatment improves the outcome of prenatally diagnosed complete atrioventricular block without structural heart disease. Circulation 2004;110(12):1542–8.

20. Trucco SM, Jaeggi E, Cuneo B, et al. Use of intravenous gamma globulin and corticosteroids in the treatment of maternal autoantibody-mediated cardiomyopathy. J Am Coll Cardiol 2011;57(6):715–23.

21. Kelly EN, Sananes R, Chiu-Man C, et al. Prenatal anti-Ro antibody exposure, congenital complete atrioventricular heart block, and high-dose steroid therapy: impact on neurocognitive outcome in school-age children. Arthritis Rheumatol 2014;66(8):2290–6.

22. Hutter D, Silverman ED, Jaeggi ET. The benefits of transplacental treatment of isolated congenital complete heart block associated with maternal anti-Ro/SSA antibodies: a review. Scand J Immunol 2010;72(3):235–41.

23. Epstein AE, DiMarco JP, Ellenbogen KA, et al. ACC/AHA/HRS 2008 guidelines for device-based therapy of cardiac rhythm abnormalities: a report of the American College of Cardiology/American Heart Association Task Force on Practice Guidelines (Writing Committee to Revise the ACC/AHA/NASPE 2002 Guideline Update for Implantation of Cardiac Pacemakers and Antiarrhythmia Devices) developed in collaboration with the American Association for Thoracic Surgery and Society of Thoracic Surgeons. J Am Coll Cardiol 2008;51(21):e1–62.

24. Lopes LM, Tavares GM, Damiano AP, et al. Perinatal outcome of fetal atrioventricular block: one-hundred-sixteen cases from a single institution. Circulation 2008;118(12):1268–75.

25. Jaeggi ET, Hamilton RM, Silverman ED, et al. Outcome of children with fetal, neonatal or childhood diagnosis of isolated congenital atrioventricular block. A single institution's experience of 30 years. J Am Coll Cardiol 2002;39(1):130–7.

26. Jaeggi ET, Carvalho JS, De Groot E, et al. Comparison of transplacental treatment of fetal supraventricular tachyarrhythmias with digoxin, flecainide, and sotalol: results of a nonrandomized multicenter study. Circulation 2011;124(16):1747–54.

27. Simpson JM, Sharland GK. Fetal tachycardias: management and outcome of 127 consecutive cases. Heart 1998;79(6):576–81.

28. Gilljam T, Jaeggi E, Gow RM. Neonatal supraventricular tachycardia: outcomes over a 27-year period at a single institution. Acta Paediatr 2008;97(8):1035–9.

29. Jaeggi E, Fouron JC, Drblik SP. Fetal atrial flutter: diagnosis, clinical features, treatment, and outcome. J Pediatr 1998;132(2):335–9.

Recent Advances in the Treatment of Preterm Newborn Infants with Patent Ductus Arteriosus

Hannes Sallmon, MD[a], Petra Koehne, MD, PhD[a],
Georg Hansmann, MD, PhD, FESC[b],*

KEYWORDS

- Patent ductus arteriosus • Preterm infant • Very low birth weight • Ibuprofen
- Indomethacin • Paracetamol

KEY POINTS

- One third of all very low birth weight infants are diagnosed with a patent ductus arteriosus (PDA) during their neonatal intensive care unit stay.
- A PDA has been associated with several adverse clinical conditions; however, data on the potential benefits of PDA treatment on short-term neonatal and long-term neurodevelopmental outcomes are sparse.
- Several established treatment strategies, including medical treatment with indomethacin and ibuprofen, and surgical/interventional options are available.
- Recent approaches, such as oral ibuprofen, high-dose regimens, and the use of oral and intravenous paracetamol, provide new alternatives to established strategies.
- Further research is warranted in order to determine which patients require treatment and how treatment protocols should be designed and adapted to allow optimal, individualized (tailored) therapy.

INTRODUCTION

The ductus arteriosus (DA) is a fetal shunt vessel that, during prenatal life, diverts blood away from the pulmonary circulation into the systemic circulation toward the placenta. During normal postnatal adaptation, because of decreasing pulmonary

Disclosures: None.
[a] Department of Neonatology, Charité University Medical Center, Augustenburger Platz 1, Berlin 13353, Germany; [b] Department of Pediatric Cardiology and Critical Care, Hannover Medical School, Carl-Neuberg-Str. 1, Hannover 30625, Germany.
* Corresponding author. Department of Pediatric Cardiology and Critical Care, Hannover Medical School, Carl-Neuberg-Str. 1, Hannover D-30625, Germany.
E-mail address: georg.hansmann@gmail.com

Clin Perinatol 43 (2016) 113–129
http://dx.doi.org/10.1016/j.clp.2015.11.008 **perinatology.theclinics.com**
0095-5108/16/$ – see front matter © 2016 Elsevier Inc. All rights reserved.

vascular resistance and pulmonary artery (PA) pressure, and increasing systemic vascular resistance, the main ductal shunt direction changes to left to right (aorta to PA).[1] In healthy term and preterm newborn infants, the DA constricts within the first postnatal days, which is triggered by several mechanisms such as hypoxia and decreasing prostaglandin levels. The initial constriction is followed by definitive DA closure leading to vascular remodeling of the DA (discussed in detail elsewhere[2,3]). Inducible growth factors such as vascular endothelial growth factor and transforming growth factor beta, but also cellular mediators such as platelets and their paracrine effects, are most likely involved in definitive DA closure.[4–6]

When the DA fails to close within approximately the first 3 days of postnatal life it usually facilitates a left-to-right shunt that can cause pulmonary vascular and left ventricular volume overload (ie, persistently patent DA [PDA]). A large ductal left-to-right shunt (Qp/Qs >>1.5) has been associated with several adverse clinical conditions, such as pulmonary edema, decreased lung compliance, pulmonary hemorrhage, and ultimately prolonged ventilator dependence and chronic lung disease (CLD) in severe cases.[7–9] Moreover, other nonpulmonary conditions, including necrotizing enterocolitis (NEC), myocardial dysfunction, and systemic hypotension, as well as altered intracerebral blood flow (ductal steal) and hemorrhage (intracerebral hemorrhage [ICH]/intraventricular hemorrhage [IVH]), have also been associated with failed ductal constriction.[2,8,9] These observations provide the rationale for treating PDA in preterm newborn infants. However, to date, validated data regarding the benefit of PDA treatment on short-term and on long-term neurodevelopmental outcomes are sparse, and the optimal treatment strategies for neonates with PDA remain subject to several ongoing debates.[10] This article reviews current strategies for PDA treatment in neonates with a special focus on recent developments such as oral ibuprofen, high-dose regimens, and the use of oral or intravenous paracetamol.

SYMPTOMS AND HEMODYNAMIC SIGNIFICANCE OF PATENT DUCTUS ARTERIOSUS

Clinical symptoms of a hemodynamically significant PDA (hsPDA) such as a murmur, active precordium, pulsus celer et altus, poor growth, and increased work of breathing are nonspecific and might develop late in the clinical course.[11,12] The gold standard for diagnosing a PDA is transthoracic echocardiography. It allows direct visualization of the ductus, determination of its size at the pulmonary and aortic end, shunt direction and velocity, and a concomitant evaluation of ventricular volumes, mass, and function (**Fig. 1**). Several markers of hemodynamic significance have been used in order to assess a PDA. A left atrium to aortic root ratio greater than or equal to 1.4, left ventricular enlargement, increased mean and diastolic PA flow values, and reversed mitral E/A ratio are established indicators for pulmonary overcirculation (high Qp/Qs). Moreover, retrograde diastolic flow in the descending aorta and low-antegrade or retrograde diastolic flow in systemic arteries (eg, anterior cerebral artery, celiac artery, superior mesenteric artery) by pulsed wave Doppler indicate systemic hypoperfusion and ductal steal. A ductal diameter greater than or equal to 1.5 mm during the first 7 to 31 hours of life can be used to predict the development of a symptomatic DA in infants less than 29 weeks' gestational age (GA)[13,14] and is weakly associated with later PDA ligation and/or death.[15,16] However, diagnosis of hsPDA should be based on a combination of these variables. To date, there are no standardized protocols based on large trials that rigorously define echocardiographic criteria for hsPDA. Measurements of cerebral saturation by near-infrared spectroscopy and the use of urine and plasma biomarkers (eg, natriuretic peptides) might help identify patients with compromised hemodynamic status, but are beyond the scope of this article.[2,17,18]

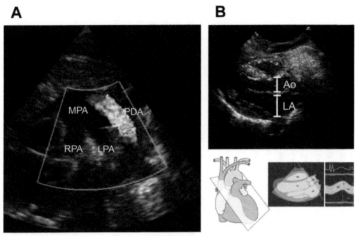

Fig. 1. Echocardiographic assessment of PDA. (*A*) Parasternal short-axis view of a PDA with left-to-right shunt. (*B*) Parasternal long-axis view and determination of left atrium (LA)/aorta (Ao) root ratio. LPA, left PA; MPA, mean PA; RPA, right PA.

CURRENT TREATMENT OPTIONS FOR PATENT DUCTUS ARTERIOSUS OF PRETERM NEWBORN INFANTS

It is estimated that one-third of all very low birth weight (VLBW) infants are diagnosed with a PDA during their neonatal intensive care unit (NICU) stays,[19] with 70% of infants less than 28 weeks GA[20] and even 80% at 24 to 25 weeks GA being affected.[21] Although spontaneous DA closure is a common observation made in one-third of all extremely low birth weight (ELBW) infants during the first week of life, up to 70% of all ELBW infants receive some kind of treatment of PDA.[22]

The question of when to treat a PDA in a preterm neonate (and when not to treat at all) is controversial. When treatment of a PDA is considered clinically, the clinician has to distinguish between 2 different general strategies: (1) prophylactic treatment (usually initiated <24 hours after birth to all infants), and (2) symptomatic treatment (usually initiated early, within 2–5 days, or late, up to 10–14 days in infants with signs of hsPDA). An intermediate third option is early asymptomatic treatment that uses echocardiographic signs of failed ductal constriction in the absence of hemodynamic significance or clinical symptoms (**Table 1**). A study from Australia (DETECT study) on early asymptomatic treatment showed a significant decrease in pulmonary hemorrhage rates in infants treated with indomethacin.[23] In addition, in a large French study enrolling 1513 extremely preterm infants (<29 weeks GA), screening echocardiography before day 3 of life was associated with lower in-hospital mortality and a reduced likelihood of pulmonary hemorrhage.[24] However, a causal relationship between echocardiographic screening and outcome was not shown in this retrospective study, there were differences between matched and unmatched cohorts, and there was a large loss of events (deaths) when performing paired analysis. Differences in NEC, severe bronchopulmonary dysplasia (BPD), or severe cerebral lesions were not observed.[24]

Treatment of a PDA includes several medical and surgical options. The current mainstay of therapy is to use the cyclooxygenase (COX) 2 inhibitors ibuprofen or indomethacin intravenously. Neither oral preparations of ibuprofen nor intravenous or oral preparations of paracetamol are licensed for the treatment of PDA in preterm infants. During the last decade, the execution of several smaller-sized randomized trials was

Table 1
Current established pharmacologic treatment strategies for PDA in preterm newborn infants

	Drug of Choice	Dosing	Comments	Pros	Cons
Prophylactic pharmacologic treatment of preterm newborn infants at risk for hsPDA (6–24 h after birth)	Indomethacin	0.1 mg/kg/dose IV every 12 h (3 doses total)	• Last dose might be omitted if echocardiography suggests ductal constriction (pressure-restrictive PDA) • Do not start treatment within the first 6 h of life • Infuse over at least 30 min • Pharmacologic treatment might be extended or repeated • It is recommended not to use ibuprofen (IV) in the first 24 h of life (PPHN risk, lack of beneficial effects on IVH rates and improved neurodevelopmental outcome in boys)	• Prevention of IVH (prophylaxis) • Risk reduction of pulmonary hemorrhage • Association with beneficial neurodevelopmental outcome in boys	Unnecessary treatment of many infants without a (hemodynamically significant) PDA
Early pharmacologic treatment of asymptomatic preterm newborn infants with PDA (<72 h after birth)	Indomethacin	0.2 mg/kg/dose IV, followed by 0.1 mg/kg/dose every 12 h (3 doses or more, total)	• Last indomethacin dose might be omitted if echocardiography suggests pressure-restrictive PDA • Infuse indomethacin over at least 30 min IV • Either treatment might be extended or repeated	• Risk reduction of pulmonary hemorrhage • Risk reduction of in-hospital mortality?	• Unnecessary treatment of some infants who have a small PDA that is hemodynamically not significant • Unclear effects on outcome
	Ibuprofen	10 mg/kg/dose PO or IV, followed by 5 mg/kg at 24 and 48 h of treatment start	• Ibuprofen PO should be followed by 2 mL/kg water or milk (hyperosmolarity) • It is recommended not to use ibuprofen (IV) in the first 24 h of life (PPHN risk)		
Pharmacologic treatment in symptomatic preterm newborn infants with hsPDA (>72 h after birth)	Ibuprofen	10 mg/kg/dose PO or IV, followed by 5 mg/kg at 24 and 48 h of treatment start	• Treatment might be extended or repeated • Higher doses can be considered • Ibuprofen PO should be followed by 2 mL/kg water or milk (hyperosmolarity)	Treatment only in infants with hsPDA	No evidence for beneficial long-term outcome

Abbreviations: IV, intravenously; PO, orally; PPHN, perinatal pulmonary hypertension of the neonate.

triggered by the still-significant failure rates of the treatment regimens discussed earlier, along with the easier application and lower costs of both oral ibuprofen and paracetamol. Surgical ligation, catheter-based interventions, and supportive conservative therapies, such as fluid restriction,[25] represent alternative or additional strategies.

INTRAVENOUS INDOMETHACIN AND IBUPROFEN
Prophylactic Treatment

Intravenous indomethacin has been extensively studied in prophylactic PDA treatment, when administered to a predefined at-risk population within the first 24 hours after birth. In a recent Cochrane meta-analysis involving 2872 infants, the ductal closure rates with either intravenous indomethacin or ibuprofen are reported to be about 75%.[26] Prophylactic indomethacin exerts short-term benefits for preterm neonates, including a decrease in the incidence of symptomatic PDA, pulmonary hemorrhage, need for surgical ligation,[27] and severe IVH. However, these findings do not clearly translate into beneficial effects on mortality or neurodevelopment. The largest trial (Trial of Indomethacin Prophylaxis in Preterms [TIPP]) included in the meta-analysis determined neurodevelopmental follow-up data after 18 months, which is likely sufficient to detect gross neurologic abnormalities, but might miss more subtle developmental differences.[28] Nevertheless, a sex-specific improvement in neurodevelopmental outcome was noted after 8 years in boys.[29] Prophylactic ibuprofen conferred similar DA closure rates, decreased the need for rescue treatment and for surgical closure, but had no effect on IVH, and led to severe pulmonary hypertension in some infants. Therefore, if prophylactic treatment is desired, indomethacin is currently the drug of choice. In general, the benefits of pharmacologic treatment have to be weighed against the potential adverse effects. When considering the high spontaneous closure rate even in ELBW infants, it can be estimated that up to 60% infants are exposed to unnecessary risks for adverse events. However, prophylaxis might be beneficial in a selected group of infants with a high likelihood of severe IVH or pulmonary hemorrhage (eg, the most immature and sick, those requiring mechanical ventilation, and male infants).

Symptomatic Treatment

Symptomatic treatment of hsPDA is the most commonly practiced treatment regimen for PDA, avoiding high rates of unnecessary drug exposure as in prophylactic treatment. Both ibuprofen and indomethacin confer similar effectiveness with respect to ductal closure (60%–80%). Nevertheless, ibuprofen currently seems to be the drug of choice because it is associated with a decreased risk for NEC and transient renal insufficiency compared with indomethacin (**Fig. 2**). Most studies examining symptomatic treatment were conducted to compare indomethacin versus ibuprofen, but usually lacked a control arm in which no treatment was administered.[30] Therefore, although widely practiced and effective in reducing PDA incidence and ligation rates, symptomatic treatment has not yet been shown to reduce any adverse outcome variables; hence, no evidence of beneficial effects of hsPDA treatment has been clearly shown. Further research on outcome and alternative regimens, including high-dose versus standard-dose comparisons,[31,32] and on continuous infusion versus intermittent bolus application[33,34] is needed in order to optimize treatment protocols.

ORAL IBUPROFEN
Effectiveness of Oral Ibuprofen

A meta-analysis of ibuprofen versus indomethacin for closing PDAs in preterm infants has been updated recently. After addition of 13 further studies, it now includes 33 trials

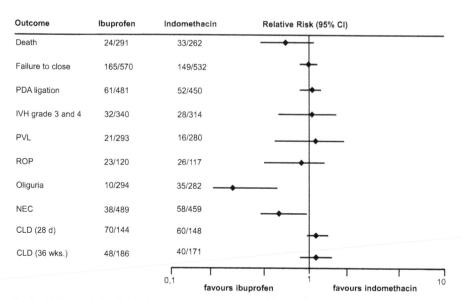

Outcome	Ibuprofen	Indomethacin	Relative Risk (95% CI)
Death	24/291	33/262	
Failure to close	165/570	149/532	
PDA ligation	61/481	52/450	
IVH grade 3 and 4	32/340	28/314	
PVL	21/293	16/280	
ROP	23/120	26/117	
Oliguria	10/294	35/282	
NEC	38/489	58/459	
CLD (28 d)	70/144	60/148	
CLD (36 wks.)	48/186	40/171	

0,1   favours ibuprofen   1   favours indomethacin   10

Fig. 2. Meta-analysis of short-term outcomes observed in randomized trials comparing indomethacin and ibuprofen for PDA treatment. CI, confidence interval; PVL, periventricular leukomalacia; ROP, retinopathy of prematurity. (*Adapted from* Ohlsson A, Walia R, Shah SS. Ibuprofen for the treatment of patent ductus arteriosus in preterm or low birth weight (or both) infants. Cochrane Database Syst Rev 2015;(2):CD000174.)

involving 2190 infants.[30] Only 1 study comparing the effectiveness of oral ibuprofen with placebo was identified.[35] Sixty-four symptomatic VLBW infants with echocardiographically confirmed PDA were enrolled. Thirty-two infants received oral ibuprofen 10 mg/kg as an initial dose within 24 hours after birth, followed by a second and a third dose of 5 mg/kg 24 and 48 hours after the initial dose. Compared with placebo, oral ibuprofen significantly reduced the closure failure rate after 3 doses (relative risk [RR] 0.26; 95% confidence interval [CI], 0.11–0.62; number needed to treat [NNT], 2). The incidences of periventricular leukomalacia and BPD were significantly lower and the durations of mechanical ventilation and hospitalization were significantly shorter in the ibuprofen group than in the placebo group. There were no significant differences in the incidence of IVH, early pulmonary hemorrhage, and NEC between the two groups.

Eight trials including 272 infants reported on failure rates for PDA closure comparing oral ibuprofen with intravenous or oral indomethacin.[36–43] There was no statistically significant difference between the two groups concerning the outcome of failure to close a PDA after 3 doses (272 infants; typical RR, 0.96; 95% CI, 0.73–1.27). Seven trials reported on NEC.[36–39,41–43] Although none of the trials showed a significant difference comparing oral ibuprofen with indomethacin, the meta-analysis showed a statistically significant reduction in NEC rates with oral ibuprofen (249 infants; typical RR, 0.41; 95% CI, 0.23–0.73; NNT, 8). In addition, there was a reduction in all-case mortality in the oral ibuprofen group compared with indomethacin.

Four studies including 304 infants reported on oral ibuprofen versus intravenous ibuprofen, both at an initial dose of 10 mg/kg, followed by 5 mg/kg at 24 and 48 hours.[44–47] Sixty-eight infants less than or equal to 2000 g, 166 VLBW infants, and 70 ELBW infants with a GA less than or equal to 32 weeks at a postnatal age between 48 and 96 hours and with echocardiographically confirmed PDA were included. There was a statistically significant reduction of the primary outcome of failure to close a PDA after 3 doses in the oral ibuprofen group in 1 of the 4 trials (102 infants); the meta-analysis showed a significantly decreased risk of failure to close a PDA with oral ibuprofen versus intravenous ibuprofen (304 infants; typical RR, 0.41; 95% CI, 0.27–0.64; NNT, 5).[45]

Adverse Events

Major concerns exist about gastrointestinal tolerance and safety of oral ibuprofen in extremely low GA preterm infants, because of the hyperosmolarity of most commercially available ibuprofen suspensions. The major concerns are gastrointestinal bleeding, NEC, and bowel perforation, although, compared with indomethacin, ibuprofen shows less impairment of mesenteric blood flow, probably because of its differential COX enzyme inhibition.[2] A recent report has shown that renal and mesenteric tissue oxygenation and oxygen extraction are preserved in preterm infants with hsPDA treated with oral ibuprofen.[48] Three studies reported on NEC,[44–47] 2 studies on intestinal perforation,[46,47] and 2 studies on gastrointestinal bleeding.[44,45] There were no statistically significant differences between oral and intravenous ibuprofen in the individual studies or in the meta-analysis. Individual variability in pharmacokinetics, composition of the ibuprofen suspension, its osmolarity, and feeding strategy may affect adverse events.

With regard to renal side effects, 2 studies (170 infants) reported on serum/plasma creatinine levels 72 hours after treatment.[44,45] There was a statistically significant reduction with oral ibuprofen compared with intravenous ibuprofen. One study reported on plasma cystatin-C level after treatment, which is a muscle mass–independent marker of glomerular filtration.[45] Cystatin-C levels increased significantly after treatment in the oral group, but did not change with intravenous ibuprofen. The need for surgical closure of the ductus was not significantly different between the oral and intravenous ibuprofen groups in any of the 4 studies. There were no significant differences between the groups regarding neurodevelopment or impairments at 18 to 24 months in the 57 infants studied to date.[49]

At present, there is only 1 study that compares the efficacy and possible adverse effects of an oral high-dose ibuprofen regimen with that of standard regimen in closing a PDA.[50] Sixty preterm infants with GA less than 37 weeks and postnatal age 3 to 7 days with echocardiographic diagnosis of hsPDA were randomly assigned to 2 treatment groups that respectively received high-dose (20-10-10 mg/kg/d) and standard-dose (10-5-5 mg/kg/d) oral ibuprofen regimen for 3 days. Complete ductal closure as confirmed by echocardiography was observed in 20 of 30 (70%) infants treated with the high-dose regimen compared with 11 of 30 (36.7%) in the standard-dose regimen group ($P = .01$). No gastrointestinal, renal, or hematological (eg, hyperbilirubinemia) adverse effects were reported. A limitation of the study is the range of the patients' GAs.

Summary

Oral ibuprofen seems to be as effective as intravenous indomethacin. A first-course orogastric administration of ibuprofen is more effective than intravenous ibuprofen for ductal closure in VLBW infants. Although high-dose oral ibuprofen seems to be more effective than the current standard-dose regimen for PDA closure in preterm neonates without increasing the adverse effects, to make further recommendations, more studies are needed, especially on pharmacokinetics in critically ill infants.

Patients with borderline renal function should be evaluated and followed closely. There is a lack of data on ibuprofen's efficacy and safety in ELBW infants, who constitute most of the patients with ductal patency in developed countries. Whether oral ibuprofen confers any important long-term advantages on development is not known.

PARACETAMOL (ACETAMINOPHEN)

Paracetamol has recently gained importance as an alternative treatment of hsPDA because of therapeutic failure and potential side effects of indomethacin and intravenous/oral ibuprofen. Few studies have been conducted on paracetamol treatment of PDA in preterm infants to date. Paracetamol was primarily not used as the drug of choice but as a supplementary medication in cases in which COX inhibitors were ineffective or contraindicated, including the first case reported in 2011.[51,52]

Clinical Pharmacology

Paracetamol has analgesic and antipyretic activity, but only modest peripheral antiinflammatory properties.[53] Although its precise mechanism of action in inhibiting prostaglandin synthetase activity remains controversial, paracetamol seems to act at the peroxidase segment of prostaglandin synthetase,[54,55] which consists of a COX and a peroxidase. Paracetamol is metabolized by the liver and subsequently eliminated by the kidneys. Extensive experience with the use of paracetamol in neonates for mild to moderate pain relief and for fever treatment has been accumulated over recent years.[56,57] A loading dose of 20 mg/kg followed by 10 mg/kg every 6 hours of intravenous paracetamol is suggested to achieve a compartment concentration of 11 mg/L in late preterm and term neonates. Aiming for the same target concentration, oral doses are similar to rectal administration of 25 to 30 mg/kg/d in preterm neonates of 30 weeks' gestation, 45 mg/kg/d in preterm infants of 34 weeks' gestation, and 60 mg/kg/d in term neonates.[58,59] Overall, these doses are well tolerated in neonates and it has been shown that neonates show less hepatotoxic effects of paracetamol than do older children when administered for a limited time (48–72 hours).[60,61] Furthermore, paracetamol seems to almost lack the adverse effects generally associated with nonsteroidal antiinflammatory drugs in preterm neonates, including peripheral vasoconstriction, gastrointestinal bleeding and perforation, weakened platelet aggregation, hyperbilirubinemia, and renal failure.[44,45,62] However, for PDA treatment, higher dosing regimens were suggested, which have not yet been sufficiently evaluated with regard to pharmacokinetic properties, efficacy, or safety.[63]

Oral Paracetamol

Since the first case report in 2011,[51] there have been many case series of PDA treatment with oral paracetamol in preterm infants. In 6 recent case series a total of 45 infants with different contraindications for the use of ibuprofen or indomethacin, with a reopened (winking) DA, or failed COX-inhibitor treatment, were included.[52,64–68] The patients' GAs ranged from 23 to 37 weeks and birth weight from 620 to 2970 g. Paracetamol 15 mg/kg/dose was administered orally every 6 to 8 hours either as a short course for 48 to 72 hours, or a long treatment of up to 6 or 7 days (if echocardiography showed DA patency). Treatment success (ie, no hsPDA by echocardiography) was seen in 39 of 45 cases (87%). One group found mildly and transiently increased gamma glutamine transferase levels in 3 patients, with most measured paracetamol blood concentrations in the range recommended for pain and fever control (10–20 mg/mL).[69]

In a recent meta-analysis of 2 randomized controlled trials that compared the efficacy of oral paracetamol and oral ibuprofen for hsPDA treatment (N = 250; ≤34 weeks GA), oral paracetamol showed clear short-term benefits versus oral ibuprofen: (1) reduction in supplementary oxygen need (mean, −12.40 days; 95% CI, −22.97 to −1.83) and (2) a lower risk of hyperbilirubinemia (RR, 0.57; 95% CI, 0.34–0.97; NNT, 7).[70–72] In the primary outcome of failure of PDA closure, paracetamol was not inferior to ibuprofen after the first course of treatment, with closure rates ranging from 72.5% to 81.2%. The paracetamol dose used in the 2 included trials was a 15 mg/kg dose every 6 hours for 3 days, which is much higher than is commonly used in extreme preterm neonates. There were no concerns in the results for mortality or common adverse neonatal outcomes. At present, there are at least 3 ongoing trials that should provide additional evidence regarding oral paracetamol use for PDA closure.

Intravenous Paracetamol

To date, no randomized controlled trial regarding the efficacy of intravenous paracetamol for the treatment of hsPDA in preterm neonates has been published. In 8 recent case series, a total of 83 infants with different contraindications to COX inhibitors (53 patients) or previously failed COX-inhibitor treatment (30 patients) were included.[73–80] The patients' GAs ranged between 23 and 34 weeks and birth weight between 365 and 1240 g. Paracetamol was administered intravenously but the dosing schemes and durations of treatment varied among the reports. PDA closure occurred in 40 of 83 patients treated with intravenous paracetamol (48%; range, 0%–100%). However, 3 reports found intravenous paracetamol to be ineffective, with success rates less than 10%.[74–76] Reports used varied time frames and closure criteria when defining response to therapy; no clear adjustment to differentiate whether success was a result of treatment or the result of spontaneous closure was made. In 2 case series, increased liver enzyme levels were reported.[74,77] Paracetamol treatment was stopped in 1 patient because of increased serum transaminase levels. No other acetaminophen-associated adverse effects were reported in any of the other case series. Thirteen patients who did not respond to paracetamol treatment required surgical ligation. Weaknesses of these case series include the single-center, open-label, uncontrolled design in an extremely limited population. Insufficient information was collected to effectively evaluate safety parameters. At present there are 2 trials registered on ClinicalTrials.gov investigating the use of intravenous paracetamol for PDA closure.

The effect of late treatment with intravenous paracetamol on hsPDA closure before possible ligation was recently investigated retrospectively.[81] All infants were unresponsive to ibuprofen; had a contraindication to common drug use; or were beyond 3 weeks of age, at which time ibuprofen is not known to be effective. Thirty-six infants with a median gestation of 26.1 weeks and a median birth weight of 773 g received paracetamol at a dose of 60 mg/kg/d in 4 divided doses at a median age of 27 days. Echocardiography was performed following 3 days of treatment and treatment was continued for an additional 3 days if the PDA remained open. Paracetamol was given for a maximum of 6 days regardless of PDA status. All infants underwent echocardiography after completion of treatment and before hospital discharge. Paracetamol was associated with immediate closure in 9 (25%) infants, none of whom reopened before discharge. There was no response to paracetamol in 4 infants (11%), all of whom subsequently underwent PDA ligation. In the remaining 23 (64%)

infants, the PDA constricted and all but 1 of this group showed complete PDA closure before discharge. There was a high incidence of NEC (31%) and CLD (81%) in survivors. In all but 1 case of NEC, the condition developed before the commencement of paracetamol. Four infants died before discharge at an age ranging between 32 and 50 days postdelivery. The median time between the receipt of paracetamol and death was 23 days. This study is limited by its retrospective nature and the lack of a control group that did not receive paracetamol. The investigators concluded that there may be a role for intravenous paracetamol in late treatment of infants with an hsPDA beyond the second week of life to avoid ligation. In contrast, another report including 20 infants after failed ibuprofen treatment showed a 0% success rate for intravenous paracetamol.[76]

The aforementioned group also retrospectively evaluated the clinical effectiveness of prolonged paracetamol on PDA closure.[82] A total of 21 infants were included in the study from 2 hospitals in Canada and Ireland. At the Canadian site paracetamol was either given orally as a short course (15 mg/kg 6 hourly for 48 hours) or a long course of 15 mg/kg/dose 6 hourly for 7 days. At the Irish site paracetamol was given intravenously, 15 mg/kg/dose 6 hourly for a minimum of 48 hours until PDA closure was confirmed on echocardiography, or up to a maximum of 6 days. In both centers, paracetamol was administered after failure of 2 courses of either ibuprofen or indomethacin or if there were contraindications to medical treatment. No changes in PDA hemodynamics were seen in the 5 infants treated with a short course of paracetamol. In 6 of the 7 infants treated with a long course ibuprofen the PDA closed. In 8 of the 9 infants treated with intravenous paracetamol the PDA closed. The investigators concluded that the efficacy of paracetamol on PDA closure may depend on the duration of treatment and the mode of administration. They also examined the in vitro effect on the murine DA, and showed a concentration-dependent constriction by paracetamol that was less potent than indomethacin-induced ductal constriction.[82]

In conclusion, oral paracetamol seems to be a promising new alternative to PDA therapy in preterm infants when indomethacin or ibuprofen are not effective or contraindicated, and thus may be considered before surgical ligation.[70,83] In view of a recent report in mice of adverse effects of paracetamol on the developing brain, and another report on the association between perinatal use of paracetamol and the development of autism or autism spectrum disorder in childhood, long-term follow-up to at least 18 to 24 months postnatal age must be incorporated in future studies of paracetamol given in the newborn population.[84–86] In addition, a target serum concentration of paracetamol during PDA treatment is unknown, and no toxicity data of high-dose paracetamol in extremely preterm neonates are available. Consequently, dose-seeking studies that also generate pharmacokinetic, pharmacodynamic, and safety data in extremely preterm neonates are needed to guide optimal dosing of paracetamol. Such trials are required before any recommendations for or against the use of paracetamol for closure of the PDA in the preterm newborn population can be made.

SURGICAL LIGATION AND CATHETER INTERVENTION OF HEMODYNAMICALLY SIGNIFICANT PATENT DUCTUS ARTERIOSUS

Surgical PDA ligation can achieve definitive DA closure but has been associated with several side effects and adverse outcomes such as resistant hypotension and hemodynamic disturbances, including a reduction in cerebral blood flow in preterm neonates.[87,88] Prophylactic ligation could not decrease BPD or death rates in premature infants and can, in view of the high spontaneous closure rates[89] and the above-mentioned adverse effects, currently not be recommended.[90] However, ligation might be useful in selected infants with a large hsPDA, who have repeatedly failed pharmacologic treatment and are highly dependent on ventilator support. A recent meta-analysis showed that, compared with medical treatment, surgical ligation was associated with increases in neurodevelopmental impairment, CLD, and high-stage retinopathy of prematurity, but with a reduction in mortality.[91] Whether such an association between PDA ligation and adverse outcomes is just an epiphenomenon in the sickest preterm infants or causally linked is unknown.

It is unclear whether and when infants with small to moderately sized PDAs require treatment. Two retrospective cohort studies showed high spontaneous closure rates in most of the preterm infants who were discharged with persistently patent DAs during the first months of life.[92,93] However, close follow-up of these infants by pediatric cardiologists is mandatory in order to identify patients who require definite DA closure. In these treatment-resistant cases, catheter intervention (which can now be performed in infants weighing 2000 g) provides an alternative to surgical approaches.[94]

SUMMARY

Several therapeutic options and different treatment strategies are available to treat PDA in preterm newborn infants. Besides the established protocols involving indomethacin and ibuprofen, more recent approaches, such as oral ibuprofen, high-dose regimens, and the use of oral and intravenous paracetamol, have recently been applied. Nevertheless, it is still unclear which long-term benefits or harms are achieved by treating PDA. Several further research questions need to be addressed in order to determine which patients require treatment and how treatment protocols should be designed to optimally benefit each patient (**Box 1**).

Box 1
Future directions of research on PDA

Further research and effort are needed on:

The establishment of standardized protocols for the diagnosis PDA and grading its hemodynamic significance

Randomized controlled multicenter trials including nontreated control groups

The natural history of PDA during NICU stay and after discharge

Long-term follow-up data with a special focus on neurodevelopment

Safety and efficacy of high-dose ibuprofen protocols (by mouth/intravenous), especially in extremely immature infants

Pharmacologic data on paracetamol in preterm newborn infants with PDA (pharmacokinetics and safety)

Data on safety and benefits of fluoroscopy or echo-guided catheter interventions compared with surgical treatment of hsPDA

Basic paracrine and cellular mechanisms during initial and permanent DA closure

---

Best practices

What is the current practice?
Persistently patent ductus arteriosus (PDA) of the preterm newborn infant

Currently, it is unclear whether and when a conservative, pharmacological, or surgical approach for PDA closure in premature infants may be advantageous. Furthermore, it is unknown if prophylactic and/or symptomatic PDA therapy will cause substantive improvements in outcome. Whether and when infants with small to moderately sized PDAs require treatment, is unknown, and according decisions are often based on local best practices. Certainly, if the diameter of a PDA is as large as or even larger than the main pulmonary artery on the 2nd day of life, then early pharmacological or surgical treatment should be strongly considered.

Major Recommendations

The current established pharmacological treatment options include:

1. Prophylactic pharmacological treatment or preterm newborn infants at risk for hsPDA with indomethacin (6 – 24 hours after birth)

2. Early pharmacological treatment of asymptomatic preterm newborn infants with PDA with either indomethacin or ibuprofen (< 72 hours after birth)

3. Pharmacological treatment in symptomatic preterm newborn infants with hsPDA with ibuprofen (> 72 hours after birth).

The benefits and caveats of each options are outlined in **Table 1** of this article.

Best Practice/Guideline/Care Path Objective(s)
What changes in current practice are likely to improve outcomes?

Unclear. However, in addition to established pharmacological treatment options, oral ibuprofen, paracetamol (p.o./i.v.), and prolonged and/or high-dose regimens represent new treatment options.

Summary Statement

It is still unclear which long-term benefits or harms are achieved by treating a PDA. Several questions need to be addressed in future studies to determine which patients require treatment at all, and how treatment protocols should be designed to optimally benefit each patient.

REFERENCES

1. Hooper SB, Polglase GR, Roehr CC. Cardiopulmonary changes with aeration of the newborn lung. Paediatr Respir Rev 2015;16(3):147–50 [Meta-analysis or review].

2. Hamrick SE, Hansmann G. Patent ductus arteriosus of the preterm infant. Pediatrics 2010;125:1020–30 [Meta-analysis or review].

3. Antonucci R, Bassareo P, Zaffanello M, et al. Patent ductus arteriosus in the preterm infant: new insights into pathogenesis and clinical management. J Matern Fetal Neonatal Med 2010;23(S3):34–7 [Meta-analysis or review].

4. Weber SC, Rheinlaender C, Sarioglu N, et al. The expression of VEGF and its receptors in the human ductus arteriosus. Pediatr Res 2008;64:340–5.

5. Echtler K, Stark K, Lorenz M, et al. Platelets contribute to postnatal occlusion of the ductus arteriosus. Nat Med 2010;16:75–82.

6. Sallmon H, Weber SC, Hüning B, et al. Thrombocytopenia in the first 24 hours after birth and incidence of patent ductus arteriosus. Pediatrics 2012;130: e623–30.
7. Clyman RI. The role of patent ductus arteriosus and its treatments in the development of bronchopulmonary dysplasia. Semin Perinatol 2013;37:102–7 [Meta-analysis or review].
8. Evans N. Preterm patent ductus arteriosus: a continuing conundrum for the neonatologist? Semin Fetal Neonatal Med 2015;20(4):272–7 [Meta-analysis or review].
9. Heuchan AM, Clyman RI. Managing the patent ductus arteriosus: current treatment options. Arch Dis Child Fetal Neonatal Ed 2014;99:F431–6 [Meta-analysis or review].
10. Clyman RI, Couto J, Murphy GM. Patent ductus arteriosus: are current neonatal treatment options better or worse than no treatment at all? Semin Perinatol 2012; 36:123–9 [Meta-analysis or review].
11. Skelton R, Evans N, Smythe J. A blinded comparison of clinical and echocardiographic evaluation of the preterm infant for patent ductus arteriosus. J Paediatr Child Health 1994;30:406–11.
12. Alagarsamy S, Chhabra M, Gudavalli M, et al. Comparison of clinical criteria with echocardiographic findings in diagnosing PDA in preterm infants. J Perinat Med 2005;33:161–4.
13. Heuchan AM, Young D. Early colour Doppler duct diameter and symptomatic patent ductus arteriosus in a cyclo-oxygenase inhibitor naïve population. Acta Paediatr 2013;102:254–7.
14. Pees C, Walch E, Obladen M, et al. Echocardiography predicts closure of patent ductus arteriosus in response to ibuprofen in infants less than 28 week gestational age. Early Hum Dev 2010;86:503–8.
15. Kluckow M, Evans N. Early echocardiographic prediction of symptomatic patent ductus arteriosus in preterm infants undergoing mechanical ventilation. J Pediatr 1995;127:774–9.
16. El Hajjar M, Vaksmann G, Rakza T, et al. Severity of the ductal shunt: a comparison of different markers. Arch Dis Child Fetal Neonatal Ed 2005;90:F419–22.
17. Kulkarni M, Gokulakrishnan G, Price J, et al. Diagnosing significant PDA using natriuretic peptides in preterm neonates: a systematic review. Pediatrics 2015; 135:e510–25 [Meta-analysis or review].
18. Lemmers PM, Toet MC, van Bel F. Impact of patent ductus arteriosus and subsequent therapy with indomethacin on cerebral oxygenation in preterm infants. Pediatrics 2008;121:142–7.
19. The Vermont-Oxford Trials Network: very low birth weight outcomes for 1990. Investigators of the Vermont-Oxford Trials Network Database Project. Pediatrics 1993;91:540–5.
20. Madan JC, Kendrick D, Hagadorn JI, et al. Patent ductus arteriosus therapy: impact on neonatal and 18-month outcome. Pediatrics 2009;123:674–81.
21. Koch J, Hensley G, Roy L, et al. Prevalence of spontaneous closure of the ductus arteriosus in neonates at a birth weight of 1000 grams or less. Pediatrics 2006; 117:1113–21.
22. Clyman RI. Ibuprofen and patent ductus arteriosus. N Engl J Med 2000;343: 728–30.
23. Kluckow M, Jeffery M, Gill A, et al. A randomised placebo-controlled trial of early treatment of the patent ductus arteriosus. Arch Dis Child Fetal Neonatal Ed 2014; 99:F99–104.

24. Rozé JC, Cambonie G, Marchand-Martin L, et al. Association between early screening for patent ductus arteriosus and in-hospital mortality among extremely preterm infants. JAMA 2015;313:2441–8.
25. Bell EF, Acarregui MJ. Restricted versus liberal water intake for preventing morbidity and mortality in preterm infants. Cochrane Database Syst Rev 2014;(12):CD000503.
26. Fowlie PW, Davis PG, McGuire W. Prophylactic intravenous indomethacin for preventing mortality and morbidity in preterm infants. Cochrane Database Syst Rev 2010;(7):CD000174. [Meta-analysis or review].
27. Alfaleh K, Smyth JA, Roberts RS, et al. Prevention and 18-month outcomes of serious pulmonary hemorrhage in extremely low birth weight infants: results from the trial of indomethacin prophylaxis in preterms. Pediatrics 2008;121: e233–8.
28. Schmidt B, Davis P, Moddemann D, et al. Long-term effects of indomethacin prophylaxis in extremely-low-birth-weight infants. N Engl J Med 2001;344: 1966–72.
29. Ment LR, Vohr BR, Makuch RW, et al. Prevention of intraventricular hemorrhage by indomethacin in male preterm infants. J Pediatr 2004;145:832–4.
30. Ohlsson A, Walia R, Shah SS. Ibuprofen for the treatment of patent ductus arteriosus in preterm or low birth weight (or both) infants. Cochrane Database Syst Rev 2015;(2):CD000174. [Meta-analysis or review].
31. Dani C, Vangi V, Bertini G, et al. High-dose ibuprofen for patent ductus arteriosus in extremely preterm infants: a randomized controlled study. Clin Pharmacol Ther 2012;91:590–6.
32. Meißner U, Chakrabarty R, Topf HG. Improved closure of patent ductus arteriosus with high doses of ibuprofen. Pediatr Cardiol 2012;33:586–90.
33. Hammerman C, Shchors I, Jacobson S, et al. Ibuprofen versus continuous indomethacin in premature neonates with patent ductus arteriosus: is the difference in the mode of administration? Pediatr Res 2008;64:291–7.
34. Lago P, Salvadori S, Opocher F, et al. Continuous infusion of ibuprofen for treatment of patent ductus arteriosus in very low birth weight infants. Neonatology 2014;105:46–54.
35. Lin XZ, Chen HQ, Zheng Z, et al. Therapeutic effect of early administration of oral ibuprofen in very low birth weight infants with patent ductus arteriosus. Chin J Contemp Pediatr 2012;14:502–5.
36. Aly H, Lotfy W, Badrawi N, et al. Oral ibuprofen and ductus arteriosus in premature infants: a randomized pilot study. Am J Perinatol 2007;24:267–70.
37. Chotigeat U, Jirapapa K, Layangkool T. A comparison of oral ibuprofen and intravenous indomethacin for closure of patent ductus arteriosus in preterm infants. J Med Assoc Thai 2003;86(Suppl 3):S563–9.
38. Salama H, Alsisi A, Al-Rifai H, et al. A randomized controlled trial on the use of oral ibuprofen to close patent ductus arteriosus in premature infants. J Neonatal Perinatal Med 2008;1:153–8.
39. Supapannachart S, Limrungsikul A, Khowsathit P. Oral ibuprofen and indomethacin for treatment of patent ductus arteriosus in premature infants: a randomized trial at Ramathibodi Hospital. J Med Assoc Thai 2002;85(Suppl 4):S1252–8.
40. Akisu M, Ozyurek AR, Dorak C, et al. Premature bebeklerde patent duktus arteriozusun tedavisinde enteral ibuprofen ve indometazinin etkinligi ve guvenilirligi. [Enteral ibuprofen versus indomethacin in the treatment of patent ductus arteriosus in preterm newborn infants]. Cocuk Sagligi ve Hastaliklari Dergisi 2001;44: 56–60 [in Turkish].

41. Fakhraee SH, Badiee Z, Mojtahedzadeh S, et al. Comparison of oral ibuprofen and indomethacin therapy for patent ductus arteriosus in preterm infants. Chin J Contemp Pediatr 2007;9:399–403.
42. Pourarian S, Pishva N, Madani A, et al. Comparison of oral ibuprofen and indomethacin on closure of patent ductus arteriosus in preterm infants. East Mediterr Health J 2008;14:360–5.
43. Yadav S, Agarwal S, Maria A, et al. Comparison of oral ibuprofen with oral indomethacin for PDA closure in Indian preterm neonates: a randomized controlled trial. Pediatr Cardiol 2014;35:824–30.
44. Erdeve O, Yurttutan S, Altug N, et al. Oral versus intravenous ibuprofen for patent ductus arteriosus closure: a randomised controlled trial in extremely low birth-weight infants. Arch Dis Child Fetal Neonatal Ed 2012;97:F279–83.
45. Gokmen T, Erdeve O, Altug N, et al. Efficacy and safety of oral versus intravenous ibuprofen in very low birth weight preterm infants with patent ductus arteriosus. J Pediatr 2011;158:549–54.
46. Cherif A, Khrouf N, Jabnoun S, et al. Randomized pilot study comparing oral ibuprofen with intravenous ibuprofen in very low birth weight infants with patent ductus arteriosus. Pediatrics 2008;122:e1256–61.
47. Pistulli E, Hamiti A, Buba S, et al. The association between patent ductus arteriosus and perinatal infection in a group of low birth weight preterm infants. Iran J Pediatr 2014;24:42–8.
48. Guzoglu N, Sari FN, Özdemir R, et al. Renal and mesenteric tissue oxygenation in preterm infants treated with oral ibuprofen. J Matern Fetal Neonatal Med 2014;27: 197–203.
49. Eras Z, Gokmen T, Erdeve O, et al. Impact of oral versus intravenous ibuprofen on neurodevelopmental outcome: a randomized controlled parallel study. Am J Perinatol 2013;30:857–62.
50. Pourarian S, Takmil F, Cheriki S, et al. The effect of oral high-dose ibuprofen on patent ductus arteriosus closure in preterm infants. Am J Perinatol 2015;32(12): 1158–63.
51. Hammerman C, Bin-Nun A, Markovitch E, et al. Ductal closure with paracetamol: a surprising new approach to patent ductus arteriosus treatment. Pediatrics 2011;128:e161821.
52. Oncel MY, Yurttutan S, Uras N, et al. An alternative drug (paracetamol) in the management of patent ductus arteriosus in ibuprofen-resistant or contraindicated preterm infants. Arch Dis Child Fetal Neonatal Ed 2013;98:F94.
53. Cuzzolin L, Antonucci R, Fanos V. Paracetamol (acetaminophen) efficacy and safety in the newborn. Curr Drug Metab 2013;14:178–85 [Meta-analysis or review].
54. Grèen K, Drvota V, Vesterqvist O. Pronounced reduction of in vivo prostacyclin synthesis in humans by acetaminophen (paracetamol). Prostaglandins 1989;37: 311–5.
55. Lucas R, Warner TD, Vojnovic I, et al. Cellular mechanisms of acetaminophen: role of cyclo-oxygenase. FASEB J 2005;19:635–7.
56. Wilson-Smith EM, Morton NS. Survey of I.V. paracetamol (acetaminophen) use in neonates and infants under 1 year of age by UK anesthetists. Paediatr Anaesth 2009;19:329–37.
57. Agrawal S, Fitzsimons JJ, Horn V, et al. Intravenous paracetamol for postoperative analgesia in a 4-day-old term neonate. Pediatr Anaesth 2007;17:70–1.
58. Allegaert K, Murat I, Anderson BJ. Not all intravenous paracetamol formulations are created equal. Paediatr Anaesth 2007;17:811–2.

59. Bartocci M, Lundeberg S. Intravenous paracetamol: the 'Stockholm protocol' for postoperative analgesia of term and preterm neonates. Paediatr Anaesth 2007; 17:1120–1.
60. Jacqz-Aigrain E, Anderson BJ. Pain control: non-steroidal anti-inflammatory agents. Semin Fetal Neonatal Med 2006;11:251–9 [Meta-analysis or review].
61. Allegaert K, Naulaers G. Haemodynamics of intravenous paracetamol in neonates. Eur J Clin Pharmacol 2010;66:855–8.
62. Rheinlaender C, Helfenstein D, Walch E, et al. Total serum bilirubin levels during cyclooxygenase inhibitor treatment for patent ductus arteriosus in preterm infants. Acta Paediatr 2009;98:36–42.
63. Pacifici MG, Allegaert K. Clinical pharmacology of paracetamol in neonates: a review. Curr Ther Res Clin Exp 2015;77:24–30 [Meta-analysis or review].
64. Sinha R, Negi V, Dalal SS. An interesting observation of PDA closure with oral paracetamol in preterm neonates. J Clin Neonatol 2013;2:30–2.
65. Jasani B, Kabra N, Nanavati RN. Oral paracetamol in treatment of closure of patent ductus arteriosus in preterm neonates. J Postgrad Med 2013;59:312–4.
66. Özdemir OM, Dogan M, Kücüktasci K, et al. Paracetamol therapy for patent ductus arteriosus in premature infants: a chance before surgical ligation. Pediatr Cardiol 2014;35:276–9.
67. Nadir E, Kassem E, Foldi S, et al. Paracetamol treatment of patent ductus arteriosus in preterm infants. J Perinatol 2014;34:748–9.
68. Kessel I, Waisman D, Lavie-Nevo K, et al. Paracetamol effectiveness, safety and blood level monitoring during patent ductus arteriosus closure: a case series. J Matern Fetal Neonatal Med 2014;27:1719–21.
69. Arana A, Morton NS, Hansen TG. Treatment with paracetamol in infants. Acta Anaesthesiol Scand 2001;45:20–9.
70. Ohlsson A, Shah PS. Paracetamol (acetaminophen) for patent ductus arteriosus in preterm or low-birth-weight infants. Cochrane Database Syst Rev 2015;(3):CD010061. [Meta-analysis or review].
71. Oncel MY, Yurttutan S, Erdeve O, et al. Oral paracetamol versus oral ibuprofen in the management of patent ductus arteriosus in preterm infants: a randomized controlled trial. J Pediatr 2014;164:510–4.
72. Dang D, Wang D, Zhang C, et al. Comparison of oral paracetamol versus ibuprofen in premature infants with patent ductus arteriosus: a randomized controlled trial. PLoS One 2013;8:e77888.
73. Oncel MY, Yurttutan S, Degirmencioglu H, et al. Intravenous paracetamol treatment in the management of patent ductus arteriosus in extremely low birth weight infants. Neonatology 2013;103:166–9.
74. Alan S, Kahvecioglu D, Erdeve O, et al. Is paracetamol a useful treatment for ibuprofen-resistant patent ductus arteriosus? Neonatology 2013;104:168–9.
75. Roofthooft DW, van Beynum IM, Helbig WA, et al. Paracetamol for ductus arteriosus closure: not always a success story. Neonatology 2013;104:170.
76. Roofthooft DW, van Beynum IM, de Klerk JC, et al. Limited effects of intravenous paracetamol on patent ductus arteriosus in very low birth weight infants with contraindications for ibuprofen or after ibuprofen failure. Eur J Pediatr 2015;174(11): 1433–40.
77. Tekgunduz KS, Ceviz N, Demirelli Y, et al. Intravenous paracetamol for patent ductus arteriosus in premature infants: a lower dose is also effective. Neonatology 2013;104:6–7.
78. Terrin G, Conte F, Scipione A, et al. Efficacy of paracetamol for the treatment of patent ductus arteriosus in preterm neonates. Ital J Pediatr 2014;40:21.

79. Pérez Dominguez ME, Rivero Rodriguez S, Garcia-Munoz Rodrigo F. El paracetamol podria ser útil en el tratamiento del ductus arterioso persistente en el recién nacido de muy bajo peso. An Pediatr (Barc) 2015;82:362–3.

80. Memisoglu A, Alp Ünkar Z, Cetiner N, et al. Ductal closure with intravenous paracetamol: a new approach to patent ductus arteriosus treatment. J Matern Fetal Neonatal Med 2015;16:1–4.

81. El-Khuffash A, James AT, Cleary A, et al. Late medical therapy for patent ductus arteriosus using intravenous paracetamol. Arch Dis Child Fetal Neonatal Ed 2015; 100:F253–6.

82. El-Khuffash A, Jain A, Corcoran D, et al. Efficacy of paracetamol on patent ductus arteriosus closure may be dose dependent: evidence from human and murine studies. Pediatr Res 2014;76:238–44.

83. Le J, Gales MA, Gales BJ. Acetaminophen for patent ductus arteriosus. Ann Pharmacother 2015;49:241–6 [Meta-analysis or review].

84. Viberg H, Eriksson P, Gordh T, et al. Paracetamol (acetaminophen) administration during neonatal brain development affects cognitive function and alters its analgesic and anxiolytic response in adult male mice. Toxicol Sci 2014;138:139–47.

85. Brandlistuen RE, Ystrom E, Nulman I, et al. Prenatal paracetamol (exposure and child neurodevelopment: a sibling-controlled cohort study. Int J Epidemiol 2013; 42:1702–13.

86. Bauer AZ, Kriebel D. Prenatal and perinatal analgesic exposure and autism: an ecological link. Environ Health 2013;12:41.

87. Clyman RI, Wickremasinghe A, Merritt TA, et al. Hypotension following patent ductus arteriosus ligation: the role of adrenal hormones. J Pediatr 2014;164: 1449–55.

88. Lemmers PM, Molenschot MC, Evens J, et al. Is cerebral oxygen supply compromised in preterm infants undergoing surgical closure for patent ductus arteriosus? Arch Dis Child Fetal Neonatal Ed 2010;95:F429–34.

89. Rolland A, Shankar-Aguilera S, Diomandé D, et al. Natural evolution of patent ductus arteriosus in the extremely preterm infant. Arch Dis Child Fetal Neonatal Ed 2015;100:F55–8.

90. Mosalli R, Alfaleh K. Prophylactic surgical ligation of patent ductus arteriosus for prevention of mortality and morbidity in extremely low birth weight infants. Cochrane Database Syst Rev 2008;(1):CD006181. [Meta-analysis or review].

91. Weisz DE, More K, McNamara PJ, et al. PDA ligation and health outcomes: a meta-analysis. Pediatrics 2014;133:e1024–46 [Meta-analysis or review].

92. Herrman K, Bose C, Lewis K, et al. Spontaneous closure of the patent ductus arteriosus in very low birth weight infants following discharge from the neonatal unit. Arch Dis Child Fetal Neonatal Ed 2009;94:F48–50.

93. Weber SC, Weiss K, Buhrer C, et al. Natural history of patent ductus arteriosus in very low birth weight infants after discharge. J Pediatr 2015;167:1149–51.

94. Lam JY, Lopushinsky S, Ma I, et al. Treatment options for the pediatric patent ductus arteriosus: systematic review and meta-analysis. Chest 2015;148(3):784–93 [Meta-analysis or review].

Nutrition in the Cardiac Newborns

Evidence-based Nutrition Guidelines for Cardiac Newborns

Heidi E. Karpen, MD

KEYWORDS

- Congenital heart disease • Neonates • Nutrition • Necrotizing enterocolitis • Growth
- Feeding • Breast milk

KEY POINTS

- Both protein and energy malnutrition are common in neonates and infants with congenital heart disease (CHD).
- Neonates with CHD are at increased risk of developing necrotizing enterocolitis (NEC), particularly the preterm population.
- Mortality in patients with CHD and NEC is higher than for either disease process alone.
- Standardized feeding protocols may affect both incidence of NEC and growth failure in infants with CHD.
- The roles of human milk and probiotics have not yet been explored in this patient population.

NUTRITIONAL REQUIREMENTS IN NEONATES WITH CONGENITAL HEART DISEASE

In the simplest terms, malnutrition is result of inadequate energy intake or an increase in energy expenditure, resulting in an energy imbalance. Studies of critically ill children have estimated that energy requirements may increase by 30% for mild to moderate stress and up to 50% in severe stress.[1] Suboptimal nutrition during periods of critical illness, resulting in energy and protein deficits, has been associated with poor clinical outcomes in both pediatric and adult populations.[2] Poor nutrition exacerbates the stress-induced catabolic responses during surgery or severe illness and has been associated with poor wound healing, myocardial dysfunction, impaired vascular

Disclosure: None.
Department of Pediatrics, Emory University School of Medicine, 2015 Uppergate Drive Northeast, Atlanta, GA 30322, USA
E-mail address: hkarpen@emory.edu

Clin Perinatol 43 (2016) 131–145
http://dx.doi.org/10.1016/j.clp.2015.11.009   perinatology.theclinics.com

endothelial integrity, reduced muscle function, and an increased risk of postoperative pneumonia.[3]

These deficits often compound throughout the course of an illness and are difficult to overcome.[4,5] Children are particularly disadvantaged by malnutrition during periods of critical illness and surgery because of the concomitant metabolic requirements for growth, cognitive development, and motor development. Within this population, neonates represent a uniquely vulnerable subset, because the first 12 months of life are a period of critical growth and development that often portends lifelong consequences. Growth failure in infancy has been correlated with long-term cognitive deficiencies such as attention deficit disorder, aggressive behavior, and poor social and emotional development.[6-8]

Most infants born with congenital heart disease (CHD) are of normal weight for gestational age at birth but develop nutritional and growth deficiencies during the first few months of life. Both cardiac and extracardiac factors contribute to the development of malnutrition in infants with CHD. Sources of increased metabolic demand in CHD include increase in resting oxygen consumption, left-to-right shunts increasing cardiac workload, increased pulmonary pressures, and increased catecholamine secretion.[9] Associated genetic conditions such as Down syndrome, DiGeorge syndrome, Turner syndrome, and trisomies 13 and 18, in particular, may also influence energy intake, gastrointestinal absorption, expenditure, and growth expectations.

Abnormalities in the use of nutritional resources also play a role in malnutrition of patients with CHD. The hormonal stress response and the therapeutic administration of catecholamines in the perioperative period shift metabolism toward fatty acid oxidation and impaired carbohydrate use.[10] Increased resting energy expenditure (REE) in patients with CHD has been directly associated with increased inflammation and higher cardiac output and inversely associated with antiinflammatory strategies.[11]

Patients with both single-ventricle and biventricle repairs in the neonatal period have persistently low weight for age z-scores at 3 months of age, primarily because of a lack of fat mass (FM). This lack of FM, as opposed to fat-free mass, most likely stems from insufficient energy intake necessary to support a state of positive energy balance, which is needed to increase fat stores.

PROTEIN STUDIES IN SICK/PRETERM NEONATES

Critical illness, including CHD and surgical conditions, leads to increased protein catabolism and turnover. A constant flow of amino acids is necessary for the synthesis of new proteins and for tissue repair and growth. The goals of nutrition in critically ill patients are to provide sufficient dietary protein to enable adequate new protein synthesis, facilitate wound healing, modulate inflammatory responses, and preserve skeletal muscle mass.

In addition to poor caloric intake, critically ill infants and children are predisposed to the effects of accumulating negative nitrogen balance and protein malnutrition, with these deficits exacerbated in the preterm population (**Fig. 1**).[5] A study of critically ill, mechanically ventilated infants showed a significant association between the adequacy of enteral protein intake and 60-day mortality that was independent of the enteral energy adequacy.[12]

In infants with CHD, the prevalence of acute and chronic protein energy malnutrition has been documented in nearly half of the patients, with only 68% of energy and 40% of protein requirements met on day of life (DOL) 7, despite an "evidence-based feeding protocol" and the daily presence of a nutritionist on rounds.[13] There are disparate data regarding the amount of protein and energy intake needed to produce anabolism in

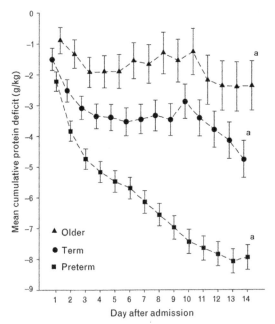

Fig. 1. Mean cumulative protein deficits for preterm neonates. All values expressed as mean ± standard error of the mean; data were analyzed using analysis of variance. [a] Cumulative protein deficits on day 14 were significantly different between all age groups. The graph has previously been published in Ref.[4] (*From* Hulst JM, Joosten KF, Tibboel D, et al. Causes and consequences of inadequate substrate supply to pediatric ICU patients. Curr Opin Clin Nutr Metab Care 2006;9(3):299; with permission.)

critically ill patients. One study documented anabolism with more than 58 kcal/kg/day and more than 1.5 g/kg/day of protein; however, these patients were intubated, sedated, and many were under muscle blockade, which significantly decreases REE,[14] is not applicable to spontaneously breathing children, and does not account for the increased demands placed by CHD.

At present, there are no precise clinical indicators or biomarkers to accurately assess REE, and indirect calorimetry is not feasible in many units. The most recent American Society for Parenteral and Enteral Nutrition (ASPEN) Clinical Guidelines for Nutrition in the Critically Ill Child set the protein requirements at 2 to 3 g/kg/d for infants 0 to 2 years of age. Preterm infants have even greater protein requirements at 3.5 to 4 g/kg/d to meet their needs and promote growth during this critical period.[15,16]

NECROTIZING ENTEROCOLITIS IN CARDIAC NEWBORNS

Necrotizing enterocolitis (NEC) is the most common surgical emergency among premature neonates but is generally a rare event in term infants without CHD. Congenital heart defects are often associated with cyanosis, decreased cardiac output, or pulmonary overcirculation/congestive heart failure, often in combination. Each of these risk factors has been independently associated with the genesis of bowel ischemia.[17] In contrast with the preterm population, in which NEC typically develops at 2 to 4 weeks of age, term infants with CHD are most likely to develop NEC in the first 7 days of life, although disease localization to the terminal small bowel does not seem to differ between the two groups.[18] As with the preterm population, NEC in term infants with CHD is likely a multifactorial disease.

Hypoplastic left heart syndrome (HLHS), total anomalous pulmonary venous return, truncus arteriosus, tetralogy of Fallot, patent ductus arteriosus, and secundum atrial septal defects have all been associated with the development of NEC, although the risk associated with any one lesion has been difficult to accurately establish. The risk of NEC, however, appears to be highest in those with cyanotic or single ventricle physiology, particularly HLHS, with an incidence reported between 11% and 20%. Diastolic flow reversal in the superior mesenteric artery is common before and immediately after the stage I palliation for a Norwood and may be associated with an increased risk of NEC.[19–21] In a study by Miller and colleagues,[22] patients who developed NEC had a lower abdominal aorta pulsatility index compared with those without NEC on both stage I preoperative and postoperative echocardiograms, despite similar ventricular function and operative risk. The investigators postulated that patients with HLHS may have abnormalities in their systemic vasculature placing them at increased risk of NEC.

Roles for low cardiac output, diastolic runoff from shunts, and aggressive postoperative feeding regimens have all been implicated in the genesis of NEC. NEC in patients with HLHS is associated with a high risk of mortality that approaches 40%, and has been reported as high as 71% in those with cyanotic CHD.[23] Several studies have shown some improvement in survival between stage I and II surgical palliation by implementing a home monitoring system of daily weights and oxygen saturations, although this approach has not been validated in a larger trial.[24]

Concern for NEC and its consequences makes many clinicians uneasy about initiating feeds in patients on prostaglandins, with low cardiac output, cyanosis, or shunts. Delay in feeding, however, may actually increase the risk and severity of NEC.[25] Lack of enteral feeding leads to the rapid atrophy of the intestinal mucosa with loss of critical barrier function. Exposure to antibiotics alters gut flora, replacing normal commensal organisms with potentially pathogenic bacterial strains.[26] Minimal enteral nutrition (MEN), typically defined as 10 to 20 mL/kg/d, aids in intestinal mucosa development and maturation of its associated immune system[25] and has been associated with a decreased incidence of NEC in this population.

NECROTIZING ENTEROCOLITIS IN PRETERM NEONATES WITH CONGENITAL HEART DISEASE

Preterm infants with CHD represent a uniquely vulnerable population with regard to NEC. Fisher and colleagues[17] performed a large prospective VON (Vermont Oxford Network) database review of 235,643 infants, 1931 of whom had CHD (0.8%). Of those infants with CHD, 13% developed NEC compared with 9% NEC in those without CHD (adjusted odds ratio [AOR], 1.8). Concordant with the literature on NEC in preterm infants, NEC in neonates without CHD was associated with younger mean gestational age, lower mean birth weight, and lower mean Apgar scores. In comparison, infants with CHD involving low systemic output (AOR, 1.79), cyanotic defects (AOR, 1.82), and lesions producing pulmonary overcirculation (AOR, 2.36) had increased odds of developing NEC. As with preterm infants without CHD, there was a nearly linear inverse relationship between birth weight and incidence of NEC (**Fig. 2**). In addition, there was an increased incidence of NEC in patients with CHD compared with those without CHD at each weight grouping. When examining NEC rates by diagnosis in the very low birth weight (VLBW) population, atrioventricular canal defect, with or without

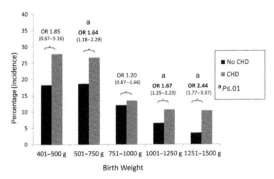

Fig. 2. Incidence of NEC without and with CHD by birth weight category. Values in parentheses are 95% confidence intervals. [a] $P \leq .01$. OR, adjusted odds ratio. (*From* Fisher JG, Bairdain S, Sparks EA, et al. Serious congenital heart disease and necrotizing enterocolitis in very low birth weight neonates. J Am Coll Surg 2015;220(6):1021.e14; with permission.)

trisomy 21, was the only lesion with NEC incidence greater than the baseline rate for infants with CHD.

Similar to data in term neonates, preterm infants with a spectrum of cardiac lesions seem to have a higher risk of developing NEC than age-matched/weight-matched premature infants without CHD. In addition, the combination of CHD and NEC portends a higher mortality than either disease alone in this population. Mortality in infants with NEC and CHD was significantly higher overall (55%) compared with both those infants with NEC without CHD (28%; AOR, 4.14) and CHD without NEC (34%; AOR, 2.58). Unlike the typical trend in mortality for VLBW neonates with NEC without CHD, which decreases with increasing birth weight, the mortality in those with NEC and CHD was independent of birth weight (**Fig. 3**).

As with NEC in the non-CHD preterm population, this is likely a multifactorial disease process. Immaturity in barrier function, immune defense mechanisms, disordered motility, digestion, and absorption has been well described in preterm neonates.[25] Poor control of circulatory regulation may be exacerbated with CHD lesions and place preterm infants at substantially increased risk of intestinal injury.[27]

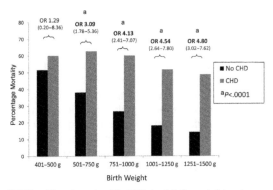

Fig. 3. Mortality of NEC without and with CHD by birth weight category. [a] $P<.0001$. (*From* Fisher JG, Bairdain S, Sparks EA, et al. Serious congenital heart disease and necrotizing enterocolitis in very low birth weight neonates. J Am Coll Surg 2015;220(6):1022.e14; with permission.)

STANDARDIZED FEEDING PROTOCOLS

Because of the concern for feeding intolerance and NEC, many clinicians are uncomfortable feeding patients with CHD preoperatively while on prostaglandins, although there is scant evidence to support or refute this practice. Many of these patients are gravely ill, requiring prolonged mechanical ventilation and vasoactive infusions, and have indwelling umbilical or central catheters. Surgical repair often requires cardiopulmonary bypass and deep hypothermic circulatory arrest. Postoperatively, it is common for these patients to have an open sternotomy for some time and experience extracardiac complications such as respiratory failure, chylothorax, renal failure, and neurologic impairment. These issues compound the concern for enteral feeding, and because there are few data associating feeding practices and outcomes in these patients, this leads to anecdotal and institution-based practices on the initiation and advancement of feeding.

Several studies have documented frequent feeding interruptions in these patients, many for routine procedures such as cardiac catheterization, imaging studies such as MRI or echocardiograms, planned extubations, and placement of chest tubes or central lines. Feedings are often withheld for clinical deterioration and for gastrointestinal issues such as abdominal distention, bilious residuals, and bloody/guaiac positive stools.[28] Fluid restriction has also been documented as a major limiting factor in achieving adequate nutritional intake in these patients and is the primary driver for the need for increased caloric density of feeds.[29]

These issues are not substantially different from those encountered when examining feeding issues in preterm infants or patients with short bowel syndrome (SBS) and underscore the need for evidence-based feeding protocols in this patient population. This issue can be divided into 2 main compartments: standardized feeding protocols and defining clear, medically sound reasons for withholding or discontinuing feeds. The preterm literature has well-documented evidence for the benefits of gut priming with MEN, and this likely holds significant benefit in this patient population both in the preoperative and immediate postoperative periods, even during times of clinical instability.

A study from Schwalbe-Terilli and colleagues[28] examined the outcomes of their feeding regimen in infants with CHD. Their practice was to typically advance feeds slowly over a period of 48 to 72 hours to a volume of 100 mL/kg/d then increasing caloric density to 24 to 27 kcal/oz with a goal of 120 to 150 mL/kg/d. These feeds were initiated via the bolus nasogastric route before attempting oral feeding. Results of their feeding regimen showed that a caloric intake of 100 kcal/kg was achieved on 48.4% of feeding days and 120 kcal/kg was achieved in only 19.7% of feeding days. They reported a median weight change in this group of −20 g, which was likely affected by their practice of discontinuing parenteral nutrition (PN) at 100 mL/kg/d of enteral nutrition or when the central venous line was removed.[28]

Boston Children's examined the effect of implementation of a standardized feeding regimen plan. Before initiation of the feeding plan, they found that many feeding interruptions lacked a clear and uniform definition of feeding intolerance, and were associated with prolonged feeding lapses surrounding routine procedures and mechanical problems with feeding tubes. After initiation of their feeding regimen, they achieved a significant decrease in the number of avoidable episodes of enteral nutrition interruption (3 vs 51; $P<.0001$), decreased the median time to reach energy goal from 4 days to 1 day ($P<.0001$), and a higher proportion of patients reached this goal (99% vs 61%; $P = .01$).[30] Standardized feeding protocols in preterm populations have been well documented to decrease the incidence of NEC or death, decrease episodes of sepsis, and shorten length of stay.[31,32] A standard approach to feeding initiation, advancement, and caloric goals, with clear definitions for feeding intolerance and limitations of feeding interruptions, and close assessment of growth and nutritional parameters is likely to substantially benefit this group of patients. Many institutions have developed their own feeding protocols.[33,34] Some key points to such an approach are outlined here.

Standardized feeding regimen:

PN

- Begin PN (preferably central) on DOL 1 with 2 g/kg/d of protein and at least 1 g/kg/d fat
- Advance PN daily to reach goals:
  - Glucose infusion rate 12 to 14 mg/kg/h
  - Protein: 3 g/kg/d protein in term infants and 4 g/kg/d in preterm
  - Fat: 2 to 3 g/kg/d in both preterm and term
  - Calories: 100 to 130 kcal/kg/d term, 120 to 140 kcal/kg/d preterm
- Use birth weight for the first 7 days of age to prevent inappropriate weigh loss (>10% in term infants, >15% in preterms)
- If patient is edematous, use a dry weight, which can be estimated by using the appropriate weight for length or the 50th percentile
- Use concentrated glucose solutions for drip medications such as pressors
- Concentrate PN substrates (glucose, amino acids, electrolytes) as much as feasible to decrease fluid intake

Enteral nutrition

- Begin MEN at 10 to 20 mL/kg/d, ideally via bolus gravity, with breast milk or 20 cal/oz formula
- Consider use of a formula enriched in medium chain triglycerides if there is chylothorax
- MEN has been shown to be well tolerated even in patients on prostaglandins and with shunts
- MEN is typically not included in the caloric goals, which may be up to 145 kcal/kg/d in patients with CHD
- Although rapid advancement in caloric density has been associated with favorable weight gain, the risk of NEC may be increased, particularly in the preterm population
- Advancements in feeds are typically 20 mL/kg/d in preterm infants and 20 to 30 mL/kg/d in term infants
- Monitor for feeding intolerance (abdominal distention, bilious residuals, and bloody stools)
- Hold feeds at 100 mL/kg/d while increasing caloric density stepwise to 24 to 27 kcal/oz before advancing to full volume (typically 150–170 mL/kg/d, but may be less if fluid restricted)
- Consider fortification to 24 kcal/oz at 60 mL/kg/d if using human milk–based fortifier
- Wean PN stepwise to maintain overall daily caloric intake of 120 to 130 kcal/kg/d and goal protein and fat intake outlined earlier
- Discontinue PN only after achieving full volume/caloric density of feeds
- Follow weight gain closely and consider increasing to 30 kcal/oz if required to achieve adequate growth
- Plot weekly weight, length, and head circumference to assess adequacy of nutritional intake

- Follow blood urea nitrogen, albumin, prealbumin, calcium, phosphorus and alkaline phosphatase levels as markers of nutritional status

BREAST MILK STUDIES

Breast milk is considered the ideal source of nutrition for all infants. Human milk feeding has been associated with a greatly reduced incidence of NEC,[35] gastroenteritis,[36] otitis media, respiratory illnesses,[37] and allergic and autoimmune disease[38] and is recommended as the exclusive diet for infants less than 6 months of age. Despite overwhelming evidence supporting the benefits of human milk, there have been no studies on the benefits of a human milk diet on outcomes in infants with CHD. Some barriers to providing human milk to these infants are separation of mother and infant after delivery, stress of having a sick infant, lack of lactation support, and clinician opinion.

Admission to an intensive care unit has been shown to affect initiation of pumping, volume of milk pumped per day, and rates of breastfeeding at discharge. A recent study from the Children's Hospital of Philadelphia examined these issues in their cardiac intensive care unit. Rates of pumping and initiation of pumping were higher among mothers whose babies were inborn (96%) versus mothers who were separated from their infants after birth because of transport to a tertiary care center (67%).[39] A large study from Norway, where 84% of healthy infants receive predominantly breast milk at 1 month of age, showed that infants with CHD were fed with breast milk less frequently than healthy controls from the second to the sixth month of life and that this percentage decreased even further if there were comorbid conditions in addition to CHD.[40]

The impact of an exclusive human milk diet in the preterm population has been well documented. Multiple randomized studies of formula feeding or human milk supplemented with cow milk–based fortifier versus an exclusive human milk diet, which includes the use of donor human milk and donor milk–based fortifier, have shown a significant reduction in the incidence of NEC.[35,41] One case of NEC could be prevented if 10 infants received an exclusive human milk diet, and 1 case of NEC requiring surgery or resulting in death could be prevented if 8 infants received an exclusive human milk diet.[41]

To date, however, there have been no clinical trials assessing the impact of a predominantly human milk diet on key outcomes such as feeding tolerance, time to full enteral nutrition, NEC, episodes of sepsis, chylothorax, and death in patients with CHD. Donor human milk is a limited and expensive resource and most hospitals have protocols for the use of human milk/human milk–based fortifier, which typically limit the use of these products to infants of 1500 g and 34 weeks' gestational age. There is a clear opportunity for studies examining the impact of an exclusive human milk diet on medical outcomes as well as quality improvement initiatives to increase rates of pumping and breastfeeding in patients with CHD.

INTESTINAL MICROBIOTA AND PROBIOTICS

Examination of the role of the fecal microbiota in the genesis and propagation of NEC has become an area of intense interest in the past decade. Numerous studies in the preterm population have associated alterations in gut immunity and intestinal microbial dysbiosis, colonization of the neonatal intestine with pathogenic bacteria that differ markedly from the flora in a healthy term newborn, with the development of NEC.[42–44] A recent Cochrane Review examined high-quality data from 24 randomized trials involving more than 5000 preterm infants, assessing the efficacy of probiotics in the prevention of NEC and/or death.[45] The conclusion of this meta-analysis was that there was sufficient evidence in the preterm population to change practice regarding the routine administration of probiotics for the prevention of NEC.

Probiotics are postulated to affect the development of NEC through a variety of mechanisms, including promotion of growth of commensal organisms, rebalancing of the inflammatory cascade promoting the secretion of antiinflammatory cytokines and decreasing production of inflammatory cytokines, competitive inhibition of pathogen adhesion receptor–binding sites, modulation of cellular apoptosis, and proliferation via induction of genes such as transforming growth factor beta, as well as induction of innate immune, hormonal, and neuroendocrine responses.[46]

Although babies with CHD lesions, such as left-sided obstructive lesions and severe left-to-right shunts, are at increased risk of developing NEC, some investigators think that this is a consequence of bowel ischemia and does not involve a primary inflammatory process that characterizes typical NEC.[47] Although hypoperfusion is postulated to be the inciting event driving the development of NEC in infants with CHD, the process is still likely multifactorial with contributions from broad-spectrum antibiotics, altered intestinal flora, indwelling feeding tubes, and central lines. Vascular dysregulation of the mesenteric bed has also been documented in these infants[48] and potentiate changes in gut permeability, barrier function, and inflammation. CHD is associated with a systemic inflammatory response both preoperatively and postoperatively, which is increased in patients undergoing cardiopulmonary bypass.[49]

To date, there are scant data on the intestinal microbiota of infants with CHD compared with healthy babies, and no large-scale, randomized controlled trials of probiotics in neonates with CHD has been undertaken. A small study from Turkey[50] compared outcomes in patients given a symbiotic preparation (*Bifidobacterium lactis* plus inulin) versus placebo in 100 patients with CHD. They showed a reduction in nosocomial sepsis, NEC, and death. Although these results are promising and may hold physiologic plausibility, the data are currently insufficient to mandate a change in practice. Probiotics are not licensed by regulatory authorities in many countries, including the United States, hence the wide variation in the potency and source of bacteria/yeast. Because these products are readily available to the public, and are likely to leak into practice by either clinicians or parents, a well-designed trial examining the safety, efficacy, and mechanisms of action of probiotics would be of great interest.

POSTDISCHARGE NUTRITION AND GROWTH

After discharge, growth failure in infants with CHD is a complex problem with contributions from a variety of issues (**Fig. 4**). These physical limitations are common features in infants with CHD and likely contribute to inadequate energy intake with resultant poor weight gain and linear growth.[51] Multiple studies have documented a high rate of growth failure at hospital discharge following neonatal surgery for infants with both single-ventricle and biventricle physiology.[52,53]

Schwalbe-Terilli and colleagues[28] evaluated the postoperative enteral caloric intake in 100 neonates following cardiac surgery. The patient groups were separated into biventricular cardiac defects (n = 52) and functional single ventricle (n = 48). It was the practice in this center not to feed infants on prostaglandins or with umbilical arterial catheters. A goal of 100 kcal/kg/d was achieved for 48.4% of patient days and 120 kcal/kg for only 19.7% of patient days during the period of enteral feeding after neonatal cardiac surgery, leading to a median weight loss overall for the group.[28] Similarly disturbing results were found in a study by Natarajan and colleagues,[54] with nearly a third of infants discharged at less than their birth weight despite increased caloric density feeds (24–30 cal/oz) in 70% of patients at discharge.

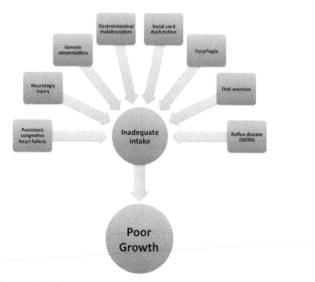

Fig. 4. Causes of growth failure in neonates/infants with CHD. GERD, gastroesophageal reflux disease.

Although surgical repair of CHD lesions in the neonatal period usually results in improved weight within a few months, longitudinal growth and head circumference often lag for a year or more. REE is usually normalized by 3 months of age and is comparable with healthy, age-matched infants so much of this growth delay is attributable to severe nutritional deficits accrued in the presurgical and postsurgical periods.[55,56]

Clearly these studies, along with many others, underscore the critical need for close attention to the intake and growth in these patients. Given the unique nutritional needs of these patients, clinicians must tailor the caloric goals and feeding strategies to the individual patient. Close attention to progress on age-appropriate growth charts is the best method for determining adequacy of nutritional interventions.

NEED FOR GAVAGE FEEDING AT DISCHARGE

A variety of factors have been associated with risk of poor rates of oral feeding at discharge in patients with CHD, including vocal cord injury, duration of postoperative intubation, weight at time of surgery, use of transesophageal echocardiography, and prematurity.[57,58] Kogon and colleagues[59] found that 44.6% infants with CHD required feeding tubes at discharge for an inability to transition or a delay in the transition to oral feeds. Prolonged intubation and a higher risk-adjusted congenital heart surgery score were associated with increased risk of adverse feeding outcomes.[59] Note that risk factors typically associated with poor feeding, such as gestational age, weight, specific cardiac lesion, intubation at the time of surgery, requirement for and length of cardiopulmonary bypass, use of transesophageal echocardiography, and surgical proximity to the aortic arch were not found to have an effect on postoperative feeding in this study. Other studies have shown a correlation between infants who died or developed feeding morbidities in those with ductal-dependent lesions, specifically hypoplastic left heart, and those infants requiring prostaglandins or cardiopulmonary bypass, despite feeds being initiated while on prostaglandins preoperatively.[54] Despite a more favorable feeding outcome in those with early initiation and achievement of feeds, a significant percentage continued to require gavage feeds at discharge, with approximately 20% of all patients with HLHS received gastrostomy (GT) tubes before discharge.[33,60]

Several sites have examined the effect of preemptive placement of GT tubes in infants with serious CHD, particularly those undergoing Norwood procedure. A retrospective review of preemptive GT placement in patients with HLHS and related disorders showed improved survival to stage 2 after a Norwood operation, but GT placement was not associated with shorter hospitalization or improved growth.[61]

The rate of poor postnatal growth, with discharge at less than birth weight, and feeding difficulties remains abysmal despite advances in neonatal/cardiac intensive care.

Clearly evidence-based strategies for feeding initiation, advancement, caloric goals, and feeding method are critical for improving outcomes in this very-high-risk population.

Best practices

What is the current practice?

There are few published data regarding nutritional guidelines and feeding protocols in neonates with CHD. Current practice on feeding preoperatively, especially while on prostaglandin infusions, and advancement of feeding postoperatively varies widely by center.

Best practice objective: improve the nutritional status of neonates/infants with CHD while minimizing risk of NEC.

What changes in current practice are likely to improve outcomes?

Any standardized feeding protocol that includes clear definitions for feeding intolerance, acceptable reasons for withholding of feeds, minimization of interruptions for routine procedures, and clear caloric goals with frequent growth assessment is likely to improve care overall.

Is there a Clinical Algorithm?

Major recommendations

- Detailed nutritional guidelines are discussed earlier
- Begin MEN at 10 to 20 mL/kg/d, ideally on DOL 1
- Prostaglandin infusions and presence of umbilical lines are not contraindications to MEN
- Encourage and support mothers in breastfeeding/pumping
- Use human milk whenever possible; consider use of donor breast milk if available/feasible
- Monitor feeding tolerance and advance feeds slowly
- Closely monitor growth parameters and adjust caloric goals accordingly

Rating for the strength of the evidence: grade III; mostly nonrandomized cohort studies with contemporaneous controls.

Summary statement

Malnutrition is common in neonates/infants with CHD and has significant impacts on morbidity, mortality, and neurologic outcome. The substantially higher risk of NEC in this patient population presents increased nutritional challenges. Clear feeding protocols and caloric goals, with frequent assessments of growth, are key to improving outcomes.

REFERENCES

1. Skillman HE, Mehta NM. Nutrition therapy in the critically ill child. Curr Opin Crit Care 2012;18(2):192–8.
2. Mikhailov TA, Kuhn EM, Manzi J, et al. Early enteral nutrition is associated with lower mortality in critically ill children. JPEN J Parenter Enteral Nutr 2014;38(4): 459–66.
3. Agus MSD, Jaksic T. Nutritional support of the critically ill child. Curr Opin Pediatr 2002;14(4):470–81.
4. Hulst JM, Joosten KF, Tibboel D, et al. Causes and consequences of inadequate substrate supply to pediatric ICU patients. Curr Opin Clin Nutr Metab Care 2006; 9(3):297–303.
5. Hulst J, Joosten K, Zimmermann L, et al. Malnutrition in critically ill children: from admission to 6 months after discharge. Clin Nutr 2004;23(2):223–32.
6. Black MM, Dubowitz H, Krishnakumar A, et al. Early intervention and recovery among children with failure to thrive: follow-up at age 8. Pediatrics 2007;120(1): 59–69.
7. Dykman RA, Casey PH, Ackerman PT, et al. Behavioral and cognitive status in school-aged children with a history of failure to thrive during early childhood. Clin Pediatr (Phila) 2001;40(2):63–70.
8. Neubauer V, Griesmaier E, Pehböck-Walser N, et al. Poor postnatal head growth in very preterm infants is associated with impaired neurodevelopment outcome. Acta Paediatr 2013;102(9):883–8.
9. Radman M, Mack R, Barnoya J, et al. The effect of preoperative nutritional status on postoperative outcomes in children undergoing surgery for congenital heart defects in San Francisco (UCSF) and Guatemala City (UNICAR). J Thorac Cardiovasc Surg 2014;147(1):442–50.
10. Gebara BM, Gelmini M, Sarnaik A. Oxygen consumption, energy expenditure, and substrate utilization after cardiac surgery in children. Crit Care Med 1992; 20(11):1550–4.
11. Floh AA, Nakada M, La Rotta G, et al. Systemic inflammation increases energy expenditure following pediatric cardiopulmonary bypass. Pediatr Crit Care Med 2015;16(4):343–51.
12. Mehta NM, Bechard LJ, Zurakowski D, et al. Adequate enteral protein intake is inversely associated with 60-d mortality in critically ill children: a multicenter, prospective, cohort study. Am J Clin Nutr 2015;102(1):199–206.
13. Toole BJ, Toole LE, Kyle UG, et al. Perioperative nutritional support and malnutrition in infants and children with congenital heart disease. Congenit Heart Dis 2014;9(1):15–25.
14. Jotterand Chaparro C, Laure Depeyre J, Longchamp D, et al. How much protein and energy are needed to equilibrate nitrogen and energy balances in ventilated critically ill children? Clin Nutr 2015. http://dx.doi.org/10.1016/j.clnu.2015.03.015.
15. Mehta NM, Compher C, ASPEN Board of Directors. A.S.P.E.N. Clinical Guidelines: nutrition support of the critically ill child. JPEN J Parenter Enteral Nutr 2009;33(3):260–76.
16. Wong JJM, Cheifetz IM, Ong C, et al. Nutrition support for children undergoing congenital heart surgeries: a narrative review. World J Pediatr Congenit Heart Surg 2015;6(3):443–54.
17. Fisher JG, Bairdain S, Sparks EA, et al. Serious congenital heart disease and necrotizing enterocolitis in very low birth weight neonates. J Am Coll Surg 2015;220(6):1018–26.e14.

18. Cozzi C, Aldrink J, Nicol K, et al. Intestinal location of necrotizing enterocolitis among infants with congenital heart disease. J Perinatol 2013;33(10):783–5.
19. Harrison AM, Davis S, Reid JR, et al. Neonates with hypoplastic left heart syndrome have ultrasound evidence of abnormal superior mesenteric artery perfusion before and after modified Norwood procedure. Pediatr Crit Care Med 2005;6(4):445–7.
20. McElhinney DB, Hedrick HL, Bush DM, et al. Necrotizing enterocolitis in neonates with congenital heart disease: risk factors and outcomes. Pediatrics 2000;106(5): 1080–7.
21. Mukherjee D, Zhang Y, Chang DC, et al. Outcomes analysis of necrotizing enterocolitis within 11 958 neonates undergoing cardiac surgical procedures. Arch Surg 2010;145(4):389–92.
22. Miller TA, Minich LL, Lambert LM, et al. Abnormal abdominal aorta hemodynamics are associated with necrotizing enterocolitis in infants with hypoplastic left heart syndrome. Pediatr Cardiol 2014;35(4):616–21.
23. Cheng W, Leung MP, Tam PK. Surgical intervention in necrotizing enterocolitis in neonates with symptomatic congenital heart disease. Pediatr Surg Int 1999;15(7): 492–5.
24. Golbus JR, Wojcik BM, Charpie JR, et al. Feeding complications in hypoplastic left heart syndrome after the Norwood procedure: a systematic review of the literature. Pediatr Cardiol 2011;32(4):539–52.
25. Neu J, Walker WA. Necrotizing enterocolitis. N Engl J Med 2011;364(3):255–64.
26. Alexander VN, Northrup V, Bizzarro MJ. Antibiotic exposure in the newborn intensive care unit and the risk of necrotizing enterocolitis. J Pediatr 2011;159(3): 392–7.
27. Stapleton GE, Eble BK, Dickerson HA, et al. Mesenteric oxygen desaturation in an infant with congenital heart disease and necrotizing enterocolitis. Tex Heart Inst J 2007;34(4):442.
28. Schwalbe-Terilli CR, Hartman DH, Nagle ML, et al. Enteral feeding and caloric intake in neonates after cardiac surgery. Am J Crit Care 2009;18(1):52–7.
29. Rogers EJ, Gilbertson HR, Heine RG, et al. Barriers to adequate nutrition in critically ill children. Nutrition 2003;19(10):865–8.
30. Hamilton S, McAleer DM, Ariagno K, et al. A stepwise enteral nutrition algorithm for critically ill children helps achieve nutrient delivery goals*. Pediatr Crit Care Med 2014;15(7):583–9.
31. Patole SK. Impact of standardised feeding regimens on incidence of neonatal necrotising enterocolitis: a systematic review and meta-analysis of observational studies. Arch Dis Child Fetal Neonatal Ed 2005;90(2):F147–51.
32. McCallie KR, Lee HC, Mayer O, et al. Improved outcomes with a standardized feeding protocol for very low birth weight infants. J Perinatol 2011;31(Suppl 1): S61–7.
33. Toms R, Jackson KW, Dabal RJ, et al. Preoperative trophic feeds in neonates with hypoplastic left heart syndrome. Congenit Heart Dis 2015;10(1):36–42.
34. del Castillo SL, McCulley ME, Khemani RG, et al. Reducing the incidence of necrotizing enterocolitis in neonates with hypoplastic left heart syndrome with the introduction of an enteral feed protocol. Pediatr Crit Care Med 2010;11(3): 373–7.
35. Quigley M, McGuire W. Formula versus donor breast milk for feeding preterm or low birth weight infants. Cochrane Database Syst Rev 2014;(4):CD002971.
36. Ballard O, Morrow AL. Human milk composition: nutrients and bioactive factors. Pediatr Clin North Am 2013;60(1):49–74.

37. Jakaitis BM, Denning PW. Human breast milk and the gastrointestinal innate immune system. Clin Perinatol 2014;41(2):423–35.
38. Section on Breastfeeding. Breastfeeding and the use of human milk. Pediatrics 2012;129(3):e827–41.
39. Torowicz DL, Seelhorst A, Froh EB, et al. Human milk and breastfeeding outcomes in infants with congenital heart disease. Breastfeed Med 2015;10(1):31–7.
40. Tandberg BS, Ystrom E, Vollrath ME, et al. Feeding infants with CHD with breast milk: Norwegian Mother and Child Cohort Study. Acta Paediatr 2010;99(3):373–8.
41. Sullivan S, Schanler RJ, Kim JH, et al. An exclusively human milk-based diet is associated with a lower rate of necrotizing enterocolitis than a diet of human milk and bovine milk-based products. J Pediatr 2010;156(4):562–7.e1.
42. Neu J, Mshvildadze M, Mai V. A roadmap for understanding and preventing necrotizing enterocolitis. Curr Gastroenterol Rep 2008;10(5):450–7.
43. Wang Y, Hoenig JD, Malin KJ, et al. 16S rRNA gene-based analysis of fecal microbiota from preterm infants with and without necrotizing enterocolitis. ISME J 2009;3(8):944–54.
44. Gritz EC, Bhandari V. The human neonatal gut microbiome: a brief review. Front Pediatr 2015;3:17.
45. AlFaleh K, Anabrees J. Probiotics for prevention of necrotizing enterocolitis in preterm infants. Evid Based Child Health 2014;9(3):584–671.
46. Ellis CL, Rutledge JC, Underwood MA. Intestinal microbiota and blue baby syndrome: probiotic therapy for term neonates with cyanotic congenital heart disease. Gut Microbes 2010;1(6):359–66.
47. Neu J. Probiotics and necrotizing enterocolitis. Clin Perinatol 2014;41(4):967–78.
48. DeWitt AG, Charpie JR, Donohue JE, et al. Splanchnic near-infrared spectroscopy and risk of necrotizing enterocolitis after neonatal heart surgery. Pediatr Cardiol 2014;35(7):1286–94.
49. Giannone PJ, Luce WA, Nankervis CA, et al. Necrotizing enterocolitis in neonates with congenital heart disease. Life Sci 2008;82(7–8):341–7.
50. Dilli D, Aydin B, Zenciroğlu A, et al. Treatment outcomes of infants with cyanotic congenital heart disease treated with synbiotics. Pediatrics 2013;132(4):e932–8.
51. Trabulsi JC, Irving SY, Papas MA, et al. Total energy expenditure of infants with congenital heart disease who have undergone surgical intervention. Pediatr Cardiol 2015. http://dx.doi.org/10.1007/s00246-015-1216-3.
52. Anderson JB, Marino BS, Irving SY, et al. Poor post-operative growth in infants with two-ventricle physiology. Cardiol Young 2011;21(4):421–9.
53. Medoff-Cooper B, Irving SY, Marino BS, et al. Weight change in infants with a functionally univentricular heart: from surgical intervention to hospital discharge. Cardiol Young 2011;21(2):136–44.
54. Natarajan G, Reddy Anne S, Aggarwal S. Enteral feeding of neonates with congenital heart disease. Neonatology 2010;98(4):330–6.
55. Nydegger A, Bines JE. Energy metabolism in infants with congenital heart disease. Nutrition 2006;22(7–8):697–704.
56. Irving SY, Medoff-Cooper B, Stouffer NO, et al. Resting energy expenditure at 3 months of age following neonatal surgery for congenital heart disease. Congenit Heart Dis 2013;8(4):343–51.
57. Einarson KD, Arthur HM. Predictors of oral feeding difficulty in cardiac surgical infants. Pediatr Nurs 2003;29(4):315–9.
58. Kohr LM, Dargan M, Hague A, et al. The incidence of dysphagia in pediatric patients after open heart procedures with transesophageal echocardiography. Ann Thorac Surg 2003;76(5):1450–6.

59. Kogon BE, Ramaswamy V, Todd K, et al. Feeding difficulty in newborns following congenital heart surgery. Congenit Heart Dis 2007;2(5):332–7.
60. Jeffries HE, Wells WJ, Starnes VA, et al. Gastrointestinal morbidity after Norwood palliation for hypoplastic left heart syndrome. Ann Thorac Surg 2006;81(3):982–7.
61. Garcia X, Jaquiss RDB, Imamura M, et al. Preemptive gastrostomy tube placement after Norwood operation. J Pediatr 2011;159(4):602–7.e1.

Developmental Care Rounds

An Interdisciplinary Approach to Support Developmentally Appropriate Care of Infants Born with Complex Congenital Heart Disease

Amy Jo Lisanti, PhD, RN, CCNS[a], Jeanne Cribben, MSOT[a],
Erin McManus Connock, MA[a], Rachelle Lessen, MS, RD[a],
Barbara Medoff-Cooper, PhD, RN[b],*

KEYWORDS

- Developmental care • Congenital heart disease • Infant • Rounds

KEY POINTS

- Infants born with complex congenital heart disease can benefit from developmentally supportive care practices before and after cardiac surgery.
- Developmental care is a safe and feasible practice in cardiac intensive care units.
- Interdisciplinary developmental care rounds can be used to promote cultural change in cardiac intensive care units to support developmental care practices.

INTRODUCTION

Progress in neonatal cardiothoracic surgery has increased survival for infants with complex congenital heart disease (CHD). For most newborn infants admitted to the cardiac intensive care unit (CICU), palliative or corrective surgery is performed during the first week of life. During the infant's postoperative period, their care is often complicated by an open chest incision, multiple indwelling devices, significant levels of opioids, and/or restraints. This complex scenario makes it almost impossible to provide routine, normal newborn infant care. In neonatal intensive care, with predominately preterm infants, the balance between highly specialized medical care and normal newborn care has been addressed within a developmental care framework.

Disclosures: None.
[a] Children's Hospital of Philadelphia, 3401 Civic Center Boulevard, Philadelphia, PA 19104, USA;
[b] University of Pennsylvania, School of Nursing, 418 Curie Boulevard, Claire Fagin Hall, Philadelphia, PA 19104, USA
* Corresponding author.
E-mail address: medoff@nursing.upenn.edu

The developmental care framework is based on a maturation paradigm with the assumption that premature infants will show increasing behavioral organizational skills over time. The developmental care framework is composed of a broad category of interventions designed to minimize the stress of an intensive care environment[1] with the goal to provide a structured care environment that supports, encourages, and guides the developmental organization of critically ill infants. Developmental care recognizes the physical, psychological, and emotional vulnerabilities of critically ill infants and their families. The focus is on minimizing potential short-term and long-term complications associated with the intensive care environment.[2] The objectives of developmental care interventions are to reduce neurodevelopmental delay, poor weight gain, length of hospital stay, length of mechanical ventilation, and physiologic stress, and increase parental involvement in care.[3,4]

Recent MRI studies have reported evidence of brain dysmaturation in infants with CHD before surgery, which highlights the influence of nonphysiologic conditions on in-utero brain development.[5] Furthermore, long-term developmental outcomes for these infants are similar those of infants born prematurely, including executive function challenges; academic struggles; behavioral issues, including hyperactivity; and other delays with speech, fine motor, and gross motor skills.[6] Given these findings, the developmental care paradigm seems to be appropriate for infants with complex CHD requiring neonatal medical care.

COMPONENTS OF DEVELOPMENTAL CARE
Infant Care

The practice of development care has evolved over recent decades with the overarching primary goal of improving short-term neurodevelopmental outcomes. Recognition of the physiologic impact of environmental noise and frequent stimuli has been the impetus for environmental modifications in a critical care setting.[7] Although there are many definitions of developmental care, Lubbe and colleagues[8] describe 7 categories that include knowledge of infant development, individualization of care, positioning, handling techniques, feeding methods, management of pain, and management of external environments. Individualized care is based on the relationships between an infant and caregiver (health care professionals or parents) and must be a central tenet of all aspects of care.[9] Caregiving approaches must be flexible and responsive to an infant's cues and behaviors communicated during interactions. The overall goal is to create an environment that supports infant behavioral organization. Some basic principles of caregiving are described in **Table 1**.

Table 1 Basic principles of caregiving	
Positioning	Infant in a contained flexed position with firm boundaries; neck neutral, shoulders protracted
Holding and skin-to-skin holding	Encourage holding whenever safe; skin-to-skin options provided to both parents
Clustering care	Provides periods of rest, decreases infant stress during procedures
Nonpharmacologic pain management	Strategies to decrease pain, such as pacifiers, sucrose dips, position containment during procedures
Environmental management	Cycled light and dark periods, decreasing surrounding noise levels
Feeding	Cue-based feeding

Family-centered Care

Developmental care cannot be implemented without a family-centered focus. The goal of family-centered care is to encourage parents to develop care skills within the context of parenting their infants. Inclusion of parents in daily caregiving has been shown to reduce maternal stress and increase self-esteem.[10] Coughlin and colleagues[2] described 3 core care measures for ensuring that family needs are addressed. These measures include providing opportunities to be actively involved in their infant's care whenever possible, assessing a family's level of emotional status with documentation and access to resources, and providing support that assists in parental well-being.

INTERDISCIPLINARY DEVELOPMENTAL CARE ROUNDS

In our center, the developmental care framework was introduced into the CICU by a clinical nurse specialist (CNS), who led a nursing developmental care committee, spearheaded unit-wide education, and initiated nursing developmental care rounds (DCR). This project to stimulate cultural change in the CICU has been described previously.[11] In order to promote the continuation of developmental care practices, our unit has continued weekly DCR and has expanded participation to an interdisciplinary team. The rounding team includes a CNS, occupational therapist (OT), speech-language pathologist (SLP), international board-certified lactation consultant (IBCLC), and nurse scientist. Each member of the team brings a unique perspective and expertise, allowing a holistic approach during rounds with each family. Patients in the CICU are screened each week for inclusion in DCR. Inclusion criteria include infants born with CHD (6 months of age or less) who are not undergoing end-of-life care. Goals for DCR include:

1. Promoting developmental care practices in the CICU for all infants born with CHD.
2. Educating parents and families on the various components of developmental care and which aspects they are able to participate in based on their infant's current clinical condition in the CICU.
3. Enhancing individualized care through interdisciplinary discussion at the infant's bedside with the nurse and family.

Clinical Nurse Specialist Role

The role of the CNS during DCR is to serve as the leader for rounds and ensure a well-rounded, consistent approach. Before approaching an infant's family for rounds, the CNS consults with the patient's bedside nurse to screen for appropriateness. Families are excluded from rounds if it is determined that the infant's condition is too critical for a developmental conversation with the family or if the family is overwhelmed with meeting many other care teams or consult services.

The CNS approaches the family and asks whether they would like to participate in DCR. Rounds are described to families as an informal discussion in which the team meets the family to talk about the infant's development. Most families voice their interest in participating and appreciate the opportunity to discuss the nonmedical issues and aspects of their parenting experience thus far. Once permission is granted, the CNS invites the rest of the rounding team to the patient's bedside. The bedside nurse is encouraged to join the team for DCR as well.

The CNS has each member of the team introduce themselves to the family. Families are asked to tell the team about their infant. Although the parents are sharing their story and their infant's story, the team is able to assess the family's learning needs, any knowledge deficits, or topics that should be further discussed. Typical parent-centered subject matter addressed during rounds includes timing of diagnosis; type of delivery; where delivery occurred; recovery from labor and delivery; initiation of lactation; and parents' sleep, eating habits, and stress. Infant-centered issues that the team discusses on rounds include behavior state, organization, self-comforting behaviors, pain, positioning, feeding, holding, and environmental stimulation. The CNS also screens for any nursing care issues, such as thermoregulation, hemody-namic assessment, nutritional status, day/night cycling, and skin care, including risk for pressure injury, diaper dermatitis, and wound management. Discussions at the bedside are tailored to the individual needs of the infant and family. Areas of improve-ment are addressed and plans of care initiated with the family and the bedside nurse. The CNS collaborates and communicates any recommendations for changes in the patient's plan of care with the front-line ordering clinician as well as the attending physician responsible for the care of the patient.

Nurse Scientist Role

As a researcher with expertise in infancy, developmental outcomes, and developmental care of the newborn, the nurse scientist serves as a mentor to the CNS and a resource during DCR. As the developmental care initiative has progressed from exclusively nursing participation to an interdisciplinary group, the nurse scientist has worked closely with the CNS to enhance the scope of developmental care in the CICU. On a weekly ba-sis, the nurse scientist identifies the infants and families who are eligible to be included in weekly rounds. The list of patients is communicated to the team, allowing team mem-bers time to consult with their colleagues and identify any potential issues that need to be addressed on DCR. This task allows clinicians to become familiar with the families on the unit before beginning the bedside rounds with the parents and the bedside nurse. Once DCR begins, the nurse scientist assists the team in addressing normal newborn concerns that families often have. The nurse scientist also assumes leadership respon-sibility for developmental rounds when the CNS is not available.

Occupational Therapist Role

The OT serves as the representative for both occupational and physical therapies. In our institution, infants who are developmentally equal to or less than 3 months of age receive a primary therapist from occupational therapy or physical therapy, unless comorbidities exist that indicate both services are needed. The OT on DCR serves as a liaison to the primary therapist assigned to the infant and communicates any specific questions that the family verbalizes on rounds regarding their infant's plan of care as well as any recommendations made by the team at the infant's bedside dur-ing rounds. In this way, DCR assist in streamlining communication between the pa-tient's family and the primary therapist.

If OT and physical therapist consults have not yet been ordered, the team requests that these orders be placed. The OT explains the role of the primary therapist, high-lighting the components of development and developmental care addressed by the primary therapist. These components typically include assessing the infant's state control, behavioral organization, movement patterns in available positions (depending on timing of surgery), range of motion, muscle tone, and reflexes, all within the context of the critical care environment and the infant's current condition. The OT uses parent-friendly language to explain these concepts. For example, the OT discusses state con-trol by telling parents, "Your infant's therapist will note how your infant moves back and forth between being asleep, awake, or upset. Does she do this quickly or slowly? What is her energy like when moving between these states?" The OT explains the concept of behavioral organization in terms of baby coping skills, explaining that the primary therapist watches for cues indicating whether their infant is ready to interact, already trying to hold themselves together, or overwhelmed (**Table 2**). For musculoskeletal components of the evaluation, the OT explains that the primary therapist assesses how the infant moves independently, how the infant's joints move when the therapist moves them, and whether the muscles feel stiff, tight, or floppy. Treatment plans are based on the strengths and weaknesses identified during the evaluation process as well as what the family identifies as priorities.

The OT assures the family that the primary therapist will educate them about expected developmental progression as the infant recovers from surgery. This progression includes demonstration of good state and behavioral organization skills, visual and social engagement, and foundational fine and gross motor skills (eg, head control and belly time). The OT reinforces that the goal of the primary therapist is to help families maximize their infant's developmental potential within the constraints of the infant's postoperative course.

In addition, the OT informs families that their primary therapist will review postoperative handling and holding techniques that will maximize the safety of their infant's healing sternum without sacrificing family bonding opportunities or developmental potential. Families are told they will also receive training from the primary therapist on scar massage, which will be performed after the incision has healed at approximately 6 weeks postsurgery. Because scar massage often occurs postdischarge, families enjoy learning about a skill that they can use in the future, providing a sense of hopefulness in the midst of a stressful situation.

The position of the infant at the time of rounds is routinely addressed during DCR. The OT comments when an infant is positioned well, identifies the components that make the positioning adequate (eg, midline orientation, alignment of limbs, use of boundaries, tucked posture), and explains why the infant should be positioned in this manner (eg, to provide and support appropriate musculoskeletal alignment, promote self-regulatory behaviors, lay the foundation for future fine and gross motor milestones). Infants who are positioned improperly are repositioned in partnership with the bedside nurse. However, infants who may be sleeping are not disturbed. The team creates a repositioning plan with the bedside nurse according to the infant's schedule and often the CNS returns to the bedside after rounds to provide assistance as needed. Families with infants showing poorly organized behaviors are given strategies for touch, containment, bundling, and boundary supports. Positioning suggestions are provided for infants showing gravity-dependent postures or postural preferences. The OT may also suggest environmental changes to address positioning concerns. For example, alternating the infant's position in the crib between the head

Table 2	
Examples of infant cues as explained to families	
Infant's Readiness Level	**Sample Cues**
1. Ready	Stable vital signs Calm, relaxed face or body Eye contact (depending on age)
2. Coping	Bringing hands to face or cheek Grasping a finger or blanket edge
3. Overwhelmed	"Stop" sign with hand Arching away Becoming limp

and foot of the crib addresses head preferences while still accommodating medical equipment and devices like ventilators and infusion pumps.

In addition, the OT introduces a component of discharge planning during rounds. Some families are aware of the developmental risks associated with CHD and the potential for long-term neurodevelopmental issues. Families are assured that developmental support can continue after the infant's hospitalization. Their primary therapist will assist with the transition to home and discuss community-based options for developmental services depending on their infant's particular needs. Options include follow-up in our cardiac neurodevelopmental clinic, early intervention services, Early Head Start programs, and outpatient services, if needed.

Speech-Language Pathologist Role

The SLP's role in the DCR team is focused on the feeding and swallowing skills of infants. During rounds, the SLP reviews the infant's oral feeding experiences and feeding readiness skills. Some infants may never have had the opportunity to feed orally. Other infants may have been orally fed preoperatively but are not ready to resume oral feeding. Some infants may currently be orally feeding.

Required prefeeding skills are discussed, including the ability to maintain an awake and alert state, the ability to maintain a stable cardiorespiratory status at rest, good secretion management, and the demonstration of adequate feeding cues. When infants are orally feeding, the SLP counsels families on feeding readiness cues, including rooting, bringing hands to mouth, and sucking on a pacifier. When infants are not orally feeding, the SLP identifies those that are good candidates for trialing pleasant, nonnutritive, oral stimulation. For mothers of infants who are candidates for oral stimulation and who wish to breastfeed, the SLP discusses potential oral stimulation strategies during rounds. Infants may practice nonnutritive sucking at the breast following pumping. Infants may also be able to tolerate single tastes of expressed breast milk or formula dipped on a pacifier.

The family is encouraged to share their preference for breastfeeding or bottle-feeding for their infant. The SLP shares common feeding issues with infants diagnosed with CHD, including fatigue, need for supplementing oral feeding with tube feeding, and the possibility of swallowing difficulties. The SLP encourages families to focus on the quality of the oral feeding experience rather than the quantity of intake, as measured by the infant staying calm, organized, and swallowing safely.

The SLP also uses rounds as a forum to discuss the role of the SLP consult in the CICU. Speech consults are indicated when parents or the medical team are having concerns about the baby's oral feeding skills or swallowing safety. If the infant is already being followed for speech therapy, the specific feeding issues, goals, and plan of care are discussed. The SLP reinforces that the goal is to help promote successful, safe, and efficient oral feeding skills.

Lactation Role

Lactation care in our institution is provided by an IBCLC. An IBCLC is a health care professional who specializes in the clinical management of breastfeeding and is certified by the International Board of Lactation Consultant Examiners. They are knowledgeable about the latest evidence-based practices in lactation, are experienced in a wide variety of complex breastfeeding situations, and are competent to assist mothers with establishing and sustaining breastfeeding even in difficult and high-risk situations while being sensitive to the needs of the mothers and infants to help mothers reach their goals.

Mothers of infants with CHD often plan to breastfeed and have many questions and concerns about how their child's cardiac surgery and hospital admission will affect their breastfeeding goals. It is essential that these mothers receive adequate support and information so that they will be successful in achieving their personal goals. Each week during DCR, the lactation consultant listens to the mother's concerns related to her breastfeeding experience in the CICU. There are challenges that are unique for mothers of infants with CHD. The postpartum period can be exhausting and overwhelming for any new mother but a mother of an infant hospitalized in the CICU has additional stress and anxiety related to the infant's diagnosis and care. Mothers may need gentle reminders regarding the importance of adequate nutrition and fluid intake along with sufficient rest to help with milk production.

Mothers are often eager to hold their infants and start breastfeeding. During DCR, the lactation consultant assures the mother that not only is it good for the mother to hold her infant but it is important for the infant's growth and development to be held skin to skin. The team assesses the infant's eligibility for holding based on the infant's lines and medical devices. The lactation consultant encourages the mother to request assistance from the infant's nurse and CNS, who can assist the mother in safely holding her infant skin to skin.

However, not every mother desires to breastfeed. The lactation consultant supports the mother's decision and encourages her to consider pumping so that the infant may be given breast milk via a bottle during the infant's hospitalization. This method allows the infant to receive the beneficial immune factors and nutrients that are present only in colostrum and breast milk. Pumping is essential for mothers to establish and maintain milk production. The lactation consultant listens carefully to any concerns the mother is having related to pumping milk for her infant. Mothers are instructed to pump every 2 to 3 hours during the day and at least once between 10 PM and 3 AM, when prolactin levels are highest. The lactation consultant encourages mothers to record their milk production at each pumping and also to tally their total daily volumes in log books provided to ensure sufficient milk for their infants' needs. Mothers often request for the lactation consult to review their pumping log during DCR. Milk production is typically low for the first few days of life. It is critical to assure mothers that even drops of colostrum are often adequate.

If an infant's feeding advance is greater than the mother's milk production, supplementation may be necessary. Parents have a choice of pasteurized donor milk or infant formula. An information sheet and a consent form for use of donor milk are given to the families and all questions are answered so that families can make an informed decision. Pasteurized donor milk is encouraged because of the risks associated with formula use.[12,13]

One concern that mothers often express during rounds is the inability to know the volume their infant is receiving during breastfeeding. Support is provided for mothers who desire to directly breastfeed rather than pump and bottle-feed. There is evidence that bottle-feeding is physiologically more stressful than breastfeeding, resulting in increased oxygen desaturation during feeding.[14] Use of an electronic scale for before and after feeding weights is encouraged to measure intake at the breast. During rounds, if an infant is approaching discharge, the lactation consultant encourages the mother to be present for as many of the infant's feedings as possible, including staying overnight for nighttime feedings. This approach increases a mother's confidence in her ability to successfully breastfeed, giving her increased familiarity with her infant's feeding patterns and behaviors. If unable to transfer adequate volumes at each feeding, the infant goes home with a feeding tube. Parents are instructed on the use of the tube and the mother's breast milk is used to supplement feedings at the breast. The lactation consultant assists the family in obtaining a breast pump for home. If necessary, a scale can also be rented for home use to continue before and after weights after discharge. The lactation consultant continues to follow the mother until discharge and addresses any other concerns or issues, such as breast engorgement, nipple pain, or low milk supply.

BARRIERS TO IMPLEMENTING DEVELOPMENTAL CARE

Although developmental care practices can be integrated into the care model within CICUs, barriers exist that must be addressed (**Table 3**). Staff may perceive developmental care practice as superfluous rather than essential. Time and effort in care are focused on the physiologic needs of the infant rather than the developmental needs. Culture change can be supported by education and weekly interdisciplinary DCR.

CASE EXAMPLE
Developmental Care Rounds: Week 1

Baby Boy L was a full-term infant prenatally diagnosed with hypoplastic left heart syndrome. At birth, he was admitted to the CICU for stabilization and evaluation for cardiac surgery. At 2 days of age, the DCR team visited the patient and family. The goal of this first DCR visit was to introduce team members, explain developmental care, and to hear about the birth and the family's immediate concerns related to the infant's diagnosis and upcoming surgery. The infant's mother verbalized her desire to breastfeed. The team confirmed that she was pumping at least 8 times a day and encouraged her to continue pumping even though she should not expect to produce much milk for another day or two. The mother was relieved to learn this because she was feeling frustrated about pumping and not producing more than a few drops of breast milk. The nurse reported that Baby Boy L was sleepy and not feeding well. The team assisted the mother to hold her baby skin to skin, which Baby Boy L tolerated without difficulty. The team explained that the sleepiness observed was normal infant behavior in the first few days of life. Nonnutritive sucking was also recommended to support Baby Boy L during procedures, ranging from diaper changes to echocardiograms.

Developmental Care Rounds: Week 2

After surgery, Baby Boy L had a cardiac arrest and was placed on extracorporeal membrane oxygenation (ECMO), sedated, and paralyzed. The family was devastated. The team focused on positive activities that they could do during this difficult time both for the infant and for themselves. Parents were encouraged to eat regular meals and to take breaks from the bedside to get fresh air. The mother's pumping, milk production, and equipment needs were reviewed. The family and bedside nurse were reminded to provide mouth care to Baby Boy L using the mother's colostrum so that the risk for infection could be reduced during this critical period. Positioning suggestions were

Table 3	
Barriers to implementing developmental care in the CICU	
Barrier	**Reason**
Nursing time	Nursing care time often directed toward physiologic needs
Resources	• Infrequent educational programs to enhance nurses knowledge of developmental care • Lack of developmental care experts to mentor at the bedside with staff
Culture	Perception that developmental care is not the greatest priority for the patient, especially for the most critically ill infants
Infant acuity	Infant may not tolerate repositioning
Parental anxiety	Parents are overwhelmed and afraid to participate in care

made to support the infant's head in midline and to align and orient the extremities toward midline using supportive devices, repositioning at least every 2 hours to reduce the risk of skin breakdown.

Developmental Care Rounds: Week 3

By week 3, Baby Boy L was able to be taken off ECMO, extubated, and slowly weaned off most of the continuous infusions. After extubation, the infant began to adopt an arched position in the crib, especially when irritable. During rounds, the DCR team supported the nurse to position the infant to reduce the arching and cervical extension. The infant's side-lying position was adjusted to side lying diagonally across an elevated head of bed, using gravity to promote a neutral head and spinal position. A bean bag support was placed between his legs to maintain alignment of hips, knees, and ankles, and his hands were placed together at midchest level. Baby Boy L had transitioned to bolus feeds via nasogastric tube and was showing feeding readiness cues at feed times, including waking, rooting, and sucking on his pacifier. Therefore, he was permitted to attempt breastfeeding. He was able to latch and engage in feeding for several minutes before becoming drowsy. Baby Boy L's mother did not report any signs concerning for swallowing dysfunction during feeds. Oral feeding was being supplemented via nasogastric tube. The team educated the mother on the importance of using the nasogastric tube for nutrition when Baby Boy L was showing disengagement cues. The mother was encouraged to be present for as many of his feedings as possible and to do skin to skin when he was too sleepy to breastfeed. Support and guidance were given regarding continued pumping to ensure adequate milk production for nasogastric feeds.

SUMMARY

Family-centered developmental care is an essential component of care for high-risk infants and is appropriate for this population of infants born with complex CHD. Weekly interdisciplinary DCR have been successfully integrated into CICU. In combination with other developmental care efforts and education, interdisciplinary DCR can provide additional support to enhance developmental care practices for infants with complex CHD.

Best practices

What is the current practice?

The current practice in our unit is for developmental rounds to take place once a week. The goal is for bedside nurses and families to implement principles of developmental care throughout the week.

What changes in current practice are likely to improve outcomes?

The consistent use of developmental care practices would enhance infants' neurodevelopmental organization.

With increased organization, infant feeding skills, response to stress, and family bonding may improve.

Summary statement

Developmental care can be safely implemented in CICUs caring for medically fragile newborn infants with CHD.

Interdisciplinary developmental rounds enhance individualization in care for infants and families.

REFERENCES

1. Als H. Neurobehavioral organization of the newborn: opportunity for assessment and intervention. NIDA Res Monogr 1991;114:106–16.
2. Coughlan MT, Gibbin S, Hoath S. Core measures for developmentally supportive care in neonatal intensive care units: theory, precedence and practice. J Adv Nurs 2009;65(10):2239–48.
3. Symington A, Pinelli J. Developmental care for promoting development and preventing morbidity in preterm infants. Cochrane Database Syst Rev 2006;2: CD001814.
4. McGrath JM, Conliffe-Torres S. Integrating family-centered developmental assessment and intervention into routine care in the neonatal intensive care unit. Nurs Clin North Am 1996;31(2):367–86.
5. Counsell SJ. New imaging approaches to evaluate newborn brain injury and their role in predicting developmental disorders. Curr Opin Neurol 2014;27(2):168–75.
6. Wernovsky G. Current insights regarding neurological and developmental abnormalities in children and young adults with complex congenital cardiac disease. Cardiol Young 2006;16(Suppl 1):92–104.
7. Browne JV. Developmental care for high-risk newborns: emerging science, clinical application, and continuity from newborn intensive care unit to community. Clin Perinatol 2011;38(4):719–29.
8. Lubbe W, Van de Walt C, Klopper H. Integrative literature review defining evidenced-based neurodevelopmental supportive care of the preterm infant. J Perinat Neonatal Nurs 2012;26(3):251–8.
9. Lawhon G. Providing developmentally supportive care in the newborn intensive care unit: an evolving challenge. Journal of Perinatal & Neonatal Nursing 1997; 19(4):48–61.
10. Galarza-Winton M, Dicky T, O'Leary L, et al. Implementing family-integrated care in the NICU. Adv Neonatal Care 2013;13(5):335–40.
11. Torowicz D, Lisanti AJ, Rim J-S, et al. A developmental care framework for a cardiac intensive care unit: a paradigm shift. Adv Neonatal Care 2012;12(5): 28–32.
12. Arnold L. The cost-effectiveness of using banked donor milk in the neonatal intensive care unit: prevention of necrotizing enterocolitis. J Hum Lact 2002;18(2): 172–6.
13. McGuire W, Anthony M. Donor human milk versus formula for preventing necrotising enterocolitis in preterm infants: systematic review. Arch Dis Child Fetal Neonatal Ed 2003;88:F11–4.
14. Marino BL, O'Brien P, LoRe H. Oxygen saturations during breast and bottle feedings in infants with congenital heart disease. J Pediatr Nurs 1995;10(6):360–4.

Management of the Preterm Infant with Congenital Heart Disease

David M. Axelrod, MD[a],*, Valerie Y. Chock, MD[b],
V. Mohan Reddy, MD[c]

KEYWORDS

- Prematurity • Low birth weight • Congenital heart disease • Congenital heart surgery
- Cardiopulmonary bypass • Neonate

KEY POINTS

- Premature neonates are more likely to be born with congenital heart disease (CHD), and neonates with CHD are more likely to be born premature.
- Prematurity imparts significant morbidity and mortality risk in the neonate with CHD.
- Premature neonates with CHD may encounter hemodynamic instability during fetal transition as well as in the perioperative period.
- Management of premature neonates with CHD requires the collaboration of highly specialized providers from multiple disciplines.

INTRODUCTION

Premature newborns with CHD require unique considerations for optimal management. Despite obstetric advances and improvements in antenatal care, the rate of preterm delivery in the United States has increased in the past 20 years, and premature neonates have a more than 2-fold higher risk of cardiovascular abnormalities.[1,2] As antenatal diagnosis of CHD improves and fetal interventions expand, preterm infants with CHD will be a growing population.

The authors have nothing to disclose.
The authors have no financial conflicts to report and have no funding to report for this article.
[a] Division of Pediatric Cardiology, Department of Pediatrics, Stanford University Medical Center, 750 Welch Road, Suite 321, Palo Alto, CA 94304, USA; [b] Division of Neonatology, Department of Pediatrics, Stanford University Medical Center, 750 Welch Road, Suite 315, MC 5731, Palo Alto, CA 94304, USA; [c] Pediatric Cardiothoracic Surgery, University of California San Francisco Medical Center, 550 16th Street, Floor 5, MH5-745, San Francisco, CA 94143-0117, USA
* Corresponding author.
E-mail address: daxelrod@stanford.edu

0095-5108/16/$ – see front matter © 2016 Elsevier Inc. All rights reserved.

The standard definitions of prematurity and low birth weight (LBW) are described in **Table 1**. Infants may be LBW (due to prematurity alone) or small for gestational age (SGA). Cardiovascular abnormalities are associated with SGA[2–4] and a 2-fold risk of prematurity (<37 weeks' gestational age [GA][2]). Furthermore, congenital anomalies or genetic or chromosomal abnormalities are frequently associated with both CHD and intrauterine growth restriction.[5] Both gestational age and birth weight are important factors with regard to timing of delivery and timing of surgical repair.

TIMING OF DELIVERY AND OBSTETRIC CONSIDERATIONS

Although preterm delivery of infants with CHD may be indicated due to maternal or fetal issues, many cases of known CHD are scheduled to deliver at term gestation to facilitate coordination of care. The notion that all term babies with CHD have equivalent outcomes, however, was recently challenged by a large study of the Society of Thoracic Surgeons Congenital Heart Surgery Database.[6] This study found that outcomes were worse for neonates born at 37 to 38 weeks' gestation compared with those born at 39.5 weeks' gestation. These early-term infants had higher in-hospital mortality (adjusted odds ratio for mortality of 1.34 [1.05–1.71]), more postoperative complications, and prolonged length of stay. Other studies have confirmed a higher mortality rate[7,8] and greater resource utilization[9] with delivery of CHD infants at 39 to 40 weeks' gestation. Furthermore, Goff and colleagues[10] found that adjusted neurodevelopmental outcomes at age 4 years were significantly improved for infants with CHD born between 39 and 40 weeks' gestation compared with those born between 36 and 38 weeks' gestation. Delayed brain maturation by up to 1 month in infants with CHD has been demonstrated by fetal and postnatal MRI[11–13] and may contribute to the poorer neurodevelopment seen in even late preterm infants or early-term infants compared with those born at 39 to 40 weeks' gestation.

American College of Obstetricians and Gynecologists guidelines recommend a gestational age of at least 39 weeks for all elective deliveries, even in infants without CHD,[14] due to the increased risk for mortality and morbidity.[15] Therefore, unless obstetric or fetal concerns, such as preterm premature rupture of membranes, oligohydramnios, preeclampsia, hydrops, placental abnormalities, or nonreassuring fetal status exist, then elective delivery for infants with CHD ideally should be targeted for 39 to 40 weeks' gestation. Antenatal care coordination should include relocation of expectant mothers (at approximately 37 weeks' gestation) near a facility with specialized pediatric cardiac care to avoid unexpected spontaneous delivery at a more remote hospital.

Table 1
Categories for prematurity and low birth weight

	Gestational Age
Preterm	<37 wk
Extremely preterm	<28 wk
Late preterm	34–36 6/7 wk
Early term	37–38 6/7 wk
	Birth Weight
LBW	<2500 g
VLBW	<1500 g
ELBW	<1000 g

PREOPERATIVE CONSIDERATIONS

Abnormal hemodynamics may create a vulnerable period for preoperative, preterm infants with CHD. Common complications of prematurity may have a further impact on infants with CHD. Timing (or even the utility) of surgical intervention for an infant's CHD may be altered based on the presence of intraventricular hemorrhage (IVH), necrotizing enterocolitis (NEC), or evolving respiratory distress syndrome (RDS). Increased risk of infection, anemia, and hyperbilirubinemia have a further impact on the typical management of an infant with CHD with regard to threshold for initiating antibiotics, transfusing blood products, or initiating phototherapy. Specific preoperative considerations in the preterm infant are outlined in **Table 2**.

Timing of Cardiac Surgery

Having considered the important transition from fetal to postnatal physiology, the clinician must then consider the implications of surgical palliation or repair of the congenital heart defect. Historically, pediatric cardiovascular surgeons were unable to repair even simple cardiac defects in small or preterm neonates. As appropriate-sized instruments were developed and surgical techniques for CHD improved, surgeons began to consider the elective palliation or repair of these challenging patients.[16,17] Today, although a surgical approach to most congenital heart defects is technically possible, debate remains regarding the appropriate timing of referral for congenital heart surgery in the preterm neonate.

Most studies of preterm, LBW, or SGA newborns with CHD have demonstrated higher morbidity and mortality after congenital heart surgery.[18–22] One study, however, of 102 patients found that emergency surgery and low cardiac output syndrome (but not prematurity or SGA, among other factors) increased the risk of mortality,[23] and the importance of LBW alone in relation to mortality has been questioned.[24] Retrospective outcome analyses have influenced clinicians to delay cardiac surgery until a newborn matures, allowing for weight gain and organ maturity. Delaying surgery, however (to achieve weight gain, for example), has not improved outcomes and in most cases exposes the neonate to a significant hemodynamic burden. Although individual centers have reported success with a delayed surgical approach to the management of preterm congenital heart defects,[25,26] no randomized study has demonstrated superior results to early primary repair or palliation. Hickey and colleagues[20] identified 2 kg as an "inflection point," below which mortality from CHD significantly increases. Although their study found no mortality difference between a delayed approach to allow maturation compared with an immediate surgical approach, the complication rate was significantly higher in the group with a delayed surgical repair. Because delayed repair or initial palliation may impose unacceptable hemodynamics and equal risk of mortality,[20] many centers advocate for early primary repair of premature or LBW neonates, despite the inherent risks.[27–29] The appropriate timing for intervention remains unclear due to the heterogeneous patient population, the center-specific surgical approaches, and the unclear impact that timing plays on neurodevelopmental outcome.

The specific anatomic diagnosis has a significant impact on outcomes in preterm neonates with CHD.[30] In a meta-analysis of 6 studies, including 356 LBW neonates, cardiac diagnosis was the most important predictor of mortality, and a complete physiologic repair demonstrated slightly improved survival compared with surgical palliation.[30] Selected individual congenital cardiac lesions have been retrospectively studied to determine the optimal approach for each lesion in the preterm (or LBW) infant.

Table 2
Physiologic challenges for management of the premature neonate with congenital heart disease

System	Physiologic Challenges	Considerations for Preoperative Management
Cardiac development	• Postnatal adjustment to physiology of congenital heart defect[16,31] • Neonatal sarcoplasmic reticulum is poorly developed. • Neonatal myocardium uses glucose for energy (compared with fat in older children). • Neonatal ventricular muscle poorly tolerant of pressure/volume load	• Anticipate significant hemodynamic changes in initial 24 h of life. • Ensure adequate ionized calcium levels for optimal cardiac contractility. • Avoid hypoglycemia because low hepatic glycogen stores and impaired gluconeogenesis may lead to cardiac dysfunction. • Cardiac output reliant on heart rate; may not tolerate pressure/volume load
Fluids and electrolytes	• Increased fluid/caloric requirements and excessive heat loss from thin stratum corneum • Immature renal function • Acidosis due to elevated lactate or renal bicarbonate loss	• Maintain adequate fluid and caloric intake; consider careful diuretic use to reduce pulmonary edema/volume overload. • Monitor closely for electrolyte derangement (especially hyponatremia). • Careful consideration of bicarbonate use to correct acidosis and avoid cardiac dysfunction (increased risk of IVH in preterm neonates)[32,33]
Cerebral blood flow and hemodynamics	• Adequate blood pressure for organ perfusion is necessary. • Preterm infants have impaired cerebral autoregulation[34] and are at greater risk for IVH/hypoxic brain injury.	• Goal mean arterial pressure above a value equivalent to the gestational age (or >30 mm Hg) has been utilized[35,36]; CHD may warrant different blood pressure thresholds. • Preserve cerebral blood flow by minimizing hypotension, hypocarbia, or anemia. • Near-infrared spectroscopy monitoring[37] may help with assessment of end organ perfusion.
Feeding and nutrition	• Higher-energy expenditure and greater risk for failure to thrive • Increased risk of NEC due to immature gut, altered intestinal microbiome, decreased gut perfusion, infection/inflammation	• Consider early initiation of trophic feeds; monitor tolerance closely given increased risk for NEC with CHD.[38,39] • Data lacking for preoperative enteral feeding in preterm infant, especially when requiring prostaglandins or pressors[40,41]

(continued on next page)

Table 2 (continued)

System	Physiologic Challenges	Considerations for Preoperative Management
RDS, apnea of prematurity	• RDS may contribute to poor oxygenation.	• Intubation and surfactant/ positive pressure ventilation may be necessary
	• Oxygenation goals not well defined in preterm	• SUPPORT trial found lower oxygenation goals reduced BPD and ROP but increased mortality.[43]
	• Permissive hypercapnia reduces BPD in preterm infants[42] but may alter hemodynamics in CHD patient.	• Consider ventilator strategies utilizing permissive hypercapnia.
	• Premature neonates at risk for apnea	• Utilize caffeine for apnea due to improved survival without neurodevelopmental impairment in VLBW infants.[44] Aminophylline prevents apnea in term neonates on prostaglandin[45] but not studied in premature neonates.
Preoperative genetic testing	• Genetic abnormalities more common in infants with CHD (especially trisomy 13, 18, 21 and 22q11.1 deletions)[5] • DiGeorge syndrome occurs in 12% of infants with CHD; common in conotruncal lesions[46]	• Karyotype and/or specific testing for 22q11.2 deletion (DiGeorge syndrome) may be warranted.
Neurologic Imaging	• Up to 50% with preoperative white matter injury or stroke[47–49]	• Obtain early cranial ultrasound.
	• Risk factors are hypoxemia and time to surgery.[35]	• Preoperative MRI when indicated/feasible

Specific Lesions in the Premature Neonate

Coarctation of the aorta

Aortic coarctation represents a surgically correctable lesion in the premature or LBW neonate. Although balloon angioplasty remains an option for certain populations, the high rate of restenosis remains an unacceptable outcome in most native aortic coarctation.[50] Small studies of newborns weighing less than 2 kg with uncomplicated, isolated coarctation of the aorta have demonstrated a high surgical success rate with acceptable mortality rates, but mortality increases with addition of associated left-sided cardiac abnormalities. Recoarctation has been reported in 15% to 40% of patients[51–54]; although contemporary results may reflect a lower recurrence rate (Reddy VM, unpublished data, 2015), patients must be closely followed for growth of the aortic arch and coarctation site. Recoarctation may not relate to LBW but rather the anatomy of the aortic arch and coarctation site.[55] Based on these studies, there seems little indication for delaying surgical repair for the premature patient with an isolated coarctation. For a complicated premature or LBW newborn or for patients with significant surgical contraindications (such as extracardiac complications), a hybrid approach with initial stenting of the aortic coarctation followed by subsequent surgical repair has been reported.[56]

Transposition of the great arteries

Premature neonates with transposition of the great arteries (TGA) require surgical correction with an arterial switch operation, which includes transfer of the coronary arteries to the neoaortic (native pulmonary) root. Historically, surgery was delayed with continuous prostaglandin infusion to maintain ductal patency, in conjunction with a balloon atrial septostomy (Rashkind procedure) to promote atrial mixing. With the advent of neonatal surgery, however, repair within the first week of life prevents muscular involution of the left ventricle and is now the standard of care. Data suggest that longer time to surgery relates to preoperative brain injury for a neonate with TGA.[57] A premature neonate with TGA, however, is likely to experience a prolonged length of stay in the postoperative ICU[58] and still has a higher risk of early postoperative mortality compared with a normal birth weight neonate.[59,60] Although the operative mortality may approximate 15% to 20% for premature or LBW neonates after arterial switch operation, Roussin and colleagues[60] found that both surgical palliation (not repair) and age greater than 30 days at the time of surgery increased the mortality risk. Therefore, data suggest that early primary repair for TGA represents a high-risk but optimal surgical approach.

Hypoplastic left heart syndrome

Hypoplastic left heart syndrome (HLHS) represents one of the most complex and challenging congenital heart lesions to manage, even in term neonates with normal birth weight. With a mortality rate of 25% to 30% in the first year after staged single-ventricle palliation, pediatric cardiologists and cardiothoracic surgeons continue to study optimal surgical approaches.[61] In premature neonates, the important morbidity and mortality of HLHS are amplified, especially after stage I palliation (Norwood procedure). Even late preterm birth imposes significant risk of death for newborns with HLHS; compared with term neonates, late preterm birth was associated with an almost 3-fold odds of hospital death in HLHS patients.[62] Newborns with HLHS are also more likely to be born premature and LBW, both factors that increase the risk of early death.[63] A recent evaluation of 47 patients after surgical palliation for HLHS reported 49% mortality, with SGA and noncardiac abnormalities representing significant risk factors for death.[64] An earlier study of 27 neonates with HLHS reported similar mortality but found that pulmonary vein and coronary artery anomalies were related to poor patient outcome (not prematurity, weight, or SGA).[65]

Aortic arch obstruction (2-ventricle surgical repair)

The complexity of the single-ventricle reconstruction inherent in the stage I palliation is underscored by the contrasting outcomes in premature neonates with aortic arch obstruction and ventricular septal defect who undergo a 2-ventricle repair. Haas and colleagues[66] studied 21 newborns with variants of aortic arch obstruction/ventricular septal defect and found a mortality of only 14%; these data suggest that early complete anatomic repair can significantly reduce mortality in preterm and LBW newborns. Underlying anatomy influences both surgical decision making and patient outcome. Neonates with all types of single-ventricle physiology (including HLHS, unbalanced atrioventricular canal, and tricuspid atresia) all experience higher rates of preterm birth, low birth rate, and SGA,[67] emphasizing the need to further study and address this important preoperative risk factor for this complex population.

Tetralogy of Fallot

Tetralogy of Fallot (TOF) is the most common cyanotic heart defect and was the first cyanotic lesion palliated with congenital heart surgery.[68] Historically, TOF was palliated with a surgical aortopulmonary shunt to augment pulmonary blood flow, followed by complete intracardiac repair before 1 year of age. With advances in neonatal surgical and cardiopulmonary bypass (CPB) techniques, however, many centers advocate for early primary repair. Referral for surgery typically occurs at approximately 3 to 6 months of age, before right ventricular and infundibular hypertrophy worsens enough to induce a hypercyanotic episode. Hypercyanotic episodes (tet spells) define an indication for immediate surgery. Therefore, for symptomatic neonates, some centers perform a complete intracardiac repair of TOF.

Unlike other congenital cardiac surgeries, however, repair of TOF increases the combined ventricular volume compared with the preoperative state. Neonatal repair also may lead to a relatively larger right ventriculotomy scar and more frequent use of a transannular patch (leading to more severe pulmonary insufficiency). Neonates have noncompliant ventricular muscle that is resistant to volume loading and, therefore, may struggle to recover from early primary repair. Studies of the surgical approach to TOF indicate that early primary repair (at 6–8 weeks of age) is technically feasible and may not be associated with increased morbidity or mortality. Even though prematurity and LBW increase the time of mechanical ventilation, length of stay, and cost,[69,70] surgical repair (with maintenance of a postoperative patent foramen ovale to allow decompression of the noncompliant right ventricle) may be a better option than the alternative, a surgically created aortopulmonary shunt. Systemic to pulmonary shunts are difficult to size appropriately in LBW and premature neonates, and may pose a higher mortality risk in neonates in general. One study of surgical aortopulmonary shunts in patients less than 3 kg described acceptable overall survival but increased reintervention with smaller (3-mm) shunts required for the LBW and premature patients.[71] One case series described interventional stenting of the right ventricular outflow tract in patients who were not surgical candidates[72]; this approach may be attractive in specific subpopulations (eg, LBW neonates with contraindications to cardiopulmonary bypass).

Postoperative Considerations

After cardiac surgery, premature neonates are at risk for complications inherent to the intraoperative course. CPB imposes significant hemodynamic and inflammatory insults that have been well described in varied populations.[73,74] Strategies to mitigate the inflammatory cascade, such as intraoperative ultrafiltration and steroid administration, are common at most institutions. Systemic heparinization is essential during CPB, and any preoperative bleeding concerns may be magnified in the postoperative period. Although heparinization can be safely performed without significant morbidity in this population,[75] clinicians should consider the risks in patients with preoperative intraventricular or gastrointestinal bleeding.

Optimal management of postsurgical cardiac neonates requires a dedicated team approach. These complex patients require the resources of multiple disciplines, and an organized handoff process can prevent errors. Specifically, neonatologists, cardiologists, (cardiac) intensivists, cardiothoracic surgeons, anesthesiologists, bedside nurses, and the frontline providers must all communicate the important preoperative clinical status (eg, duration of preoperative intubation and preoperative lung compliance) and intraoperative details (such as arrhythmias or residual lesions). Interdisciplinary consultation is appropriate in both the preoperative and postoperative settings; it is not uncommon for neonatologists at the authors' institution to provide postoperative guidance in the cardiovascular ICU.

OUTCOMES: MORTALITY AND COMMON COMPLICATIONS OF PREMATURITY

Several multicenter studies have confirmed a mortality rate between 1.5 and 4 times higher in LBW,[76] very LBW (VLBW),[77] and extremely LBW (ELBW)[78] infants with CHD compared with their counterparts of similar birth weight without CHD. A description of the most common and important morbidities after surgical repair of CHD follows.

Bronchopulmonary Dysplasia

VLBW infants with CHD were found more than 4 times as likely to develop bronchopulmonary dysplasia (BPD) compared with those without CHD,[79] likely due to prolonged mechanical ventilation and pulmonary edema. BPD has significant impact on the morbidity of neonates with CHD, especially in patients with single-ventricle physiology.[80] Clinicians must pay careful attention to the goals of mechanical ventilation, to avoid the development of ventilator-induced lung injury. The goal of low tidal volume (4–6 mL per kilogram), shorter inspiratory time, and permissive hypercapnia can be achieved in some neonates, but hypercapnia may alter cardiopulmonary hemodynamics by elevating pulmonary vascular resistance, causing dilation of the systemic vascular bed, and impairing cardiac contractility. Nitric oxide may mitigate the effects of hypercapnia and elevated pulmonary vascular resistance, but data in premature neonates with CHD are lacking.

Postoperative management of premature or LBW neonates with CHD may also present a unique challenge when titrating fraction of inspired oxygen concentration (Fio_2). The detrimental effects of hyperoxygenation should be emphasized in managing the ventilator, because reactive oxygen species have been implicated in retinopathy of prematurity (ROP) and also BPD.[43] Therefore, the authors' postoperative management includes administering the minimum Fio_2 to achieve the goals for the cardiac repair. Patients with single-ventricle disease are rapidly titrated to minimal oxygen levels but may still require supplemental oxygen (Fio_2 approximately 0.3) to overcome pulmonary venous desaturation common after CPB.[81] Patients with fully septated intracardiac anatomy should be maintained at an oxygen level adequate to oxygenate tissues and allow organ recovery; neonates rarely require a Pao_2 greater than 100, even in the setting of right ventricular dysfunction or pulmonary hypertension. The authors' general approach is to target a Pao_2 and $Paco_2$ of 50 mm Hg to optimize postoperative ventilation (rather than increasing ventilator pressure or respiratory rates to achieve a lower $Paco_2$ or higher Pao_2). In select patients, high-frequency oscillation has been used in an attempt to minimize of ventilator-induced lung injury.

Sepsis

Small studies have demonstrated a greater than 2-times higher incidence of sepsis in preterm infants with CHD compared with those without CHD[82] as well as higher rates of nosocomial infections in preterm infants with CHD compared with those born at 39 weeks' gestation.[21] These findings may be attributable to longer durations of hospital stay, mechanical ventilation, and central venous catheter placement in preterm infants with CHD. Premature and LBW newborns are also at significantly increased risk of invasive fungal infections.[83] Fungal infections in neonates with CHD impart a mortality risk as high as 21%[84]; some clinicians opt for early antifungal prophylaxis in a high-risk premature neonate (eg, delayed sternal closure). Many patients require stable preoperative vascular access, such as a peripherally inserted central catheter or an umbilical venous catheter for medication administration (such as prostaglandin). These catheters put patients at risk for central line–associated blood stream infections and should be attentively managed with bundled care protocols. The authors' preference is to place a right atrial Broviac catheter at the time of chest closure in the operating room or with subsequent sternal closure.

Necrotizing Enterocolitis

NEC is a known complication of prematurity, and CHD is a risk factor for development of NEC. A large study of VLBW infants from the Vermont Oxford Network (VON) found a higher incidence of NEC when CHD was also present (adjusted odds ratio 1.8; $P<.0001$). Although lower birth weight typically is a predictor of higher mortality in VLBW infants with NEC, this study did not demonstrate an effect of birth weight on mortality for patients with both CHD and NEC. Although splanchnic ischemia and associated intestinal tissue hypoxia are contributing risks, a different pathophysiologic mechanism for NEC in preterm infants with CHD may predominate. Different specific cardiac lesions, including HLHS[85] and atrioventricular canal defect,[38] have been associated with increased risk for NEC, but no consistent cardiac pathophysiology has been identified (See Karpen HE: Nutrition in the Cardiac Newborn Evidence-based Nutrition Guidelines for the Cardiac Newborn, in this issue).

Intraventricular Hemorrhage and Periventricular Leukomalacia

Both preterm infants without CHD and term infants with CHD are susceptible to white matter injury in the brain. The selective vulnerability of developing oligodendrocytes in an environment of both ischemia and inflammation may contribute to injury,[86] but no studies have specifically focused on unique patterns of brain injury with the combined risks of prematurity and CHD. Literature also remains inconsistent regarding increased risk for IVH in preterm infants with CHD.[21,77] Intraoperative variables may also contribute to the risk of neurologic injury. Specifically, hemodilution of hematocrit (caused by the priming volume of the CPB circuit) may contribute to lower oxygen delivery to the brain.[87] Similarly, the hypothermia required to perform complex cardiac repairs may alter cerebral autoregulation and blood flow; many pediatric centers use a pH-stat management during CPB to correct for this alteration.[88] Finally, the choice of anesthetic agent has become increasingly scrutinized, because animal models have demonstrated neurotoxicity with certain drug combinations.[89] No human data have confirmed these findings, and there is consensus that inadequate analgesia during cardiac surgery results in important negative hemodynamic and behavioral changes. To optimize the treatment of premature neonates, further study of specific anesthetic agents is warranted.

Retinopathy of Prematurity

Disturbances in retinal perfusion, increased VEGF (vascular endothelial growth factor) expression from hypoxia, and ensuing neovascularization potentially lead to worsening ROP in preterm infants with CHD. A large study of ELBW infants found that the ROP rate was not significantly different between infants with and without CHD, but the infants with CHD had an increased risk of bilateral blindness (relative risk 7.8; CI, 2.5–23.9). It is unclear if this increased risk was due to central nervous system injury of the visual cortex or due to increased abnormalities specific to the lens or retina of the eyes.[78] Limitation of Fio_2 during mechanical ventilation (as described previously) may also prevent hypervascularization of the retina and ROP.

Neurodevelopmental Outcomes and Follow-up Needs

Close neurodevelopmental follow-up and engagement with early intervention services as needed for infants with CHD are recommended and particularly necessary in premature infants due to inherent neurodevelopmental risk associated with prematurity alone. A large study of ELBW infants in the National Institute of Child Health and Human

Development Neonatal Research Network centers found increased mortality and risk for neurodevelopmental impairment at 18 to 22 months of age in infants with isolated CHD compared with those without CHD (relative risk 1.43; CI, 1.29–1.58).[78] This study found poorer growth parameters and longer length of hospital stay in the infants with CHD. Delayed brain maturation of infants with CHD may further predispose these infants to neurodevelopmental impairment.[12,13] Specific evaluation of gross and fine motor skills, speech and language, executive functioning, and behavior is necessary with formal developmental testing and early referral for services.

SUMMARY

In summary, premature neonates with CHD require the collaborative effort of highly specialized teams to manage the perioperative course. Preoperative complications of prematurity are amplified in the setting of hemodynamic disturbances that are common with CHD. The decision to proceed with surgery and the surgical procedure performed are important determinants of postoperative hemodynamics. Postoperative complications may arise in virtually every organ system and require the close attention of clinicians. As more is learned about the management of these comorbidities, improved outcomes will follow for premature neonates with CHD.

Best practices

What is the current practice?

Best practice/guideline/care path objective(s):

In the absence of maternal or fetal indications for early delivery, the fetus with CHD should be delivered at term.

The premature neonate with CHD should be managed by a multidisciplinary team with experience in complex neonatal and cardiac care.

When technically possible (and in the absence of morbidities or contraindications), early primary surgical repair should be performed for congenital heart lesions with significant hemodynamic abnormalities; a delayed surgical approach may allow for weight gain in anticipation of subsequent repair but may lead to unacceptable cardiac pressure and volume load.

What changes in current practice are likely to improve outcomes?

The continued improvement in fetal diagnosis may provide an opportunity for optimal timing of delivery (39–40 weeks' gestation).

Early surgical repair of hemodynamically significant cardiac lesions may lead to improved cardiac physiology.

The impact of CPB and congenital heart surgery on the premature developing brain and subsequent neurodevelopmental outcomes, however, is unclear. Further study of these outcomes is warranted.

Continued collaboration of multidisciplinary teams, including neonatologists, cardiologists, anesthesiologists, cardiac surgeons, intensivists, nurses, and advanced practice providers, will be critical in the management of postoperative complications in this fragile population.

Summary statement

Premature neonates with CHD represent a complex and high-risk population that requires highly specialized medical care. When unable to achieve term delivery, a neonate with CHD provides important challenges to the clinician. A collaborative approach to the surgical decision making and postoperative management of complications is required.

REFERENCES

1. Blencowe H, Cousens S, Oestergaard MZ, et al. National, regional, and worldwide estimates of preterm birth rates in the year 2010 with time trends since 1990 for selected countries: a systematic analysis and implications. Lancet 2012;379(9832):2162–72.
2. Tanner K, Sabrine N, Wren C. Cardiovascular malformations among preterm infants. Pediatrics 2005;116(6):e833–8.
3. Rosenthal GL, Wilson PD, Permutt T, et al. Birth weight and cardiovascular malformations: a population-based study. The baltimore-Washington infant study. Am J Epidemiol 1991;133(12):1273–81.
4. Archer JM, Yeager SB, Kenny MJ, et al. Distribution of and mortality from serious congenital heart disease in very low birth weight infants. Pediatrics 2011;127(2): 293–9.
5. Hartman RJ, Rasmussen SA, Botto LD, et al. The contribution of chromosomal abnormalities to congenital heart defects: a population-based study. Pediatr Cardiol 2011;32(8):1147–57.
6. Costello JM, Pasquali SK, Jacobs JP, et al. Gestational age at birth and outcomes after neonatal cardiac surgery: an analysis of the society of thoracic surgeons congenital heart surgery database. Circulation 2014;129(24):2511–7.
7. Cnota JF, Gupta R, Michelfelder EC, et al. Congenital heart disease infant death rates decrease as gestational age advances from 34 to 40 weeks. J Pediatr 2011; 159(5):761–5.
8. Costello JM, Polito A, Brown DW, et al. Birth before 39 weeks' gestation is associated with worse outcomes in neonates with heart disease. Pediatrics 2010; 126(2):277–84.
9. Bishop NB, Zhou TX, Chen JM, et al. The impact of gestational age on resource utilization after open heart surgery for congenital cardiac disease from birth to 1 year of age. Pediatr Cardiol 2013;34(3):686–93.
10. Goff DA, Luan X, Gerdes M, et al. Younger gestational age is associated with worse neurodevelopmental outcomes after cardiac surgery in infancy. J Thorac Cardiovasc Surg 2012;143(3):535–42.
11. Limperopoulos C, Tworetzky W, McElhinney DB, et al. Brain volume and metabolism in fetuses with congenital heart disease: evaluation with quantitative magnetic resonance imaging and spectroscopy. Circulation 2010;121(1):26–33.
12. Miller SP, McQuillen PS, Hamrick S, et al. Abnormal brain development in newborns with congenital heart disease. N Engl J Med 2007;357(19):1928–38.
13. Licht DJ, Shera DM, Clancy RR, et al. Brain maturation is delayed in infants with complex congenital heart defects. J Thorac Cardiovasc Surg 2009;137(3): 529–36 [discussion: 536–7].
14. ACOG Committee on Practice Bulletins – Obstetrics. ACOG practice bulletin No. 107: induction of labor. Obstet Gynecol 2009;114(2 Pt 1):386–97.
15. Morse SB, Zheng H, Tang Y, et al. Early school-age outcomes of late preterm infants. Pediatrics 2009;123(4):e622–9.
16. Reddy VM. Cardiac surgery for premature and low birth weight neonates. Semin Thorac Cardiovasc Surg Pediatr Card Surg Annu 2001;4:271–6.
17. Reddy VM, Hanley FL. Cardiac surgery in infants with very low birth weight. Semin Pediatr Surg 2000;9(2):91–5.
18. Kalfa D, Krishnamurthy G, Duchon J, et al. Outcomes of cardiac surgery in patients weighing <2.5 kg: affect of patient-dependent and -independent variables. J Thorac Cardiovasc Surg 2014;148(6):2499–506.e1.

19. Alsoufi B, Manlhiot C, Mahle WT, et al. Low-weight infants are at increased mortality risk after palliative or corrective cardiac surgery. J Thorac Cardiovasc Surg 2014;148(6):2508–14.e1.
20. Hickey EJ, Nosikova Y, Zhang H, et al. Very low-birth-weight infants with congenital cardiac lesions: is there merit in delaying intervention to permit growth and maturation? J Thorac Cardiovasc Surg 2012;143(1):126–36, 136.e1.
21. Cheng HH, Almodovar MC, Laussen PC, et al. Outcomes and risk factors for mortality in premature neonates with critical congenital heart disease. Pediatr Cardiol 2011;32(8):1139–46.
22. Oppido G, Pace Napoleone C, Formigari R, et al. Outcome of cardiac surgery in low birth weight and premature infants. Eur J Cardiothorac Surg 2004;26(1):44–53.
23. Seo D-M, Park J-J, Yun T-J, et al. The outcome of open heart surgery for congenital heart disease in infants with low body weight less than 2500 g. Pediatr Cardiol 2011;32(5):578–84.
24. Wernovsky G, Rubenstein SD, Spray TL. Cardiac surgery in the low-birth weight neonate. New approaches. Clin Perinatol 2001;28(1):249–64.
25. Shepard CW, Kochilas LK, Rosengart RM, et al. Repair of major congenital cardiac defects in low-birth-weight infants: is delay warranted? J Thorac Cardiovasc Surg 2010;140(5):1104–9.
26. Jennings E, Cuadrado A, Maher KO, et al. Short-term outcomes in premature neonates adhering to the philosophy of supportive care allowing for weight gain and organ maturation prior to cardiac surgery. J Intensive Care Med 2012;27(1):32–6.
27. Azakie A, Johnson NC, Anagnostopoulos PV, et al. Cardiac surgery in low birth weight infants: current outcomes. Interact Cardiovasc Thorac Surg 2011;12(3):409–13 [discussion: 414].
28. Reddy VM. Low birth weight and very low birth weight neonates with congenital heart disease: timing of surgery, reasons for delaying or not delaying surgery. Semin Thorac Cardiovasc Surg Pediatr Card Surg Annu 2013;16(1):13–20.
29. Ades AM, Dominguez TE, Nicolson SC, et al. Morbidity and mortality after surgery for congenital cardiac disease in the infant born with low weight. Cardiol Young 2010;20(1):8–17.
30. Abrishamchian R, Kanhai D, Zwets E, et al. Low birth weight or diagnosis, which is a higher risk?–a meta-analysis of observational studies. Eur J Cardiothorac Surg 2006;30(5):700–5.
31. Rudolph AM. Congenital diseases of the heart?: clinical-physiological considerations. Hoboken (NJ): Wiley-Blackwell; 2009.
32. Papile LA, Burstein J, Burstein R, et al. Relationship of intravenous sodium bicarbonate infusions and cerebral intraventricular hemorrhage. J Pediatr 1978;93(5):834–6.
33. Aschner JL, Poland RL. Sodium bicarbonate: basically useless therapy. Pediatrics 2008;122(4):831–5.
34. Soul JS, Hammer PE, Tsuji M, et al. Fluctuating pressure-passivity is common in the cerebral circulation of sick premature infants. Pediatr Res 2007;61(4):467–73.
35. Report of working group of the British Association of Perinatal Medicine and Neonatal Nurses Association on categories of babies requiring neonatal care. Arch Dis Child 1992;67(7):868–9.
36. Dempsey EM, Barrington KJ. Treating hypotension in the preterm infant: when and with what: a critical and systematic review. J Perinatol 2007;27(8):469–78.
37. Johnson BA, Hoffman GM, Tweddell JS, et al. Near-infrared spectroscopy in neonates before palliation of hypoplastic left heart syndrome. Ann Thorac Surg 2009;87(2):571–7.

38. Fisher JG, Bairdain S, Sparks EA, et al. Serious congenital heart disease and necrotizing enterocolitis in very low birth weight neonates. J Am Coll Surg 2015;220(6):1018–26.

39. McElhinney DB, Hedrick HL, Bush DM, et al. Necrotizing enterocolitis in neonates with congenital heart disease: risk factors and outcomes. Pediatrics 2000;106(5):1080–7.

40. Natarajan G, Reddy Anne S, Aggarwal S. Enteral feeding of neonates with congenital heart disease. Neonatology 2010;98(4):330–6.

41. Willis L, Thureen P, Kaufman J, et al. Enteral feeding in prostaglandin-dependent neonates: is it a safe practice? J Pediatr 2008;153(6):867–9.

42. Ryu J, Haddad G, Carlo WA. Clinical effectiveness and safety of permissive hypercapnia. Clin Perinatol 2012;39(3):603–12.

43. SUPPORT Study Group of the Eunice Kennedy Shriver NICHD Neonatal Research Network, Carlo WA, Finer NN, et al. Target ranges of oxygen saturation in extremely preterm infants. N Engl J Med 2010;362(21):1959–69.

44. Schmidt B, Roberts RS, Davis P, et al. Long-term effects of caffeine therapy for apnea of prematurity. N Engl J Med 2007;357(19):1893–902.

45. Lim DS, Kulik TJ, Kim DW, et al. Aminophylline for the prevention of apnea during prostaglandin E1 infusion. Pediatrics 2003;112:e27–9.

46. Botto LD, May K, Fernhoff PM, et al. A population-based study of the 22q11.2 deletion: phenotype, incidence, and contribution to major birth defects in the population. Pediatrics 2003;112:101–7.

47. Mahle WT, Tavani F, Zimmerman RA, et al. An MRI study of neurological injury before and after congenital heart surgery. Circulation 2002;106(12 Suppl 1):I109–14.

48. van Houten JP, Rothman A, Bejar R. High incidence of cranial ultrasound abnormalities in full-term infants with congenital heart disease. Am J Perinatol 1996; 13(1):47–53.

49. McQuillen PS, Barkovich AJ, Hamrick SEG, et al. Temporal and anatomic risk profile of brain injury with neonatal repair of congenital heart defects. Stroke 2007; 38(2 Suppl):736–41.

50. Rothman A, Galindo A, Evans WN, et al. Effectiveness and safety of balloon dilation of native aortic coarctation in premature neonates weighing < or = 2,500 grams. Am J Cardiol 2010;105(8):1176–80.

51. Karamlou T, Bernasconi A, Jaeggi E, et al. Factors associated with arch reintervention and growth of the aortic arch after coarctation repair in neonates weighing less than 2.5 kg. J Thorac Cardiovasc Surg 2009;137(5):1163–7.

52. Bacha EA, Almodovar M, Wessel DL, et al. Surgery for coarctation of the aorta in infants weighing less than 2 kg. Ann Thorac Surg 2001;71(4):1260–4.

53. Sudarshan CD, Cochrane AD, Jun ZH, et al. Repair of coarctation of the aorta in infants weighing less than 2 kilograms. Ann Thorac Surg 2006;82(1):158–63.

54. Burch PT, Cowley CG, Holubkov R, et al. Coarctation repair in neonates and young infants: is small size or low weight still a risk factor? J Thorac Cardiovasc Surg 2009;138(3):547–52.

55. McElhinney DB, Yang S-G, Hogarty AN, et al. Recurrent arch obstruction after repair of isolated coarctation of the aorta in neonates and young infants: is low weight a risk factor? J Thorac Cardiovasc Surg 2001;122(5):883–90.

56. Gorenflo M, Boshoff DE, Heying R, et al. Bailout stenting for critical coarctation in premature/critical/complex/early recoarcted neonates. Catheter Cardiovasc Interv Off J Soc Card Angiogr Interv 2010;75(4):553–61.

57. Petit CJ, Rome JJ, Wernovsky G, et al. Preoperative brain injury in transposition of the great arteries is associated with oxygenation and time to surgery, not balloon atrial septostomy. Circulation 2009;119(5):709–16.

58. Wheeler DS, Dent CL, Manning PB, et al. Factors prolonging length of stay in the cardiac intensive care unit following the arterial switch operation. Cardiol Young 2008;18(1):41–50.
59. Fricke TA, d'Udekem Y, Richardson M, et al. Outcomes of the arterial switch operation for transposition of the great arteries: 25 years of experience. Ann Thorac Surg 2012;94(1):139–45.
60. Roussin R, Belli E, Bruniaux J, et al. Surgery for transposition of the great arteries in neonates weighing less than 2,000 grams: a consecutive series of 25 patients. Ann Thorac Surg 2007;83(1):173–7 [discussion: 177–8].
61. Ohye RG, Sleeper LA, Mahony L, et al. Comparison of shunt types in the Norwood procedure for single-ventricle lesions. N Engl J Med 2010;362(21):1980–92.
62. Attar MA, Dechert RE, Schumacher RE. The effect of late preterm birth on mortality of infants with hypoplastic left heart syndrome. Am J Perinatol 2012;29(8):593–8.
63. Hirsch JC, Copeland G, Donohue JE, et al. Population-based analysis of survival for hypoplastic left heart syndrome. J Pediatr 2011;159(1):57–63.
64. Gelehrter S, Fifer CG, Armstrong A, et al. Outcomes of hypoplastic left heart syndrome in low-birth-weight patients. Pediatr Cardiol 2011;32(8):1175–81.
65. Pizarro C, Davis DA, Galantowicz ME, et al. Stage I palliation for hypoplastic left heart syndrome in low birth weight neonates: can we justify it? Eur J Cardiothorac Surg 2002;21(4):716–20.
66. Haas F, Goldberg CS, Ohye RG, et al. Primary repair of aortic arch obstruction with ventricular septal defect in preterm and low birth weight infants. Eur J Cardiothorac Surg 2000;17(6):643–7.
67. Williams RV, Ravishankar C, Zak V, et al. Birth weight and prematurity in infants with single ventricle physiology: pediatric heart network infant single ventricle trial screened population. Congenit Heart Dis 2010;5(2):96–103.
68. Taussig HB, Blalock A. The tetralogy of Fallot; diagnosis and indications for operation; the surgical treatment of the tetralogy of Fallot. Surgery 1947;21(1):145.
69. Peer SM, Zurakowski D, Jonas RA, et al. Early primary repair of tetralogy of Fallot does not lead to increased postoperative resource utilization. Ann Thorac Surg 2014 Dec;98(6):2173–9 [discussion: 2179–80].
70. Kirsch RE, Glatz AC, Gaynor JW, et al. Results of elective repair at 6 months or younger in 277 patients with tetralogy of Fallot: a 14-year experience at a single center. J Thorac Cardiovasc Surg 2014;147(2):713–7.
71. Myers JW, Ghanayem NS, Cao Y, et al. Outcomes of systemic to pulmonary artery shunts in patients weighing less than 3 kg: analysis of shunt type, size, and surgical approach. J Thorac Cardiovasc Surg 2014;147(2):672–7.
72. Castleberry CD, Gudausky TM, Berger S, et al. Stenting of the right ventricular outflow tract in the high-risk infant with cyanotic teratology of Fallot. Pediatr Cardiol 2014;35(3):423–30.
73. Allan CK, Newburger JW, McGrath E, et al. The relationship between inflammatory activation and clinical outcome after infant cardiopulmonary bypass. Anesth Analg 2010;111(5):1244–51.
74. Bronicki RA, Backer CL, Baden HP, et al. Dexamethasone reduces the inflammatory response to cardiopulmonary bypass in children. Ann Thorac Surg 2000;69(5):1490–5.
75. Reddy VM, McElhinney DB, Sagrado T, et al. Results of 102 cases of complete repair of congenital heart defects in patients weighing 700 to 2500 grams. J Thorac Cardiovasc Surg 1999;117(2):324–31.

76. Curzon CL, Milford-Beland S, Li JS, et al. Cardiac surgery in infants with low birth weight is associated with increased mortality: analysis of the society of thoracic surgeons congenital heart database. J Thorac Cardiovasc Surg 2008;135(3): 546–51.
77. Anderson AW, Smith PB, Corey KM, et al. Clinical outcomes in very low birth weight infants with major congenital heart defects. Early Hum Dev 2014;90(12):791–5.
78. Pappas A, Shankaran S, Hansen NI, et al. Outcome of extremely preterm infants (<1,000 g) with congenital heart defects from the national institute of child health and human development neonatal research network. Pediatr Cardiol 2012;33(8): 1415–26.
79. Polito A, Piga S, Cogo PE, et al. Increased morbidity and mortality in very pre-term/VLBW infants with congenital heart disease. Intensive Care Med 2013; 39(6):1104–12.
80. McMahon CJ, Penny DJ, Nelson DP, et al. Preterm infants with congenital heart disease and bronchopulmonary dysplasia: postoperative course and outcome after cardiac surgery. Pediatrics 2005;116(2):423–30.
81. Taeed R, Schwartz SM, Pearl JM, et al. Unrecognized pulmonary venous desatu-ration early after Norwood palliation confounds Gp:Gs assessment and compro-mises oxygen delivery. Circulation 2001;103(22):2699–704.
82. Hadzimuratovic E, Dinarevic SM, Hadzimuratovic A. Sepsis in premature new-borns with congenital heart disease. Congenit Heart Dis 2010;5(5):435–8.
83. Kaufman D, Fairchild KD. Clinical microsbiology of bacterial and fungal sepsis in very-low-birth-weight infants. Clin Microbiol Rev 2004;17(3):638–80.
84. Ascher SB, Smith PB, Clark RH, et al. Sepsis in young infants with congenital heart disease. Early Hum Dev 2012;88:S92–7.
85. Mukherjee D, Zhang Y, Chang DC, et al. Outcomes analysis of necrotizing entero-colitis within 11 958 neonates undergoing cardiac surgical procedures. Arch Surg 2010;145(4):389–92.
86. Back SA, Han BH, Luo NL, et al. Selective vulnerability of late oligodendrocyte progenitors to hypoxia-ischemia. J Neurosci 2002;22(2):455–63.
87. Jonas RA, Wypij D, Roth SJ, et al. The influence of hemodilution on outcome after hypothermic cardiopulmonary bypass: results of a randomized trial in infants. J Thorac Cardiovasc Surg 2003;126(6):1765–74.
88. Williams GD, Cohen RS. Perioperative management of low birth weight infants for open-heart surgery. Paediatr Anaesth 2011;21(5):538–53.
89. Durrmeyer X, Vutskits L, Anand KJS, et al. Use of analgesic and sedative drugs in the NICU: integrating clinical trials and laboratory data. Pediatr Res 2010;67(2):117–27.

Neurodevelopmental Outcomes of the Child with Congenital Heart Disease

Beatrice Latal, MD, MPH

KEYWORDS

- Congenital heart disease • Development • Impairment • Outcome • School-age
- Genetic disorder • Examination

KEY POINTS

- Noncardiac complications and comorbidities play a critical role for lifelong quality of life and academic achievement in children born with congenital heart disease (CHD).
- A significant proportion of children with CHD manifest neurodevelopmental impairments, affecting cognition, motor and language development, and higher-order cognitive functions.
- Impairments are often of mild to moderate severity; however, they may occur in conjunction and significantly affect school performance, integration, and academic achievement.
- Developmental problems seem not to diminish, but rather become more apparent as demands on the developing child, in particular the school-age child, increase.
- Major risk factors for impaired development are genetic disorders, delayed preoperative brain development, a complicated postoperative course, and a poor socioeconomic environment.

INTRODUCTION

Moderate and severe congenital heart disease (CHD) occurs in about 6 per 1000 live births[1] and constitutes the most frequent congenital malformation in childhood. Around half of all newborns with a CHD require immediate surgical intervention to survive. With dramatic improvements in neonatal, perioperative care, and surgical management, survival rates have increased and reached rates of 80% to 90% even for the most complex forms of CHD.[2] In addition, cardiac outcome is often good or even excellent, allowing these children to survive into adulthood. This has led to the

Disclosure Statement: The author has nothing to disclose.
Child Development Center, University Children's Hospital Zurich, Steinwiesstrasse 75, Zurich 8032, Switzerland
E-mail address: Bea.Latal@kispi.uzh.ch

Clin Perinatol 43 (2016) 173–185
http://dx.doi.org/10.1016/j.clp.2015.11.012
0095-5108/16/$ – see front matter

situation where more adults are alive now with CHD than children.[3] With this development from a childhood disease to an adult disease, it is critical to address potential cardiac and noncardiac complications. Restrictions in cardiac function, but also impairments in cognitive and academic performance, are associated with lifelong individual psychological and societal financial burdens.[4] The description of noncardiac consequences, such as neuropsychological and psychoemotional problems, becomes even more critical in this view. Only with this information can clinicians sensitize primary care providers and specialists, inform patients and parents, develop programs for early detection, and ultimately develop therapeutic strategies to reduce or prevent these sequelae.

This article addresses the spectrum, severity, and evolution of potential neurodevelopmental and neuropsychological problems associated with CHD. Furthermore, in every chronic childhood disorder including CHD, child and parental quality of life are affected. It is beyond the focus of this article to also cover this important topic, but see referenced review articles.[5,6]

GENETIC COMORBIDITY

When discussing neurodevelopmental impairments in children with CHD, one has to consider that about one-third of all newborns and children operated for CHD have an underlying genetic disorder.[7] The most frequent disorders include trisomy 21 syndrome, 22q11 microdeletion syndrome, and CHARGE syndrome. With more sophisticated and readily available genetic screening options, the proportion of children born with CHD who are diagnosed with a genetic comorbidity will likely increase.[7] Thus, when describing the neurodevelopmental outcome in association with CHD, keep in mind that outcome in children with a genetic comorbidity is even poorer[8,9] and is strongly determined by that specific genetic aberration. There is still a large variability in outcome (eg, intelligence quotient [IQ]) within a given genetic disorder, but the IQ distribution is significantly shifted even more leftward than for CHD alone. Importantly, these children are being operated for their CHD, but often are faced with a variety of noncardiac medical problems, such as leukemia or immunodeficiency, and hearing and visual impairments. Therefore, these children need particular attention and an interdisciplinary approach that cannot be provided by the cardiologist or primary care provider alone. In addition, when following children with CHD, the diagnosis or suspicion of a genetic disorder may only arise during follow-up after children show poorer development progress with lower IQ scores than expected or explained by the CHD or the perioperative course. In combination with subtle facial or other minor dysmorphisms or other organ disorders, evaluation for a genetic disorder must then be initiated. Often a diagnosis of a genetic disorder is then made, which is essential in the view of prognosis, family counseling, and search for other organ malfunctions.

Fig. 1 shows a schematic overview of IQ outcome curves compared with norms in children with CHD and in those with genetic comorbidities. Importantly, the graph illustrates the significant overlap of performance despite differing mean IQs between these groups and despite higher proportions of children in each category performing below clinically relevant cut-off values, such as an IQ of 70 or 85 (-2 standard deviation and -1 standard deviation of the mean, respectively). This also translates into clinical experience: children with CHD may perform well within the norm or even in a high-normal level. In addition, clinical parameters during the neonatal period and surgical treatment variables very rarely help to predict outcome in an individual child. Little is still known about the factors that lead to a poor performance in one child and to

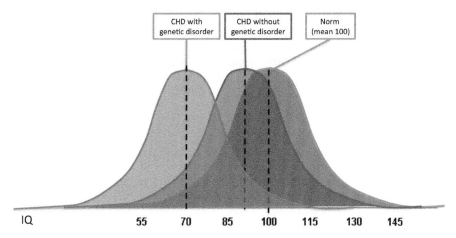

CHD with genetic disorder

CHD without genetic disorder

Norm (mean 100)

| IQ | 55 | 70 | 85 | 100 | 115 | 130 | 145 |

Fig. 1. Schematic overview of IQ outcome curves compared with norms in children with CHD and in those with genetic comorbidities and those suspected of having a genetic comorbidity.

good performance in another child even if both children have the same cardiac diagnosis and hospital course.

Therefore, it remains of importance to examine these children because they constitute an at-risk population, similar to those born at a premature gestational age.

PERIOPERATIVE NEUROLOGIC FINDINGS
Clinical Examination and Electrocardiogram

Many neurodevelopmental impairments that manifest later in life, independent of the cause, have neonatal or early infancy markers on detailed neurodevelopmental examination. Despite the increased use of neuroimaging and functional tools assessing brain structure (cerebral ultrasound and cerebral MRI) and function (electrocardiogram [EEG], amplitude integrated EEG) the value of a well-performed neurologic assessment performed by an experienced physician remains high. This has been demonstrated in high-risk populations, such as preterm infants, where the assessment of general movements has a strong predictive value for later motor disabilities,[10] but also for other neurodevelopmental domains.[11] Furthermore, the clinical assessment of the severity of hypoxic-ischemic encephalopathy, such as the Sarnat score or Thomson score, remains an important tool in the outcome prediction of these patients, particularly in the era of therapeutic hypothermia.[12] It is therefore not surprising that the neurodevelopmental and neurobehavioral abnormalities in infants with CHD are very strong predictors of later neurodevelopmental impairments.[13] Importantly, abnormal neurologic findings not only occur after the surgical procedure, but also before surgery.[14] A total of 20% to 60% of all newborns and infants undergoing early bypass surgery show neurobehavioral problems before surgery,[15] which often persist and predict later neurodevelopmental performance.[16] Neurologic findings, mostly muscular hypotonia, have been shown to correlate with MRI findings.[17] Poor feeding may also be a sign not only of cardiac failure but also of neurologic comorbidity[15] and therefore should be carefully examined. Other neurologic symptoms include seizures, which may occur preoperatively, but more frequently postoperatively. Importantly, they are often not detected clinically because infants are sedated and seizures may be subtle. A study by Clancy and colleagues[18] demonstrated that 11.5% of all infants who underwent bypass surgery had electrographic seizures without a clinical visible correlate. Importantly, clinical or electrographic seizures are strongly related to poorer neurodevelopmental outcome when measured by continuous EEG,[19] but also when detected by amplitude EEG[20] and remain a predictor for long-term outcome.[21] Thus, continuous EEG or amplitude EEG is a critical tool to help identify infants at greatest risk for poor outcome.

Neuroimaging

A large number of studies have examined the incidence, time course, and pattern of brain injuries using cerebral MRI (for review see Refs.[22,23]). There is consistent evidence that white matter injury is the predominant injury pattern detected in about 20% to 40% of all neonates.[15] Importantly, the occurrence of white matter injury is more likely in the presence of a less mature brain[24] and less mature brain microstructure.[25] Delayed brain maturation has been shown for newborns with complex cardiac lesions,[26,27] starting at around 30 weeks of gestation.[28] Another preoperative injury type, stroke, occurs less frequently[29,30] and is most often focal and small. It is interesting that despite the often dramatic neonatal course, particularly when no prenatal diagnosis is made and the child presents with profound hypoxia, cerebral injuries found on MRI are small in extent. It may be that these infants are protected by preconditioning mechanisms that take place before delivery. A concern is that preoperative cerebral injuries may expand or worsen during bypass surgery. So far, no study has shown that this is the case; preoperative MRI abnormalities seem not to worsen during surgery.[17,24,31] Also, the prevalence of cerebral injuries is equal for all complex cardiac lesions.[24] Postoperatively, new brain injuries occur in up to 50% of all neonates and are again predominantly found in the white matter.[24,32] Here, more complex CHD, particularly single ventricle physiology and arch repairs, are most associated with higher rates of injuries. Preoperative and postoperative brain injuries seem not to predict early neurodevelopmental outcome but brain immaturity does.[24,25]

Although cerebral ultrasound is a useful tool for the detection of overt cerebral malformations, cerebral hemorrhages, large strokes. and the evolution of cerebral abnormalities, its use for the cardiac population is limited, in particular for the detection of the white matter lesions and small strokes found in CHD neonates and particularly fails to predict early neurodevelopmental outcome.[33]

Open question: So far, no long-term outcome studies are available that could relate the previously mentioned subtle MRI abnormalities with later, possibly more complex, cognitive and motor functions. Also, the additive or combined value of cerebral function monitoring, cerebral imaging, clinical examination, and postoperative complications for outcome prediction should be analyzed, ideally providing an algorithm helping to predict neurodevelopmental outcome in these children.

DOMAINS OF NEURODEVELOPMENTAL IMPAIRMENTS

There is extensive literature describing neurodevelopmental outcomes for children with CHD and a recently published scientific statement from the American Heart Association (and approved by the American Academy of Pediatrics), comprehensively describes the evaluation and management of neurodevelopmental impairments in children with CHD.[8]

When describing neurodevelopmental impairments for children with CHD requiring open-heart surgery, note that many children develop normally. However, impairments, mostly mild to moderate, may occur in all developmental domains[8] with "a distinctive pattern of neurodevelopmental and behavioral impairments…".[4] Importantly, because certain capacities or skills (eg, memory function, abstract-logic thinking) mature during childhood, some problems may not be apparent during early childhood. This is not because clinicians fail to detect them or do not use good assessment tools, but rather because they are not yet fully developed. These skills include executive functions (Calderon and Bellinger, 2015),[34] social interaction functions, reading and writing, or mathematical skills. A significant deficit in these domains poses major disadvantages for the school child or adolescent.

Fig. 2 schematically depicts the potential areas of neurodevelopmental impairments, the approximate timing, and the estimated prevalence over a child's life with one or multiple surgical approaches.

Early Childhood

In early childhood, particularly within the first year of life, many children, even those with only one surgical procedure, may manifest delayed motor milestones, often associated with generalized muscular hypotonia,[35] which results in lower motor scores on developmental tests, such as the Bayley Scales of Infant Development.[36,37] In early childhood, motor development seems more affected than cognitive development with significantly lower motor scores than cognitive scores. This seems to change as the child becomes older with motor scores improving within the first 3 years of life.[38] During preschool age and school age, most studies report reduced overall IQ scores with impairments in language and memory functioning and slower processing speed.[39] Motor development also remains affected, but less apparent as in early childhood. Fine motor and visuomotor impairments occur frequently[40,41] and affect processing speed and school performance, leading to higher rates of educational and therapeutic support.[41] Importantly, these difficulties, also in the presence of a normal IQ, can be associated with problems in peer interaction and emotional symptoms. Language problems include delayed acquisition of language milestones resulting in predominantly expressive language impairments,[42,43] possibly mediated by problems

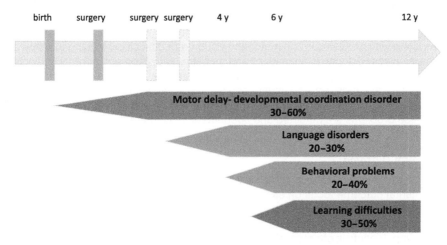

Fig. 2. Schematic overview of affected developmental domains, temporal occurrence, and estimated prevalence.

in motor aspects of speech.[40] However, when examined at older school age and adolescent age, reading abilities persist to be affected, but not more than other functional domains.[21,44]

A large body of evidence exists that overall IQ in children with CHD is lowered by around 5 to 10 IQ points[39,45,46] and that this results in learning difficulties at school age. Furthermore, behavioral problems, including externalizing symptoms, such as hyperactivity or impulsivity, and internalizing problem, such as depression or emotional problems, are described for up to 40% of all children.[41,47] The mechanisms leading to these behavioral problems are probably multifactorial and certainly involve delayed maturation of emotional control mechanisms caused by either subtle brain injuries or delayed brain maturation. Parental factors, such as maternal anxiety, maternal posttraumatic stress, and overprotection, also significantly contribute to these behavioral problems.[5]

Not all potentially affected areas of impairment are depicted in **Fig. 2**. For example, it has been shown that children with CHD may exhibit particular problems in social cognition and interaction associated with poorer cognitive and behavioral inhibition in early childhood,[48] but also in adolescents with different forms of CHD.[21,44] More evidence of the mechanisms leading to these problems needs to be accumulated to optimally support this specific, but potentially significant area of impairment, particularly when considering its consequence for adult life and social integration.

One area of specific impairment relates to executive functions.[34,49] Executive functions are higher-order cognitive functions that involve inhibitory and interference control, working memory, cognitive flexibility, verbal fluency, and planning.[50] In general, when children enter secondary school level, increasing demands are placed on executive functions from home and school as personal autonomy, independence, and planning responsibilities increase. There is evidence that children with CHD, particularly those with more severe CHD,[49] may have particular problems in executive function leading to difficulties in academic performance and in other aspects of everyday life. Importantly, delays in components of executive functioning, such as inhibition or cognitive flexibility, have been shown for children with transposition of the great arteries as early as 5 years.[51]

In clinical practice, it is often a combination of difficulties with which the school-aged child or adolescent is faced. A boy may have gross motor coordination problems, making it difficult to participate in leisure activities with peers. Sometimes this goes along with problems in fine motor and visuomotor difficulties, leading to a slower processing speed during examinations and problems with geometry or other subjects. If this is coupled with problems in planning and memory, many tasks become challenging as demands on the independence of a growing adolescent increase. Ultimately, this may lead to poorer academic achievement and poorer self-esteem unless these problems are detected and adequate educational and therapeutic support is provided.

Long-Term Outcome

As in other at-risk populations, most studies on children with CHD reporting neurodevelopmental outcome focus on early childhood or early school-age. Because of difficulties in performing long-term cohort studies (need for longitudinal funding, high patient drop-out rates), the evidence for persistent or newly emerging neurodevelopmental impairments is oftentimes sparse. However, it has been shown in very preterm born children that they may be faced with lifelong problems affecting academic achievements and social interaction.[52] Children with CHD have certain similarities in the pathomechanism of brain injury[22] and show a strikingly similar neurodevelopmental impairment profile as very premature children do (except for the frequently occurring muscular hypotonia before and after surgery). Furthermore, with the growing population of adults with CHD, it is critical to describe potential persistent problems. There is evidence that adolescents with CHD may have problems in overall intellectual performance, executive function, visuoperceptual, and fine and gross motor functioning.[21,44,53] These problems may persist into adulthood and result in a substantial social disadvantage with lower education, poorer academic achievement, and a higher unemployment rate,[54] and poorer quality of life and problems in executive functions.[55]

> Open question: It is unclear how developmental impairments evolve over time. The determinants of an improvement or decline in developmental functions are not well understood. It is conceivable that because of a delay in brain maturation and deficits in experience associated with extended hospital stays certain deficits may be outgrown, whereas others with increased demands and less brain connectivity may emerge during adolescence and become more apparent over time.

Predictors of Neurodevelopmental Outcome

Extensive effort has been undertaken to identify risk factors for adverse outcome. Here, the distinction between modifiable and nonmodifiable factors is made to define variables that can be improved. Nonmodifiable risk factors include the type of CHD, gender, genetic disorders, and socioeconomic factors.[9] Surgical techniques have been compared in various studies (eg, low-flow vs circulatory arrest), showing very little effect on long-term outcome.[21] However, the use of deep hypothermic circulatory arrest in infants with arch obstruction seems to lead to a higher rate of white matter injuries.[24] It is plausible that in the face of a tremendously large number of potential risk factors occurring before and during surgery and during the intensive care period, no single factor can be isolated as strong enough to independently predict adverse outcome. In contrast, the duration of intensive care stay, summarizing the postoperative course, remains the strongest medical risk factor for adverse outcome.[56] In addition, one has to keep in mind that over a period of a child's life, such factors as need for resuscitation or high postoperative lactate levels may fade in their significance as environmental factors, such as socioeconomic environment, and family factors become more relevant. It seems, however, that indicators of neurologic injury (eg, seizures, brain injury, and radiologically defined delayed brain development) are clearly relevant predictors of poor outcome. Also, it has to be noted that recent studies have examined new risk factors for adverse outcome, in particular fetal hemodynamic changes[57,58] and better intraoperative monitoring of brain perfusion.[4]

CLINICAL IMPLICATIONS

The clinical implications of the various neurodevelopmental impairments in children with CHD are manifold. They include raising awareness in treating physicians, other health professionals, and parent organizations about the risk of neurodevelopmental impairments. Parents may be poorly informed about potential difficulties because the link between the heart and the brain is not as apparent and they may be under the impression that by "fixing" the heart, everything will be fine. The involved medical team needs to provide information that neurodevelopmental problems may occur and that therefore neurodevelopmental follow-up is indicated. This should be similar to the well-established follow-up programs for children born very preterm and with moderate and severe hypoxic-ischemic encephalopathy.

When comparing different at-risk populations, the disease prevalence and subsequent neurodevelopment impairment rates are quite similar (**Table 1**). Hence, shared structures and resources already in place for these at-risk populations should be used, but additional financial resources need to be made available to cover the extra costs required to provide follow-up assessment for children with CHD. Importantly, these follow-up visits should take place in specialized centers, experienced with the neurodevelopmental assessment, counseling, and care of these children, comprising the expertise of various professionals, such as developmental pediatricians, neurologists, nurse practitioners, and neuropsychologists. Regional and national registries need to be established, using the same assessment tools and age intervals so that outcome research and quality control are measured.

In the consensus statement by Marino and colleagues[8] a well-defined algorithm is presented, categorizing children with CHD into higher and lower risk groups based on the need for open-heart surgery, complexity of heart lesion, and comorbidities. A detailed overview is given over the potentially affected developmental domains and the suggested, age-appropriate, and standardized assessment tools and questionnaires. Because neurodevelopmental impairments in children with CHD may only evolve during school-age, follow-up needs to be provided until school-age and ideally through adolescence. Once parents and children are familiar with the follow-up team, they will feel comfortable returning to seek counseling in the case of newly emerging school problems or behavioral and psychological concerns. This, in turn, demands an experienced and stable team of health care professionals that can establish a good relationship with the parents and child.

Because a large number of neonates and infants with CHD undergoing bypass surgery already show neurobehavioral and neuroradiologic abnormalities before surgery, a careful clinical assessment before surgery performed by an experienced neonatal neurologist or neurodevelopmental pediatrician should be considered for infants with the most complex CHD. A cerebral MRI may be considered a routine evaluation for preoperative injury; however, it is often difficult to organize and the abnormalities found on MRI may have little impact on the timing of surgery and on short-term outcome. After surgery, particularly when the postoperative course is complicated,

Table 1 Overview of major outcome categories in the largest at-risk population			
	HIE	Very Preterms	CHD
Prevalence	1–6/1000	10/1000	6/1000
Cerebral palsy	30% TH: 20%	5%–10%	2%
IQ <70	30%	10%–20%	10%–20%
Mild deficits	~50%	~50%	~30%–50%

Abbreviations: HIE, hypoxic-ischemic encephalopathy; TH, therapeutic hypothermia.

cerebral MRI should be performed in association with a discharge examination that can determine the need for therapeutic support, such as physical therapy and speech and language therapy.

SUMMARY/DISCUSSION

Children born with CHD who undergo open-heart surgery constitutes a growing population particularly vulnerable for subsequent neurodevelopmental impairments. These can occur in all developmental domains, are often of mild to moderate degree, but may occur in combination. During early childhood, motor development is predominantly affected with slower attainment of motor milestones and clinical signs of muscular hypotonia. Thereafter, children may present with slower cognitive and language development. At school-age, a variety of problems in learning, memory function, expressive language, behavior, and visuomotor functions may manifest. Importantly, complex cognitive and motor dysfunctions may emerge only as children become older and enter adolescence, leading to poorer academic achievement.

Many children with CHD have an underlying genetic disorder associated with poorer neurodevelopmental outcome. Other risk factors include comorbidities, such as preterm birth, longer intensive care stay, and poorer socioeconomic environment. There is strong evidence that intrauterine brain maturation is delayed and that the white matter is particularly affected, before and during surgical interventions. The mechanisms leading to altered brain development need to be better understood before potential interventions during the fetal or neonatal period can be implemented.[22,23] Here, the role of fetal cerebral perfusion and potential neuroprotective agents, such as erythropoietin, need to be studied using appropriate animal models.

Furthermore, the role of genetic aberrations leading to the heart defect and the impaired brain development needs to be elucidated. It is striking that a large number of genes involved in the heart formation[59] are transcriptional and signaling factors critical for early neural development and axon guidance, such as those involved in the Notch pathway and the Wnt pathway.[60]

The socioeconomic environment the child is born into and returns to after discharge from the hospital plays a critical, maybe even the most important role for the child's development and well-being. Therefore, efforts to support lower-income families and to provide early counseling need to be made because parents of chronically ill children are at risk for a variety of psychological, stress-related disorders.[61] Neurodevelopmental interventions during childhood are well established and include individually tailored motor interventions (physical therapy, occupational therapy); early intervention; and specific therapies, such as learning support, speech, and language therapy. However, little is known about interventions that aim at preventing problems before they manifest. Such therapies may include motor training during early childhood or executive function training.[34] Because the effect of these interventions is often weak in normally developing children, clinicians need to establish their effectiveness in this population. Meanwhile, follow-up networks, providing individual neurodevelopmental assessment and counseling of children and their families throughout childhood to detect emerging developmental problems early on and to provide appropriate therapies, need to be established. Finally, individual academic and psychological counseling is mandatory in the phase of adolescence and transition to adulthood.

Best practices

What is the current practice?

Congenital heart disease
  Currently, most neonates and infants with CHD undergoing bypass surgery are not routinely followed regarding their neurodevelopmental and behavioral development.

What changes in current practice are likely to improve outcomes?

Tertiary centers performing open-heart surgery in neonates and infants with severe forms of CHD need to establish a neurodevelopmental follow-up program at their institution and collaborate with clinics in other centers following these children.

Examinations need to be performed by trained specialists experienced in the care of at-risk patients and should include the administration of age-appropriate, standardized assessment tools.

This allows for individual counseling and early detection and treatment of developmental problems.

Follow-up needs to be offered until adolescence, and health care professionals responsible for the transition into adulthood also need to address academic and psychological problems.

Major recommendations
  The recommendations proposed by the American Heart Association and the American Academy of Pediatrics[8] need to be implemented and national networks need to be established not only in North America, but in all countries caring for these children.

REFERENCES

1. Hoffman JI, Kaplan S. The incidence of congenital heart disease. J Am Coll Cardiol 2002;39:1890–900.
2. Wernovsky G. The paradigm shift toward surgical intervention for neonates with hypoplastic left heart syndrome. Arch Pediatr Adolesc Med 2008;162:849–54.
3. Bhatt AB, Foster E, Kuehl K, et al. Congenital heart disease in the older adult: a scientific statement from the American Heart Association. Circulation 2015;131: 1884–931.
4. Marino BS. New concepts in predicting, evaluating, and managing neurodevelopmental outcomes in children with congenital heart disease. Curr Opin Pediatr 2013;25:574–84.
5. Latal B, Helfricht S, Fischer JE, et al. Psychological adjustment and quality of life in children and adolescents following open-heart surgery for congenital heart disease: a systematic review. BMC Pediatr 2009;9:6.
6. Spijkerboer AW, Utens EM, De Koning WB, et al. Health-related quality of life in children and adolescents after invasive treatment for congenital heart disease. Qual Life Res 2006;15:663–73.
7. Pierpont ME, Basson CT, Benson DW Jr, et al. Genetic basis for congenital heart defects: current knowledge: a scientific statement from the American Heart Association Congenital Cardiac Defects Committee, Council on Cardiovascular Disease in the Young: endorsed by the American Academy of Pediatrics. Circulation 2007;115:3015–38.
8. Marino BS, Lipkin PH, Newburger JW, et al. Neurodevelopmental outcomes in children with congenital heart disease: evaluation and management: a scientific statement from the American Heart Association. Circulation 2012;126:1143–72.
9. Wernovsky G. Current insights regarding neurological and developmental abnormalities in children and young adults with complex congenital cardiac disease. Cardiol Young 2006;16(Suppl 1):92–104.

10. Hadders-Algra M. General movements: a window for early identification of children at high risk for developmental disorders. J Pediatr 2004;145:S12–8.
11. Spittle AJ, Spencer-Smith MM, Cheong JL, et al. General movements in very preterm children and neurodevelopment at 2 and 4 years. Pediatrics 2013;132: e452–558.
12. Sabir H, Cowan FM. Prediction of outcome methods assessing short- and long-term outcome after therapeutic hypothermia. Semin Fetal Neonatal Med 2015; 20:115–21.
13. Majnemer A, Limperopoulos C, Shevell M, et al. Long-term neuromotor outcome at school entry of infants with congenital heart defects requiring open-heart surgery. J Pediatr 2006;148:72–7.
14. Limperopoulos C, Majnemer A, Shevell MI, et al. Neurologic status of newborns with congenital heart defects before open heart surgery. Pediatrics 1999;103: 402–8.
15. Khalil A, Suff N, Thilaganathan B, et al. Brain abnormalities and neurodevelopmental delay in congenital heart disease: systematic review and meta-analysis. Ultrasound Obstet Gynecol 2014;43:14–24.
16. Limperopoulos C, Majnemer A, Shevell MI, et al. Predictors of developmental disabilities after open heart surgery in young children with congenital heart defects. J Pediatr 2002;141:51–8.
17. Bertholdt S, Latal B, Liamlahi R, et al. Cerebral lesions on magnetic resonance imaging correlate with preoperative neurological status in neonates undergoing cardiopulmonary bypass surgery. Eur J Cardiothorac Surg 2014;45:625–32.
18. Clancy RR, Sharif U, Ichord R, et al. Electrographic neonatal seizures after infant heart surgery. Epilepsia 2005;46:84–90.
19. Gaynor JW, Jarvik GP, Bernbaum J, et al. The relationship of postoperative electrographic seizures to neurodevelopmental outcome at 1 year of age after neonatal and infant cardiac surgery. J Thorac Cardiovasc Surg 2006;131: 181–9.
20. Algra SO, Schouten AN, Jansen NJ, et al. Perioperative and bedside cerebral monitoring identifies cerebral injury after surgical correction of congenital aortic arch obstruction. Intensive Care Med 2015;41:2011–2.
21. Bellinger DC, Wypij D, Rivkin MJ, et al. Adolescents with d-transposition of the great arteries corrected with the arterial switch procedure: neuropsychological assessment and structural brain imaging. Circulation 2011;124:1361–9.
22. McQuillen PS, Miller SP. Congenital heart disease and brain development. Ann N Y Acad Sci 2010;1184:68–86.
23. Morton PD, Ishibashi N, Jonas RA, et al. Congenital cardiac anomalies and white matter injury. Trends Neurosci 2015;38:353–63.
24. Beca J, Gunn JK, Coleman L, et al. New white matter brain injury after infant heart surgery is associated with diagnostic group and the use of circulatory arrest. Circulation 2013;127:971–9.
25. Dimitropoulos A, McQuillen PS, Sethi V, et al. Brain injury and development in newborns with critical congenital heart disease. Neurology 2013;81:241–8.
26. Licht DJ, Shera DM, Clancy RR, et al. Brain maturation is delayed in infants with complex congenital heart defects. J Thorac Cardiovasc Surg 2009;137:529–36 [discussion: 536–7].
27. Miller SP, McQuillen PS, Hamrick S, et al. Abnormal brain development in newborns with congenital heart disease. N Engl J Med 2007;357:1928–38.
28. Limperopoulos C, Tworetzky W, McElhinney DB, et al. Brain volume and metabolism in fetuses with congenital heart disease: evaluation with

quantitative magnetic resonance imaging and spectroscopy. Circulation 2010; 121:26–33.

29. Beca J, Gunn J, Coleman L, et al. Pre-operative brain injury in newborn infants with transposition of the great arteries occurs at rates similar to other complex congenital heart disease and is not related to balloon atrial septostomy. J Am Coll Cardiol 2009;53:1807–11.

30. McQuillen PS, Hamrick SE, Perez MJ, et al. Balloon atrial septostomy is associated with preoperative stroke in neonates with transposition of the great arteries. Circulation 2006;113:280–5.

31. Block AJ, McQuillen PS, Chau V, et al. Clinically silent preoperative brain injuries do not worsen with surgery in neonates with congenital heart disease. J Thorac Cardiovasc Surg 2010;140:550–7.

32. Algra SO, Jansen NJ, van der Tweel I, et al. Neurological injury after neonatal cardiac surgery: a randomized, controlled trial of 2 perfusion techniques. Circulation 2014;129:224–33.

33. Latal B, Kellenberger CJ, Dimitropoulos A, et al. Can preoperative cranial ultrasound predict early neurodevelopmental outcome in infants with congenital heart disease? Dev Med Child Neurol, in press.

34. Calderon J, Bellinger DC. Executive function deficits in congenital heart disease: why is intervention important? Cardiol Young 2015;25:1238–46.

35. Limperopoulos C, Majnemer A, Shevell MI, et al. Neurodevelopmental status of newborns and infants with congenital heart defects before and after open heart surgery. J Pediatr 2000;137:638–45.

36. Gaynor JW, Stopp C, Wypij D, et al. Neurodevelopmental outcomes after cardiac surgery in infancy. Pediatrics 2015;135:816–25.

37. Snookes SH, Gunn JK, Eldridge BJ, et al. A systematic review of motor and cognitive outcomes after early surgery for congenital heart disease. Pediatrics 2010;125:e818–27.

38. Mussatto KA, Hoffmann RG, Hoffman GM, et al. Risk and prevalence of developmental delay in young children with congenital heart disease. Pediatrics 2014; 133:e570–7.

39. Miatton M, De Wolf D, Francois K, et al. Neurocognitive consequences of surgically corrected congenital heart defects: a review. Neuropsychol Rev 2006;16:65–85.

40. Karl TR, Hall S, Ford G, et al. Arterial switch with full-flow cardiopulmonary bypass and limited circulatory arrest: neurodevelopmental outcome. J Thorac Cardiovasc Surg 2004;127:213–22.

41. Liamlahi R, von Rhein M, Buhrer S, et al. Motor dysfunction and behavioural problems frequently coexist with congenital heart disease in school-age children. Acta Paediatr 2014;103:752–8.

42. Bellinger DC, Wypij D, Kuban KC, et al. Developmental and neurological status of children at 4 years of age after heart surgery with hypothermic circulatory arrest or low-flow cardiopulmonary bypass. Circulation 1999;100:526–32.

43. Hovels-Gurich HH, Bauer SB, Schnitker R, et al. Long-term outcome of speech and language in children after corrective surgery for cyanotic or acyanotic cardiac defects in infancy. Eur J Paediatr Neurol 2008;12:378–86.

44. Bellinger DC, Rivkin MJ, DeMaso D, et al. Adolescents with tetralogy of Fallot: neuropsychological assessment and structural brain imaging. Cardiol Young 2015;25:338–47.

45. Krueger JJ, Brotschi B, Balmer C, et al. Postoperative hyperglycemia and 4-year neurodevelopmental outcome in children operated for congenital heart disease. J Pediatr 2015;167(6):1253–8.e1.

46. Majnemer A, Limperopoulos C, Shevell MI, et al. A new look at outcomes of infants with congenital heart disease. Pediatr Neurol 2009;40:197–204.
47. Shillingford AJ, Glanzman MM, Ittenbach RF, et al. Inattention, hyperactivity, and school performance in a population of school-age children with complex congenital heart disease. Pediatrics 2008;121:e759–67.
48. Calderon J, Bonnet D, Courtin C, et al. Executive function and theory of mind in school-aged children after neonatal corrective cardiac surgery for transposition of the great arteries. Dev Med Child Neurol 2010;52:1139–44.
49. Cassidy AR, White MT, DeMaso DR, et al. Executive function in children and adolescents with critical cyanotic congenital heart disease. J Int Neuropsychol Soc 2015;21:34–49.
50. Diamond A. Executive functions. Annu Rev Psychol 2013;64:135–68.
51. Calderon J, Jambaque I, Bonnet D, et al. Executive functions development in 5- to 7-year-old children with transposition of the great arteries: a longitudinal study. Dev Neuropsychol 2014;39:365–84.
52. Hack M. Adult outcomes of preterm children. J Dev Behav Pediatr 2009;30:460–70.
53. Schaefer C, von Rhein M, Knirsch W, et al. Neurodevelopmental outcome, psychological adjustment, and quality of life in adolescents with congenital heart disease. Dev Med Child Neurol 2013;55:1143–9.
54. Zomer AC, Vaartjes I, Uiterwaal CS, et al. Social burden and lifestyle in adults with congenital heart disease. Am J Cardiol 2012;109:1657–63.
55. Tyagi M, Austin K, Stygall J, et al. What do we know about cognitive functioning in adult congenital heart disease? Cardiol Young 2014;24:13–9.
56. Newburger JW, Wypij D, Bellinger DC, et al. Length of stay after infant heart surgery is related to cognitive outcome at age 8 years. J Pediatr 2003;143:67–73.
57. Sethi V, Tabbutt S, Dimitropoulos A, et al. Single-ventricle anatomy predicts delayed microstructural brain development. Pediatr Res 2013;73:661–7.
58. Sun L, Macgowan CK, Sled JG, et al. Reduced fetal cerebral oxygen consumption is associated with smaller brain size in fetuses with congenital heart disease. Circulation 2015;131:1313–23.
59. Bruneau BG. The developmental genetics of congenital heart disease. Nature 2008;451:943–8.
60. Stoeckli ET. What does the developing brain tell us about neural diseases? Eur J Neurosci 2012;35:1811–7.
61. Werner H, Latal B, Valsangiacomo Buechel E, et al. The impact of an infant's severe congenital heart disease on the family: a prospective cohort study. Congenit Heart Dis 2014;9:203–10.

Pulmonary Hypertension and Pulmonary Vasodilators

Roberta L. Keller, MD

KEYWORDS

- Bronchopulmonary dysplasia • Congenital diaphragmatic hernia
- Echocardiography • Persistent pulmonary hypertension of the newborn
- Pulmonary vascular disease • Pulmonary vascular resistance

KEY POINTS

- Persistent pulmonary hypertension of the newborn is an acute perinatal condition with accepted clinical and echocardiographic criteria for diagnosis.
- There is limited validation for echocardiographic criteria for the diagnosis of pulmonary hypertension in infants after the acute transitional period.
- Cardiovascular comorbidities may be present in up to 50% of infants with bronchopulmonary dysplasia and pulmonary hypertension. Intervention may be necessary before or during treatment of pulmonary hypertension.
- There are no controlled studies supporting specific pulmonary vasodilator therapy for infants with pulmonary hypertension, but there are data to support specific dosing strategies for these children.

INTRODUCTION

Pulmonary hypertension (PH) in the perinatal period is often referred to as persistent PH of the newborn (PPHN). This diagnosis generally refers to the early, acute condition of systemic-to-suprasystemic pulmonary vascular resistance (PVR), with its attendant extrapulmonary right-to-left shunts and profound hypoxemia. PPHN may be transient, caused by metabolic derangements, or more persistent, most frequently in the setting of perinatal infection or lung disease. Further, with improvements in perinatal care, the increased survival of infants at risk for more chronic forms of PH, related to abnormal development of the lung and its vasculature, creates a different set of issues for providers, with assessments and treatment strategies that may differ from those that have

Conflict of interest and funding: The author has nothing to disclose.
Neonatology, Department of Pediatrics, UCSF Benioff Children's Hospital, University of California San Francisco, Box 0734, 550 16th Street, 5th Floor, San Francisco, CA 94143, USA
E-mail address: kellerr@ucsf.edu

Clin Perinatol 43 (2016) 187–202
http://dx.doi.org/10.1016/j.clp.2015.11.013   **perinatology.theclinics.com**

evolved for the acute care of infants with PPHN. This article focuses on current issues in the evaluation and management of PH in the perinatal period, including assessment and initiation of chronic therapies, with most attention to infants with bronchopulmonary dysplasia (BPD) and congenital diaphragmatic hernia (CDH).

DEFINITIONS AND CRITERIA FOR DIAGNOSIS OF PULMONARY HYPERTENSION

Older definitions of PH in predominantly adult patients were focused on an increase in mean pulmonary arterial pressure (P_{PA}) without evidence of significant left heart disease.[1] This definition was intended to identify patients with increased PVR caused by pulmonary vascular disease (PVD). However, because an increase in the pulmonary/systemic blood flow ratio (Qp/Qs) also affects the direct interpretation of the measurement of this value, the definition has been modified in children to include the assessment of PVR (normal, 1–3 Wood units $\times$ m^2)[2,3] as a better indicator of PVD. In the perinatal period, the timing of the usual transition to adult values for these parameters also needs to be considered, because term infants should reach these values by 2 to 3 months of age.[1,3] However, the transition for preterm infants is not as well defined.

Invasive Assessment of Pulmonary Hypertension: the Gold Standard

The only way to obtain direct measurements of pulmonary hemodynamic parameters is through cardiac catheterization. The hemodynamic criteria for the diagnosis of PH are:

- Mean P_{PA} greater than or equal to 25 mm Hg
- PVR greater than 3 Wood units $\times$ m^2
- Pulmonary capillary wedge pressure less than or equal to 15 mm Hg

To perform this procedure safely in any pediatric population, experienced personnel are required; serious complications from diagnostic catheterization in children with PH are uncommon (1%–3% of procedures) at experienced centers.[4,5] However, complications from cardiac catheterization may be more likely in small and ill children, particularly those with low birth weight (<2500 g).[6] Thus, catheterization is not frequently undertaken early in the course of neonatal illness (such as in the first month of life) unless complex congenital heart disease (CHD) potentially amenable to catheter-based intervention is present, and, if then, at a few experienced centers. Further, in interpretation of hemodynamic data from cardiac catheterization, therapies at the time of study need to be considered.

Cardiac magnetic resonance (MR) could supply much of the data that is obtained from cardiac catheterization, in a less invasive manner. However, there are limited validation studies for cardiac MR and diagnosis of PH in adults and none in infants.[7,8] Regardless, multiple factors may limit the application of this technology for assessment of PH:

- Transport to MR scanner and clinical management and sedation of a sick infant outside the intensive care unit or operating room
- Appropriate equipment and specialized expertise in cardiac MRI required to obtain sequences and interpret data
- Limitation of hemodynamic measurements: inability to assess the contribution of shunts, technical challenges in direct measurements with small infants

One report of cardiac MR for evaluation of CHD in infants showed a low rate of serious complications, comparable with reports on cardiac catheterization from experienced pediatric PH programs.[9]

Clinical Assessment of Pulmonary Hypertension

In the assessment of infants with concern for PPHN during the acute perinatal period, the standard physical examination and supporting radiographic and laboratory data are critical for the initial evaluation.[10]

Data that might raise concern for a significant intrapulmonary (evidence of structural or parenchymal lung disease) or extrapulmonary shunt (preductal and postductal oxygen saturation differential indicating pulmonary to systemic blood flow at the level of a patent ductus arteriosus [PDA]) are useful in the initial and ongoing assessment of infants with concern for PPHN. Variable patterns of preductal (usually right hand) and lower body oxygen saturation differences can exist, and none completely rule PPHN in or out, although trends in the preductal and postductal saturation differential can be a useful parameter to follow to assess the response to various interventions for PPHN, once the diagnosis is established. Thus, it is important to consider the potential interpretation of these patterns of oxygen saturations:

- Upper body greater than lower body
  - PPHN (suprasystemic PVR)
  - Arch obstruction with systemic circulation dependent on ductal blood flow
  - Other forms of structural heart disease with preferential streaming of blood flow (eg, total anomalous pulmonary venous return [TAPVR], septal defects)
- Upper body less than lower body
  - Transposition of the great vessels
  - Other forms of structural heart disease with preferential streaming of blood flow (eg, TAPVR)
- No difference between upper and lower body saturations
  - Bidirectional ductus arteriosus flow (systemic PVR)
  - Large intracardiac shunt equalizing saturations in right ventricle (RV) and left ventricle (LV)
  - Anomalous take-off of right subclavian artery (postductal position)
  - Closed ductus arteriosus (including premature in utero closure, often associated with PPHN)
  - Absent ductus arteriosus

If rapid, expert echocardiographic interpretation of structural CHD cannot be completed and there is any suspicion for cyanotic CHD, the early assessment should include a hyperoxic challenge test (**Fig. 1**). Regardless, clinical evidence of a genetic condition (eg, dysmorphic features, noncardiac anomalies, stigmata of Down syndrome) in an ill or hypoxic newborn, even with evidence of lung disease, should prompt transfer to a center where expert evaluation and intervention for CHD can be undertaken, because the likelihood of CHD is higher in this group of infants, and both cyanotic and acyanotic CHD can contribute to hypoxemia.

The later clinical assessment of infants at risk for PH caused by an associated underlying condition (eg, extreme prematurity, BPD, structural lung defects) includes many of the same elements of the assessment as in the acute setting. Cardiac evaluation should pay special attention to the presence of a hyperdynamic precordium or right ventricular heave, and the character of the heart sounds (eg, loud S2, fixed split S1 and S2, gallop). Liver position should be noted, and followed as a potential reflection of right atrial pressure. There should be particular attention to growth parameters and trajectory, ongoing need for support (respiratory and feeding), and developmental status and trajectory. These parameters are important for ascertaining the pediatric functional class (as proposed by Lammers and

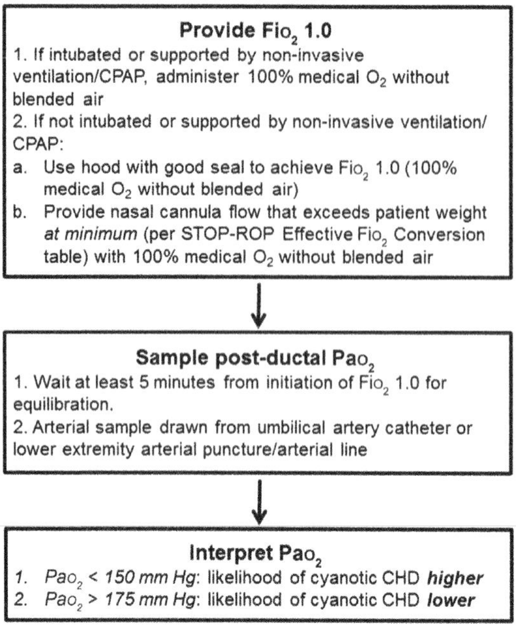

Provide Fio₂ 1.0

1. If intubated or supported by non-invasive ventilation/CPAP, administer 100% medical O₂ without blended air
2. If not intubated or supported by non-invasive ventilation/CPAP:
   a. Use hood with good seal to achieve Fio₂ 1.0 (100% medical O₂ without blended air)
   b. Provide nasal cannula flow that exceeds patient weight *at minimum* (per STOP-ROP Effective Fio₂ Conversion table) with 100% medical O₂ without blended air

↓

Sample post-ductal Pao₂

1. Wait at least 5 minutes from initiation of Fio₂ 1.0 for equilibration.
2. Arterial sample drawn from umbilical artery catheter or lower extremity arterial puncture/arterial line

↓

Interpret Pao₂

1. *Pao₂ < 150 mm Hg:* likelihood of cyanotic CHD *higher*
2. *Pao₂ > 175 mm Hg:* likelihood of cyanotic CHD *lower*

Fig. 1. Neonatal hyperoxic challenge: procedure and interpretation. CPAP, continuous positive airway pressure; Fio₂, fraction of inspired oxygen, STOP-ROP, Supplemental Therapeutic Oxygen for Prethreshold Retinopathy of Prematurity. (*Data from* STOP-ROP: Supplemental Therapeutic Oxygen for Prethreshold Retinopathy of Prematurity. Available at: http://pub. emmes.com/study/rop/. Accessed August 7, 2015. *Adapted from* Benaron DA, Benitz WE. Maximizing the stability of oxygen delivered via nasal cannula. Arch Pediatr Adolesc Med 1994;148(3):294–300.)

colleagues[11]), which may be useful to consider in the follow-up of children treated for PH.

In the acute assessment of PPHN, decreased systemic oxygen levels are prominent. However, there are multiple reasons why impaired oxygenation may not be clinically apparent, particularly later in the clinical course. As noted previously, in the absence of extrapulmonary communications, even suprasystemic PVR does not result in right-to-left shunting. In addition, the effects of near-systemic PVR may not be apparent even with communications in place, because blood may be shunting left to right. However, the persistence of intrapulmonary bronchopulmonary anastomotic pathways has recently been described from autopsy tissue in BPD and CDH,[12,13] creating another explanation for persistence of hypoxemia in infants at risk for later PH. In addition, if cardiac output is compromised by the increase in PVR, the decrease in mixed venous saturation in the presence of lung disease increases the need for supplemental oxygen.

Echocardiographic Assessment of Pulmonary Hypertension

There is no definitive standard for diagnosis of PH by echocardiography. However, it is frequently used in newborns as a diagnostic tool for PPHN with a consistent clinical setting, with broadly accepted criteria of right-to-left or bidirectional flow at the level of the ductus arteriosus or other intracardiac communication.[14,15] This approach has led to further classifications of the severity of PH based on the degree of increase in the RV or P_{PA} to systemic pressure ratio (RV or P_{PA}/systemic ratio), because it reflects increased PVR:

- Severe: greater than or equal to 1.0 (systemic to suprasystemic)
- Moderate: greater than or equal to 1:2 to 2:3 and <1.0
- None/mild/minimal: <1:2 to 2:3

These classifications are most useful when assessing infants later in their clinical course, and/or longitudinally, with the state of their systemic vascular resistance considered. Echocardiographic measurements used for these classifications are described in **Table 1**. These measurements assume that there is no RV outflow tract obstruction.

The best classification scheme to apply in clinical practice is not yet clear. Investigators have proposed using both any of these criteria[16] or a hierarchy of these criteria,[17,18] and identical classification schemes have not been widely adopted across various research groups. Further, validation of these classification schemes is limited, with respect to a confirmed diagnosis of PH, as well as the implications for outcome. In children with lung disease less than 2 years of age, Mourani and colleagues[19] found that tricuspid regurgitation (TR) jet velocity predicting RV systolic pressure (RVsp) greater than 40 mm Hg (by modified Bernoulli equation, assuming right atrial pressure [RAp] = 0) and interventricular septum (IVS) flattening had similar sensitivity (88%) but poor specificity (33%) for the diagnosis of PH by cardiac catheterization. However, TR jet velocity was only quantifiable in 61% of the children, TR was more likely to be quantifiable in children with higher measured pulmonary artery (PA) pressure, and the estimated RVsp correlated poorly with the PA pressure. Similarly, in a validation study of RV pressure estimates from concurrent TR and invasive catheterization measurements, less than 25% of potentially eligible children had quantifiable TR, agreement was moderately poor for increased RV pressure (both underestimate and overestimate), and TR lacked accuracy for classification of PH (>one-half to two-thirds systemic pressure), with ~20% misclassified, even while incorporating the measured RAp for the calculation of RVsp.[20] We similarly found that quantifiable TR was more likely to be present with a more severe classification of PH by echocardiogram.[17] Thus, these studies suggest that using TR alone is insufficient to correctly identify infants with PH, and to grade its severity.

Table 1
Echocardiographic measurements for the assessment of the presence and severity of PH, as used in published reports from neonatal patient populations

Measurement	Criteria Used for Classification
TR jet velocity[a]	RVsp >40 mm Hg (RAp = 0) RVsp/SBP ratio ≥1:2 or 2:3 (RAp = 0 or 5 mm Hg)
Nonrestrictive cardiac shunt (PDA, VSD, atrial septum)	Right-to-left or bidirectional flow RV or PA pressure ≥ one-half or two-thirds systemic
IVS position	D-shaped or convex into LV Flattened throughout cardiac cycle Any flattening

Abbreviations: IVS, interventricular septum; LV, left ventricle; PA, pulmonary artery; RAp, right atrial pressure; RVsp, right ventricular systolic pressure; SBP, systemic blood pressure; TR, tricuspid regurgitation; VSD, ventricular septal defect.
[a] RVsp calculated from peak TR jet velocity by modified Bernoulli equation: RVsp = 4 × velocity2 + RAp (assumed RAp noted).
Data from Refs.[16–19,22]

The clinical significance of PH assessed by these echocardiographic criteria is also not fully established. Khemani and colleagues[21] followed former preterm children with BPD after 2 months of age, and classified PH by IVS position only. Children with severe PH (systemic to suprasystemic) at any time during follow-up had worse survival than those with less severe PH, with only 33% of the children with severe PH alive 6 months after diagnosis. Mourani and colleagues[16] found a 10% mortality among former preterm infants with a diagnosis of PH by any echocardiographic criteria (>one-half the systemic pressure, as discussed earlier) at 36 weeks' post-menstrual age (PMA), compared with 1% mortality in children without PH. In infants with CDH, using a hierarchy of echo measurements (PDA shunt, followed by IVS position, followed by TR jet velocity), we found that persistence of PH ($\geq$two-thirds of systemic pressure) at greater than or equal to 2 weeks of age predicted poor clinical outcomes, including mortality, prolonged intubation ($\geq$28 days of age), and prolonged respiratory support ($\geq$56 days of age or home oxygen supplementation).[22] However, 2 concerns are raised by these data, in their application outside the research setting. IVS position may be subjective, with varying proportions of children classified with PH, depending on how the data are interpreted.[16] Using a more strict definition of IVS position resulted in lower PH prevalence in the study by Mourani and colleagues,[16] with prevalence estimates that approached those of Mirza and colleagues.[18] Further, these classification schemes may not be valid for infants with PH from other causes.

Echocardiography and the assessment of cardiovascular comorbidities

In addition, in the assessment of infants with suspected PH, echocardiographic evaluation needs to pay careful attention to potential cardiovascular comorbidities, which include:

- PDA
- Atrial septal defect (ASD)
- Pulmonary vein stenosis (PVS)
- Systemic-to-pulmonary collateral vessels

Each of these conditions can have a hemodynamic influence during the assessment and management of PH, and thus cardiac catheterization may be required for further assessment. del Cerro and colleagues[3] found that 65% of infants and children with BPD and PH born at or transferred to a national referral center had cardiovascular comorbidities detected by computed tomography scan or cardiac catheterization (50% for infants born at the center). In these 19 children, the most common abnormalities were PDA (n = 9), systemic-to-pulmonary collateral vessels (n = 9), PVS (n = 7), and ASD (n = 5). Catheter-based or operative intervention was undertaken for 5 children with PDA, 3 with systemic-to-pulmonary collaterals and 2 with ASD (2 ASDs closed spontaneously). Additional potential hemodynamic data that might be useful are seen with the potential response to vasodilators. Khemani and colleagues[21] described increased Qp/Qs with vasodilator challenge in 3 infants with BPD and ASD. Similarly, LV diastolic dysfunction has also been shown by cardiac catheterization in the setting of BPD, and both this condition and PVS can result in worsening pulmonary edema with initiation of pulmonary vasodilator therapy.[19]

THERAPIES FOR PULMONARY HYPERTENSION: ACUTE AND CHRONIC

The approach to management and therapy for PH in the perinatal period depends on several clinical factors; at minimum:

1. Whether PH is acute and severe (eg, PPHN) versus chronic, and
2. The cause of the PH

The cause of perinatal PH is important, because some infants with early PH are at substantial risk for prolonged, persistent, and chronic PH, whereas others are unlikely to have ongoing PH.[23] The management of PPHN is often focused on improving oxygenation, with less attention to effects of therapy on cardiac function, whereas the management of infants at risk for chronic PH needs to focus on preserving RV function, because high afterload is likely to be prolonged and persistent, putting the RV at risk for failure over time.

Treatment of Persistent Pulmonary Hypertension of the Newborn

Causes of transient PPHN include hypoxia, acidosis, hypoglycemia, hyperviscosity (usually caused by polycythemia in the perinatal period), and hypothermia. Treatment is focused on correcting these derangements, with supportive therapy during this correction. However, in the contemporary era of therapeutic hypothermia for neonatal hypoxic ischemic encephalopathy (HIE), hypothermia is continued for 72 hours from its initiation. Infants with HIE may already be at risk for PPHN, given their history of perinatal depression, which may be associated with acidosis, meconium-stained amniotic fluid, and/or infection. Although there may be increased severity of PPHN with therapeutic hypothermia, data are not consistent across studies.[24–27]

Supportive care for the underlying cause of PPHN is the mainstay of treatment, and includes providing the appropriate level of respiratory support for lung disease (including supplemental oxygen, which also acts as a pulmonary vasodilator), and direct support for impaired circulatory function. In general, infants with parenchymal lung disease, such as meconium aspiration syndrome (MAS) or respiratory distress syndrome (RDS), have improvements in oxygenation with lung recruitment maneuvers (as applied during high-frequency ventilation).[14] Other than increasing alveolar surface area, achieving functional residual capacity also decreases PVR. If clinical and laboratory information is consistent with RDS, surfactant replacement is indicated. Apart from RDS, ventilated infants with MAS and moderately impaired oxygenation may also respond to exogenous surfactant, with a decreased rate of progression to the need for extracorporeal membrane oxygenation (ECMO) support.[28] In general, in the setting of severe respiratory failure and PPHN, surfactant dosing should be undertaken with caution, when benefit clearly outweighs risk. These strategies are rarely effective in the setting of PPHN without alveolar filling.[14] Lung overdistention may increase PVR and result in further hemodynamic compromise. Thus, the optimal ventilator management in the setting of lung hypoplasia (eg, CDH) or idiopathic PPHN (when lung fields are clear and oligemic, consistent with decreased pulmonary blood flow) is also challenging, and various approaches have been proposed, including the use of low positive end-expiratory pressure.[29]

The primary goal of therapy for PPHN is to decrease PVR while maintaining or increasing cardiac output (which should result in improved systemic oxygenation). Inhaled nitric oxide (iNO), the potent pulmonary vasodilator, has been the mainstay of pharmacologic therapy for PPHN in term and near-term infants since regulatory approval was granted (1999 and 2001 in United States and Europe, respectively). iNO doses from 5 to 80 ppm are effective in improving oxygenation; however, significant decreases in P_{PA}/systemic ratio in PPHN have only been shown at greater than or equal to 20 ppm.[15,30–33] Infants with the most impaired oxygenation showed the greatest improvements in these studies, which likely represents reversal of extrapulmonary shunting. Other infants may have improved oxygenation caused by enhanced ventilation/perfusion (V/Q) matching with preferential delivery of the vasodilator to ventilated areas of the lung.[14,15,33] However, caution should be taken in initiating iNO without a full echocardiogram to rule out anatomic and physiologic conditions that might be exacerbated by pulmonary vasodilation (eg, TAPVR with obstruction or left heart dysfunction, with left-to-right flow at atrial level caused by left atrial hypertension).

In multicenter randomized controlled trials (RCTs), iNO reduced the need for ECMO by 28% to 46%.[30,32] However, use of ECMO for neonatal respiratory failure/PPHN has decreased 40% to 50% from peak levels in 1992 (Extracorporeal Life Support Organization semiannual report, July 2015). Thus, it is likely that both the availability of iNO and additional emerging technologies, such as high-frequency ventilation, have contributed to this change.[34–36] These reports also note that some populations of infants remain refractory to conventional therapies, thus several investigators have evaluated the hemodynamic effects of adjunctive therapies for refractory PPHN. One that has been more extensively studied, and increasingly used in the perinatal period, is milrinone, a phosphodiesterase (PDE)-3 inhibitor of cyclic AMP metabolism. Milrinone may potentiate the effect of iNO and endogenous pulmonary vasodilators. In uncontrolled studies, milrinone has been shown to improve oxygenation in infants with PPHN from diverse causes, with substantial decreases in estimated RVsp and improvements in RV function and cardiac output.[37–39] Effects in infants with CDH receiving iNO are less pronounced, but still promising, with improved oxygenation and RV diastolic function, which was severely impaired.[40] In these infants with right-to-left or bidirectional flow through a PDA, improvements in LV diastolic function and filling may be caused by interventricular dependence (with decreased RV load afterload) and increased pulmonary venous return, even if the PDA shunt persists, with improved systemic oxygen delivery. Milrinone in these perinatal populations is administered as a continuous infusion at 0.33 to 1 μg/kg/min, either with or without a loading dose. The half-life in newborns is 4.1 ± 1.1 hours.[41]

Preterm Infants with Persistent Pulmonary Hypertension of the Newborn

Preterm infants born after a period of oligohydramnios, frequently following premature prolonged rupture of the membranes, and without significant acute RDS, may have pulmonary vascular physiology similar to that of term and near-term infants who are treated with iNO. There are several reports describing acute improvements in oxygenation following initiation of iNO in this clinical situation.[42–44] However, there is caution around the use of iNO in preterm newborns; a summary statement from the National Institutes of Health Consensus Development Conference stated that, "the available evidence does not support use of iNO in early-routine, early-rescue, or later-rescue regimens in the care of premature infants of <34 weeks' gestation who require respiratory support," while recognizing there are insufficient data on the management of PH in preterm infants.[45] Milrinone has also been administered in this population, although there are concerns that it may increase the risk of intracranial hemorrhage.[37,46,47]

Chronic Therapies for Perinatal Pulmonary Hypertension

The medications discussed here are those that are primarily used in the chronic therapy for PH in other patient populations. In general, chronic therapies are focused on reversing pulmonary vascular remodeling, with an additional potential benefit of acute pulmonary vasodilation. However, drugs used acutely for treatment of PH in the perinatal period may also be used chronically, and vice versa.[48–50] It is important to recognize that any systemically administered vasodilator can cause systemic hypotension and decreased V/Q matching, resulting in desaturation and increasing oxygen requirement in children with lung disease. In each of the drug classes discussed, there are additional medications that do not yet have accepted doses in the perinatal population, so these are not specifically addressed.

Phosphodiesterase inhibitors: sildenafil
Sildenafil is a PDE-5 inhibitor of cyclic GMP metabolism, potentiating the effect of NO. It is available in parenteral and enteral formulations, with a stable oral suspension for pediatric administration.[51] Enteral sildenafil reduces mortality in PPHN in low-resource settings.[52] However, there are no published RCTs of the efficacy of chronic sildenafil therapy for PH in infants, although multiple case series suggest that sildenafil may improve outcomes in PH complicating BPD and CDH.[53–56] The dosing has been broad in these reports (2–8 mg/kg/d); pediatric administration and dosing are controversial, because of variable interpretation of data from the STARTS I and II trials (Sildenafil in Treatment Naive Children, Aged 1 to 17 Years, with Pulmonary Arterial Hypertension) conducted in children greater than or equal to 1 year old and 8 kg (**Table 2**).[57,58]

Based on these data, the European Medicines Agency approved sildenafil for pediatric patients, in using the medium-dose regimen (10 mg 3 times daily for 8–20 kg and 20 mg 3 times daily for >20 kg), with the rationale that increased mortality is not as pronounced in this group, and there is a good likelihood of benefit in the primary outcome and multiple secondary outcomes in this group. However, the US Food and Drug Administration (FDA) failed to approve the drug for children in the United States, based on the same data. Following the STARTS 1 data reporting, the FDA released the following statement: "…Revatio, particularly chronic use, is not recommended in children." (August 2012). This statement was later clarified to not be a contraindication but a warning that clinicians need to use their best judgment. In our center, we extrapolate the medium dose on a per-kilogram basis to infants, prescribing 2 to 3 mg/kg divided 3 to 4 times daily, up to 10 kg. Dosing is often limited in the perinatal period by side effects, particularly feeding intolerance and gastroesophageal reflux. Because this effect is dose dependent, sometimes tolerance is better with a lower dose administered 4 times daily. Gastrointestinal side effects of sildenafil in children with PH on monotherapy occur in up to 24%, with vascular and neurologic effects in 21% and 18%, respectively; rates are higher when sildenafil is combined with other PH-specific therapies.[59] In infants and young children, serious bleeding and erections are also reported.[3,54,60,61]

There is a single study of parenteral sildenafil dosing in infants with PPHN.[62] This study revealed that a continuous infusion with a slow loading dose was best tolerated, with other regimens resulting in systemic hypotension; there were modest improvements in oxygenation. In general, pharmacokinetic studies support halving an enteral dose with parenteral administration because oral sildenafil has ~40% bioavailability.[63]

Endothelin receptor antagonists: bosentan
There is good rationale for use of endothelin receptor antagonists in PH from many causes in the perinatal period, because endothelin-1 (ET1) pathways are activated in neonatal lung disease, fibrosis and inflammation are prominent in acute and chronic phases of illness, and ET1 is profibrotic and proinflammatory.[17,64–67] There

Table 2
Issues in pediatric sildenafil dosing as raised by the STARTS 1 and 2 trials

Study Design and Analysis	Comment
3 weight ranges, 3 dose groups: Low/medium/high[a]	Dose range (mg/kg/d)
≥8–20 kg: NA/10 mg/20 mg	Low: 0.6–1.5
>20–45 kg: 10 mg/20 mg/40 mg	Medium: 1.5–3
>45 kg: 20 mg/40 mg/80 mg	High: 3–6
Primary outcome VO$_2$max by CPET	Of 234 participants, only 106 able to complete CPET (≥7 y old, developmentally able)
Dose groups combined in primary outcome analysis of VO$_2$max	Marginal statistical significance in combined analysis ($P = .056$) Minimal treatment effect (NS) in low-dose group
Significant treatment effect in several secondary outcomes (dose groups combined)	Some outcomes collected in only a subset of participants (eg, invasive hemodynamic data) Minimal treatment effects in low-dose group
Dose response in multiple secondary outcomes	
Increased mortality in higher dose groups over ≥3 y of follow-up	Differences most pronounced in children >20 kg at entry Mortality also increased when analyzed by actual dose administered, because up-titration allowed Differences persist despite adjustment for imbalances in baseline prognostic factors

Abbreviations: CPET, cardiopulmonary exercise testing; NA, not applicable; NS, not significant; VO$_2$max, peak oxygen consumption.
[a] Dose administered 3 times daily.
Data from Barst RJ, Ivy DD, Gaitan G, et al. A randomized, double-blind, placebo-controlled, dose-ranging study of oral sildenafil citrate in treatment-naive children with pulmonary arterial hypertension. Circulation 2012;125(2):324–34; and Barst RJ, Beghetti M, Pulido T, et al. STARTS-2: long-term survival with oral sildenafil monotherapy in treatment-naive pediatric pulmonary arterial hypertension. Circulation 2014;129(19):1914–23.

are fewer reports of the use of bosentan in the perinatal period compared with sildenafil,[68] and pediatric dosing of bosentan has been studied, with side effects in children that are well described, occurring at lower rates than in adults.[69–71] In our center, extrapolating the dosing ranges from older children, we initiate infant bosentan dosing at 1 mg/kg twice daily, and advance to 2 mg/kg twice daily if liver enzyme levels are not increased (with ongoing monitoring). There is no stable suspension, so the drug must be prepared for each administration. We have found bosentan to be well tolerated when initiated for chronic therapy, consistent with data showing that transaminitis occurs at less than half the rate of older children and adults in young children.[70] In our experience, infants who are most likely to develop transaminitis are those with underlying liver disease or acute infection. Caution is needed in initiating bosentan in these populations.

A small RCT of bosentan for PPHN showed no beneficial effects, with low enrollment and early discontinuation (NCT01389856, clinicaltrials.gov, accessed 9/1/2015.)

Prostacyclin and its analogues

Parenteral prostacyclin formulations are the mainstay of therapy for severe PH. They have been used in the perinatal period, in both the acute period and later.[72–75] The short half-life of epoprostenol (3 minutes) allows controlled uptitration of the dose, with the ability to decrease side effects by dose reduction. However, there is a serious risk of rebound PH with abrupt discontinuation, which is mitigated with treprostinil (half-life of ~4 hours). Treprostinil allows more stable administration, with the subcutaneous route providing the potential for outpatient management in small infants without the risks of an indwelling central line.[76,77] However, because of its inherently high-risk profile, parenteral prostacyclin administration requires specific training in the inpatient setting, and extensive support in the outpatient setting. Titration of parenteral prostacyclin administration is often associated with gastrointestinal side effects (vomiting, nausea, diarrhea), requiring a decreased rate of uptitration. Pain at medication initiation and with catheter changes for subcutaneous administration, as well as local skin reactions or infection, can require additional intervention.[3,75] Some investigators have raised concerns regarding the initiation of parenteral therapy in infants; however, we and others have described successful transition to oral therapies in survivors.[74,77]

Inhaled prostacyclin analogues provide an opportunity for vasodilation along with improved V/Q matching via an "intelligent" nebulizer which is a patient-activated delivery system wherein the drug is only delivered during the inhalation phase of the respiratory cycle, ensuring full-dose delivery. Inhaled iloprost, which has a short systemic half-life of 6 to 10 minutes, can be administered via ultrasonic nebulizer, with loss of drug during exhalation.[78,79] Note that pulmonary vascular pharmacodynamic effects are more prolonged, with clinical effects seen up to 30 minutes after administration.[78] The drug is prescribed every 2 hours when awake, which usually results in 5 to 6 doses of 5 μg in 24 hours with outpatient administration. Because this dose is intended for delivery only on inspiration, the dose can be doubled when administered by nebulizer, because medication aerosolized during exhalation is not delivered. There is minimal information on potential long-term benefit of iloprost initiated in infancy, but, as an inhaled drug, it can improve V/Q matching with concurrent lung disease. However, one of the major side effects of concern is bronchoconstriction, which may require discontinuation or pretreatment with a bronchodilator.[79,80] Hemoptysis has also been described in ventilated infants.[3]

SUMMARY

After the acute perinatal period, the diagnosis of PH by echocardiography is not broadly established. Several classification schemes have been proposed, but validation studies are limited and their application outside the research setting has not been evaluated. Despite this, it is likely that many infants are treated with specific pulmonary vasodilators for PH without diagnostic confirmation. There are reasonable data to guide dosing of drugs from various classes of therapies for PH, but controlled trials of efficacy toward improving important outcomes have not been done, and drugs have significant side effects. Thus, careful evaluation and monitoring throughout treatment are critical, and confirmatory studies to evaluate the extent of PVD should be undertaken if possible. Registries of pediatric patients with PH may help clinicians to gain insight through describing the natural history of these disorders, and identify characteristics and treatment strategies for particular perinatal patient populations.[81]

> **Best practices**
>
> **What is the current practice?**
>
> Echocardiography is often used to diagnose chronic PH in the perinatal period, without confirmatory studies.
>
> **What changes in current practice are likely to improve outcomes?**
>
> Multicenter collaboration and patient registries could help identify those infants who might benefit from pulmonary vasodilator therapy.
>
> **Is there a clinical algorithm?**
>
> Although individual referral centers may have a standard approach to these high-risk populations, there is no universal algorithm or consistency across centers.
>
> **Summary statement**
>
> There is currently a lack of high-quality data to guide the chronic therapy for infants with PH.

REFERENCES

1. Ivy DD, Abman SH, Barst RJ, et al. Pediatric pulmonary hypertension. J Am Coll Cardiol 2013;62(25 Suppl):D117–26.
2. Barst RJ, McGoon MD, Elliott CG, et al. Survival in childhood pulmonary arterial hypertension: insights from the registry to evaluate early and long-term pulmonary arterial hypertension disease management. Circulation 2012;125: 113–22.
3. del Cerro MJ, Sabaté Rotés A, Cartón A, et al. Pulmonary hypertension in bronchopulmonary dysplasia: clinical findings, cardiovascular anomalies and outcomes. Pediatr Pulmonol 2014;49:49–59.
4. Zuckerman WA, Turner ME, Kerstein J, et al. Safety of cardiac catheterization at a center specializing in the care of patients with pulmonary arterial hypertension. Pulm Circ 2013;3:831–9.
5. Bobhate P, Guo L, Jain S, et al. Cardiac catheterization in children with pulmonary hypertensive vascular disease. Pediatr Cardiol 2015;36:873–9.
6. Simpson JM, Moore P, Teitel DF. Cardiac catheterization of low birth weight infants. Am J Cardiol 2001;87:1372–7.
7. Swift AJ, Rajaram S, Hurdman J, et al. Noninvasive estimation of PA pressure, flow, and resistance with CMR imaging: derivation and prospective validation study from the ASPIRE registry. JACC Cardiovasc Imaging 2013;6:1036–47.
8. Peacock AJ, Crawley S, McLure L, et al. Changes in right ventricular function measured by cardiac magnetic resonance imaging in patients receiving pulmonary arterial hypertension-targeted therapy: the EURO-MR study. Circ Cardiovasc Imaging 2014;7:107–14.
9. Rangamani S, Varghese J, Li L, et al. Safety of cardiac magnetic resonance and contrast angiography for neonates and small infants: a 10-year single-institution experience. Pediatr Radiol 2012;42:1339–46.
10. Shivananda S, Ahliwahlia L, Kluckow M, et al. Variation in the management of persistent pulmonary hypertension of the newborn: a survey of physicians in Canada, Australia, and New Zealand. Am J Perinatol 2012;29:519–26.

11. Lammers AE, Adatia I, Cerro MJ, et al. Functional classification of pulmonary hypertension in children: report from the PVRI pediatric taskforce, Panama 2011. Pulm Circ 2011;1:280–5.
12. Galambos C, Sims-Lucas S, Abman SH. Histologic evidence of intrapulmonary anastomoses by three-dimensional reconstruction in severe bronchopulmonary dysplasia. Ann Am Thorac Soc 2013;10:474–81.
13. Acker SN, Mandell EW, Sims-Lucas S, et al. Histologic identification of prominent intrapulmonary anastomotic vessels in severe congenital diaphragmatic hernia. J Pediatr 2015;166:178–83.
14. Kinsella JP, Truog WE, Walsh WF, et al. Randomized, multicenter trial of inhaled nitric oxide and high-frequency oscillatory ventilation in severe, persistent pulmonary hypertension of the newborn. J Pediatr 1997;131:55–62.
15. Roberts JD, Fineman JR, Morin FC, et al. Inhaled nitric oxide and persistent pulmonary hypertension of the newborn. N Engl J Med 1997;336:605–10.
16. Mourani PM, Sontag MK, Younoszai A, et al. Early pulmonary vascular disease in preterm infants at risk for bronchopulmonary dysplasia. Am J Respir Crit Care Med 2015;191:87–95.
17. Keller RL, Tacy TA, Hendricks-Munoz K, et al. Congenital diaphragmatic hernia: endothelin-1, pulmonary hypertension, and disease severity. Am J Respir Crit Care Med 2010;182:555–61.
18. Mirza H, Ziegler J, Ford S, et al. Pulmonary hypertension in preterm infants: prevalence and association with bronchopulmonary dysplasia. J Pediatr 2014;165:909–14.e1.
19. Mourani PM, Sontag MK, Younoszai A, et al. Clinical utility of echocardiography for the diagnosis and management of pulmonary vascular disease in young children with chronic lung disease. Pediatrics 2008;121:317–25.
20. Groh GK, Levy PT, Holland MR, et al. Doppler echocardiography inaccurately estimates right ventricular pressure in children with elevated right heart pressure. J Am Soc Echocardiogr 2014;27:163–71.
21. Khemani E, McElhinney DB, Rhein L, et al. Pulmonary artery hypertension in formerly premature infants with bronchopulmonary dysplasia: clinical features and outcomes in the surfactant era. Pediatrics 2007;120:1260–9.
22. Lusk LA, Wai KC, Moon-Grady AJ, et al. Persistence of pulmonary hypertension by echocardiography predicts short-term outcomes in congenital diaphragmatic hernia. J Pediatr 2015;166:251–6.e1.
23. Lusk LA, Wai KC, Moon-Grady AJ, et al. Fetal ultrasound markers of severity predict resolution of pulmonary hypertension in congenital diaphragmatic hernia. Am J Obstet Gynecol 2015;213:216.e1–8.
24. Thoresen M, Whitelaw A. Cardiovascular changes during mild therapeutic hypothermia and rewarming in infants with hypoxic-ischemic encephalopathy. Pediatrics 2000;106(1 Pt 1):92–9.
25. Eicher DJ, Wagner CL, Katikaneni LP, et al. Moderate hypothermia in neonatal encephalopathy: safety outcomes. Pediatr Neurol 2005;32:18–24.
26. Shankaran S, Pappas A, Laptook AR, et al. Outcomes of safety and effectiveness in a multicenter randomized, controlled trial of whole-body hypothermia for neonatal hypoxic-ischemic encephalopathy. Pediatrics 2008;122:e791–8.
27. Massaro A, Rais-Bahrami K, Chang T, et al. Therapeutic hypothermia for neonatal encephalopathy and extracorporeal membrane oxygenation. J Pediatr 2010;157:499–501.e1.
28. El Shahed AI, Dargaville PA, Ohlsson A, et al. Surfactant for meconium aspiration syndrome in term and late preterm infants. Cochrane Database Syst Rev 2014;(12):CD002054.

29. Keller RL. Management of the infant with congenital diaphragmatic hernia. In: Bancalari E, editor. The newborn lung: neonatology questions and controversies. 2nd edition. Philadelphia: Elsevier Saunders; 2012. p. 381–406.
30. Neonatal Inhaled Nitric Oxide Study Group. Inhaled nitric oxide in full-term and nearly full-term infants with hypoxic respiratory failure. N Engl J Med 1997;336: 597–604.
31. Davidson D, Barefield ES, Kattwinkel J, et al. Inhaled nitric oxide for the early treatment of persistent pulmonary hypertension of the term newborn: a randomized, double-masked, placebo-controlled, dose-response, multicenter study. The I-NO/PPHN Study Group. Pediatrics 1998;101(3 Pt 1):325–34.
32. Clark RH, Kueser TJ, Walker MW, et al. Low-dose nitric oxide therapy for persistent pulmonary hypertension of the newborn. Clinical Inhaled Nitric Oxide Research Group. N Engl J Med 2000;342:469–74.
33. Tworetzky W, Bristow J, Moore P, et al. Inhaled nitric oxide in neonates with persistent pulmonary hypertension. Lancet 2001;357:118–20.
34. Hintz SR, Suttner DM, Sheehan AM, et al. Decreased use of neonatal extracorporeal membrane oxygenation (ECMO): how new treatment modalities have affected ECMO utilization. Pediatrics 2000;106:1339–43.
35. Roy BJ, Rycus P, Conrad SA, et al. The changing demographics of neonatal extracorporeal membrane oxygenation patients reported to the Extracorporeal Life Support Organization (ELSO) registry. Pediatrics 2000;106:1334–8.
36. Karimova A, Brown K, Ridout D, et al. Neonatal extracorporeal membrane oxygenation: practice patterns and predictors of outcome in the UK. Arch Dis Child Fetal Neonatal Ed 2009;94:F129–32.
37. Bassler D, Choong K, McNamara P, et al. Neonatal persistent pulmonary hypertension treated with milrinone: four case reports. Biol Neonate 2006;89:1–5.
38. McNamara PJ, Laique F, Muang-In S, et al. Milrinone improves oxygenation in neonates with severe persistent pulmonary hypertension of the newborn. J Crit Care 2006;21:217–22.
39. James AT, Corcoran JD, McNamara PJ, et al. The effect of milrinone on right and left ventricular function when used as a rescue therapy for term infants with pulmonary hypertension. Cardiol Young 2015;1–10 [Epub ahead of print].
40. Patel N. Use of milrinone to treat cardiac dysfunction in infants with pulmonary hypertension secondary to congenital diaphragmatic hernia: a review of six patients. Neonatology 2012;102:130–6.
41. McNamara PJ, Shivananda SP, Sahni M, et al. Pharmacology of milrinone in neonates with persistent pulmonary hypertension of the newborn and suboptimal response to inhaled nitric oxide. Pediatr Crit Care Med 2013;14:74–84.
42. Peliowski A, Finer NN, Etches PC, et al. Inhaled nitric oxide for premature infants after prolonged rupture of the membranes. J Pediatr 1995;126:450–3.
43. Chock VY, Van Meurs KP, Hintz SR, et al. Inhaled nitric oxide for preterm premature rupture of membranes, oligohydramnios, and pulmonary hypoplasia. Am J Perinatol 2009;26:317–22.
44. Semberova J, O'Donnell SM, Franta J, et al. Inhaled nitric oxide in preterm infants with prolonged preterm rupture of the membranes: a case series. J Perinatol 2015;35:304–6.
45. Cole FS, Alleyne C, Barks JD, et al. NIH consensus development conference statement: inhaled nitric-oxide therapy for premature infants. Pediatrics 2011;127:363–9.
46. Danhaive O, Margossian R, Geva T, et al. Pulmonary hypertension and right ventricular dysfunction in growth-restricted, extremely low birth weight neonates. J Perinatol 2005;25:495–9.

47. James AT, Bee C, Corcoran JD, et al. Treatment of premature infants with pulmonary hypertension and right ventricular dysfunction with milrinone: a case series. J Perinatol 2015;35:268–73.

48. Kinsella JP, Parker TA, Ivy DD, et al. Noninvasive delivery of inhaled nitric oxide therapy for late pulmonary hypertension in newborn infants with congenital diaphragmatic hernia. J Pediatr 2003;142:397–401.

49. Ehlen M, Wiebe B. Iloprost in persistent pulmonary hypertension of the newborn. Cardiol Young 2003;13:361–3.

50. Noori S, Friedlich P, Wong P, et al. Cardiovascular effects of sildenafil in neonates and infants with congenital diaphragmatic hernia and pulmonary hypertension. Neonatology 2007;91:92–100.

51. Nahata MC, Morosco RS, Brady MT. Extemporaneous sildenafil citrate oral suspensions for the treatment of pulmonary hypertension in children. Am J Health Syst Pharm 2006;63:254–7.

52. Shah PS, Ohlsson A. Sildenafil for pulmonary hypertension in neonates. Cochrane Database Syst Rev 2011;(8):CD005494.

53. Keller RL, Moore P, Teitel D, et al. Abnormal vascular tone in infants and children with lung hypoplasia: findings from cardiac catheterization and the response to therapy. Pediatr Crit Care Med 2006;7:589–94.

54. Mourani PM, Sontag MK, Ivy DD, et al. Effects of long-term sildenafil treatment for pulmonary hypertension in infants with chronic lung disease. J Pediatr 2009;154:379–84, 384.e1–2.

55. Humpl T, Reyes JT, Erickson S, et al. Sildenafil therapy for neonatal and childhood pulmonary hypertensive vascular disease. Cardiol Young 2011;21:187–93.

56. Wardle AJ, Connolly GM, Stonier T, et al. Sildenafil in bronchopulmonary dysplasia: safe to use? Arch Dis Child Fetal Neonatal Ed 2015;100:F369.

57. Barst RJ, Ivy DD, Gaitan G, et al. A randomized, double-blind, placebo-controlled, dose-ranging study of oral sildenafil citrate in treatment-naive children with pulmonary arterial hypertension. Circulation 2012;125:324–34.

58. Barst RJ, Beghetti M, Pulido T, et al. STARTS-2: long-term survival with oral sildenafil monotherapy in treatment-naive pediatric pulmonary arterial hypertension. Circulation 2014;129:1914–23.

59. Siehr SL, McCarthy EK, Ogawa MT, et al. Reported sildenafil side effects in pediatric pulmonary hypertension patients. Front Pediatr 2015;3:12.

60. Gamboa D, Robbins D, Saba Z. Bleeding after circumcision in a newborn receiving sildenafil. Clin Pediatr (Phila) 2007;46:842–3.

61. Samada K, Shiraishi H, Aoyagi J, et al. Cerebral hemorrhage associated with sildenafil (Revatio) in an infant. Pediatr Cardiol 2009;30:998–9.

62. Steinhorn RH, Kinsella JP, Pierce C, et al. Intravenous sildenafil in the treatment of neonates with persistent pulmonary hypertension. J Pediatr 2009;155:841–7.e1.

63. Vachiery JL, Huez S, Gillies H, et al. Safety, tolerability and pharmacokinetics of an intravenous bolus of sildenafil in patients with pulmonary arterial hypertension. Br J Clin Pharmacol 2011;71:289–92.

64. Rosenberg AA, Kennaugh J, Koppenhafer SL, et al. Elevated immunoreactive endothelin-1 levels in newborn infants with persistent pulmonary hypertension. J Pediatr 1993;123:109–14.

65. Christou H, Adatia I, Van Marter LJ, et al. Effect of inhaled nitric oxide on endothelin-1 and cyclic guanosine 5'-monophosphate plasma concentrations in newborn infants with persistent pulmonary hypertension. J Pediatr 1997;130:603–11.

66. Husain AN, Siddiqui NH, Stocker JT. Pathology of arrested acinar development in postsurfactant bronchopulmonary dysplasia. Hum Pathol 1998;29:710–7.

67. Heerema AE, Rabban JT, Sydorak RM, et al. Lung pathology in patients with congenital diaphragmatic hernia treated with fetal surgical intervention, including tracheal occlusion. Pediatr Dev Pathol 2003;6:536–46.
68. Kinsella JP, Ivy DD, Abman SH. Pulmonary vasodilator therapy in congenital diaphragmatic hernia: acute, late, and chronic pulmonary hypertension. Semin Perinatol 2005;29:123–8.
69. Barst RJ, Ivy D, Dingemanse J, et al. Pharmacokinetics, safety, and efficacy of bosentan in pediatric patients with pulmonary arterial hypertension. Clin Pharmacol Ther 2003;73:372–82.
70. Beghetti M, Hoeper MM, Kiely DG, et al. Safety experience with bosentan in 146 children 2-11 years old with pulmonary arterial hypertension: results from the European Postmarketing Surveillance Program. Pediatr Res 2008;64:200–4.
71. Beghetti M, Haworth SG, Bonnet D, et al. Pharmacokinetic and clinical profile of a novel formulation of bosentan in children with pulmonary arterial hypertension: the FUTURE-1 study. Br J Clin Pharmacol 2009;68:948–55.
72. Eronen M, Pohjavuori M, Andersson S, et al. Prostacyclin treatment for persistent pulmonary hypertension of the newborn. Pediatr Cardiol 1997;18:3–7.
73. Golzand E, Bar-Oz B, Arad I. Intravenous prostacyclin in the treatment of persistent pulmonary hypertension of the newborn refractory to inhaled nitric oxide. Isr Med Assoc J 2005;7:408–9.
74. Melnick L, Barst RJ, Rowan CA, et al. Effectiveness of transition from intravenous epoprostenol to oral/inhaled targeted pulmonary arterial hypertension therapy in pediatric idiopathic and familial pulmonary arterial hypertension. Am J Cardiol 2010;105:1485–9.
75. McIntyre CM, Hanna BD, Rintoul N, et al. Safety of epoprostenol and treprostinil in children less than 12 months of age. Pulm Circ 2013;3:862–9.
76. Ferdman DJ, Rosenzweig EB, Zuckerman WA, et al. Subcutaneous treprostinil for pulmonary hypertension in chronic lung disease of infancy. Pediatrics 2014;134: e274–8.
77. Olson E, Lusk LA, Fineman JR, et al. Short-term treprostinil use in infants with congenital diaphragmatic hernia following repair. J Pediatr 2015;167:762–4.
78. Olschewski H, Rohde B, Behr J, et al. Pharmacodynamics and pharmacokinetics of inhaled iloprost, aerosolized by three different devices, in severe pulmonary hypertension. Chest 2003;124:1294–304.
79. Ivy DD, Doran AK, Smith KJ, et al. Short- and long-term effects of inhaled iloprost therapy in children with pulmonary arterial hypertension. J Am Coll Cardiol 2008; 51:161–9.
80. Reichenberger F, Mainwood A, Doughty N, et al. Effects of nebulised iloprost on pulmonary function and gas exchange in severe pulmonary hypertension. Respir Med 2007;101:217–22.
81. Ivy DD, Abman SH. Gaining insights into pediatric pulmonary hypertensive disorders through patient registries. Am J Respir Crit Care Med 2015;191:2–4.

Index

Note: Page numbers of article titles are in **boldface** type.

A

Clin Perinatol 43 (2016) 203–213
http://dx.doi.org/10.1016/S0095-5108(15)00150-5
0095-5108/16/$ – see front matter © 2016 Elsevier Inc. All rights reserved.

Moving?

Make sure your subscription moves with you!

To notify us of your new address, find your **Clinics Account Number** (located on your mailing label above your name), and contact customer service at:

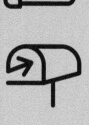

Email: journalscustomerservice-usa@elsevier.com

800-654-2452 (subscribers in the U.S. & Canada)
314-447-8871 (subscribers outside of the U.S. & Canada)

Fax number: 314-447-8029

Elsevier Health Sciences Division
Subscription Customer Service
3251 Riverport Lane
Maryland Heights, MO 63043

*To ensure uninterrupted delivery of your subscription, please notify us at least 4 weeks in advance of move.

Printed and bound by CPI Group (UK) Ltd, Croydon, CR0 4YY

03/10/2024

01040491-0005